"This book is five stars! The protocol is indispensable for any physician treating CFIDS. The text is a godsend for patients—giving them hope and a means for educating themselves and, hopefully, their doctors."

—BILL DEAN
Author, *The Immune System*

"I provide all my patients with *From Fatigued to Fantastic!* and find it a wonderful tool to open dialogue between the patient and myself. It is critical that the patient play a major role in his or her own healing. This book provides that bridge. I could not practice as effectively without this book."

—TERENCE COLLINS, M.D., MPH, MPS
Professor and Chair, Department of Preventive Medicine,
University of Kentucky

"Practical, evidence-based, and easy to read, *From Fatigued to Fantastic!* offers hope and guidance for millions of CFIDS and fibromyalgia sufferers."

—MARK W. MCCLURE, M.D., FACS
Author, *Smart Medicine for a Healthy Prostate*

"Dr. Teitelbaum's book is a 'must read' for all health-care professionals who want to understand a truly holistic method to help patients with CFS. No longer do we have to be frustrated with inadequate treatments and unscientific evidence. He gives real answers to what before were unsolvable issues."

—E. J. (LEV) LINKNER, M.D.
Clinical Instructor, University of Michigan Medical School
Founding Member, American Board of Holistic Medicine

"The first edition has already helped so many who have been unable to find help elsewhere. This edition brings us up to date with exciting new information, including new clinical research. Reading this book is a must!"

—JAMES H. BRODSKY, M.D.
Instructor, Georgetown University Medical School

"Dr. Teitelbaum's *From Fatigued to Fantastic!* is a must-read for CFS patients and health-care providers alike. There are few physicians in this country who have the scope of research and clinical experience in chronic fatigue as Dr. Teitelbaum and who have such extraordinary ability to communicate what he knows so well. He takes the reader on a friendly and yet extremely comprehensive journey into the whys and hows of this disease and its treatment, weaving in and out of the alternative, conventional, and psychological/emotional approaches, which are part of his successful program. His writing is clear, careful, and considerate. Bravo, Dr. Teitelbaum!"

—RALPH GOLAN, M.D.
Author, *Optimal Wellness*

"I am grateful for Dr. Jacob Teitelbaum's great work on FMS and CFS. His well-done, published research validates what many of us working in the trenches know: This works!"

—MARK HOCH, M.D.
Secretary, American Holistic Medicine Association

"Thank you, Jacob Teitelbaum. Your research and carefully designed program for patients suffering from CFS and fibromyalgia has given my patients relief from symptoms, improved sense of well-being, hope, and in many cases has facilitated a path to optimal health and full recovery."

—NANCY RUSSELL, M.D.
Medical Director, Combined Health Care Professionals
University of Colorado School of Medicine, Continuing Medical Education

"As a psychiatrist and acupuncturist, I frequently see patients with chronic fatigue and soft-tissue pain. Dr. Teitelbaum's book *From Fatigued to Fantastic!* has been a fantastic resource for these individuals. They uniformly report to me that they found it helpful to them on many different levels. This book has clear benefit for anyone dealing with chronic fatigue or fibromyalgia."

—SCOTT SHANNON, M.D.
President-Elect, American Holistic Medicine Association

"Dr. Teitelbaum's work and studies show us the way forward in treating this group of illnesses. They are a major advance on what we have here at present."

—ANDREW WRIGHT, M.D.
Editor, *Chronobiology* (U.K.)

"In the management of chronic fatigue syndrome, Dr. Teitelbaum's comprehensive approach is the most successful program available today. Practitioners and patients alike will find within the pages of *From Fatigued to Fantastic!* the rudiments of recovery, which offer hope to those afflicted with this disease."

—ROBERT A. ANDERSON, M.D.
President, American Board of Holistic Medicine

From Fatigued to Fantastic!

A proven program
to regain vibrant
health, based on a
new scientific study
showing effective
treatment for
chronic fatigue
and fibromyalgia

JACOB TEITELBAUM, M.D.

AVERY
a member of Penguin Putnam Inc.
New York

Most Avery books are available at special quantity discounts for bulk purchase for sales promotions, premiums, fund-raising, and educational needs. Special books or book excerpts also can be created to fit specific needs. For details, write Putnam Special Markets, 375 Hudson Street, New York, NY 10014.

a member of
Penguin Putnam Inc.
375 Hudson Street
New York, NY 10014
www.penguinputnam.com

Library of Congress Cataloging-in-Publication Data

Teitelbaum, Jacob.
From fatigued to fantastic! / by Jacob Teitelbaum.—Completely rev. and updated ed.
p. cm.
Includes bibliographical references and index.
ISBN 1-58333-097-6
1. Chronic fatigue syndrome—Popular works. 2. Fibromyalgia—Popular works. I. Title
RB150.F37 T45 2001 2001022740
616'.0478—dc21

Printed in the United States of America

1 3 5 7 9 10 8 6 4 2

Book design by Tanya Maiboroda

To Laurie, the love of my life;
my children David, Amy, Shannon, Brittany and Kelly,
who already seem to know much of what I'm trying to learn;
and my mother, Sabina, and father, David,
whose unconditional love made this book possible.
And to my patients, who have taught me more
than I can ever hope to teach them.

Acknowledgments

SO MANY SPECIAL PEOPLE HELPED MAKE THIS BOOK possible that I cannot possibly list them all. In truth, I have created nothing new; I have simply synthesized the wonderful work done by an army of hardworking and courageous physicians and healers.

I would like to extend my sincerest thanks to:

First and foremost, my staff. Their hard work, compassion, and dedication (and, I must admit, patience with me) are what made my work possible.

My research partner and lab manager, Birdie (Barbara Bird). Her sense of humor and encouragement kept me going when I got tired. Her dedication to quality showed in every facet of her work. Mary Groom, Amy Podd, Cheryl Alberto, and Lisa Pinder make everything run smoothly, no matter how much chaos I create.

The Anne Arundel Medical Center librarian, Joyce Miller. Over the last twenty years, I have often wondered when she would politely tell me to stop asking for so many studies. So far, she has not. In fact, she always smiles when I ask her for more.

My physician associates. Dr. Robert Greenfield taught me healthy skepticism, and Dr. Alan Weiss always reminded me to reclaim my sense of humor.

My publishers, Phyllis Grann and Rudy Shur, and my editors, Laura

Shepherd and Amy Tecklenburg. They guided me through unknown terrain.

My many teachers, the real heroes and heroines in their fields, whose names could fill this book. They include William Crook, Max Boverman, Brugh Joy, Janet Travell, William Jefferies, Jay Goldstein, Paul Levine, Leo Galland, Leonard Jason, George Mitchell, Lloyd Lewis, Michael Rosenbaum, Murray Susser, Charles Lapp, Paul Cheney, James Brodsky, Melvyn Werbach, Sherry Rogers, Robert Ivker, Jeff Bland and Alan Gaby.

The many chronic fatigue syndrome and fibromyalgia support groups. These are easily the best patient support groups I have ever seen.

And finally, God and the universe, for the guidance and infinite blessings I have been given and for using me as an instrument for healing.

Contents

Preface

A CURIOUS THING HAPPENED DURING THE RIGOR-
ous process I went through to become a physician. By the time I completed my formal training, I presumed that if an important treatment
existed for an illness, I had been taught about it. I understood that physicians need to keep reading to stay abreast of new information. But I *knew*
that if someone claimed he or she could effectively treat a nontreatable disease, that person was a quack. If such a treatment existed, I would surely
have been taught about it.

I was wrong.

Dr. Werner Barth, my rheumatology instructor, taught me many things.
The most important thing he taught me, though, was to spend an hour a
day reading the scientific literature. This has gotten me into all kinds of
trouble.

When I first started my practice, patients would ask me if I knew
about certain herbal or nutritional treatments for illnesses. One patient
asked me if I had ever heard about using vitamin B_6 for carpal tunnel syndrome. "That's nonsense," I answered. "If B_6 cures carpal tunnel syndrome, don't you think I would have been taught to use that instead of to
operate on people's wrists?" I said that I would look into it, however.

Joyce Miller, the Anne Arundel Medical Center librarian, has always
been happy to obtain studies for me (and she has gotten many thousands

over the years). When she did a literature search for vitamin B$_6$ and carpal tunnel syndrome, she found a number of studies showing that 250 milligrams of B$_6$ per day for three months, combined with wrist splints, often cures carpal tunnel syndrome. I thought that was curious. Over the months, this scene was played out again and again. I decided to keep notes on these rare "pearls" in a thirty-page spiral notebook. My notes are now over a thousand pages long.

After a while, I began to comprehend that, indeed, my professors had not taught me everything in medical school. As I continued my research, I realized that although our modern allopathic medical system might be the best in the world, it has its weaknesses. These days, it is rare (albeit wonderful) for a major medical development to come out of a doctor's office instead of a research center. This stems from a critical drawback in our economic system (and all systems have their drawbacks). In our current system, a treatment must be very profitable to be promoted. Experts estimate that it costs about $400,000,000 to develop a single new treatment and to get it through the Food and Drug Administration (FDA) approval process. Unless a medication or supplement is put through the FDA approval process, its manufacturer is banned from making any medical claims for the product. However, if a product is inexpensive and *nonpatentable,* its manufacturer will most likely not want to pay $400,000,000 to put it through the FDA process.

Vitamin B$_6$ used for carpal tunnel syndrome is an excellent example. Treating carpal tunnel syndrome with B$_6$ costs about nine dollars per patient. Vitamin B$_6$ manufacturers would therefore find it impossible to recoup the cost of getting FDA approval for this treatment. Because of this, most patients instead spend between $2,000 and $4,000 to have surgery. This situation is the same for hundreds of other nonpatentable, effective, inexpensive, and relatively safe treatments. The FDA has even been fighting to make it illegal for stores that sell supplements to hand out copies of well-done scientific studies on the supplements!

The treatment approach that you will learn about in *From Fatigued to Fantastic!* is well grounded in the scientific literature. Dr. Janet Travell, professor emeritus of internal medicine at George Washington University Medical School, is considered the world's leading expert on muscle disorders. She served as White House physician for presidents John F. Kennedy and Lyndon B. Johnson and authored the eight-hundred-page bible on treating muscle disorders entitled *Myofascial Pain and Dysfunction: The*

Trigger Point Manual. Although the research connecting fibromyalgia and myofascial (muscle) pain syndromes had not yet been done when she wrote her book, she investigated the perpetuating factors—that is, the conditions that keep the muscles from appropriately relaxing. In one chapter alone, she referenced 317 scientific studies that showed how important it is to treat these perpetuating factors. There is no lack of scientific basis for treatment, just a lack of awareness of the treatment, due to its relative inexpensiveness and nonpatentability.

Unfortunately, your doctor is likely to be unfamiliar with the research on effective treatment of myofascial pain and fibromyalgia. Your doctor may be hostile to the information presented in this book, considering it to be quackery because it was not covered in medical school. Or, your doctor may choose to disregard the information. On the other hand, your doctor might be open-minded (though reasonably skeptical) and will choose to explore the subject in more depth. If this last possibility is the case, the information and references in this book will give your doctor the scientific basis necessary to manage and optimize your treatment. Show your doctor Appendix A: For Physicians, which I wrote specifically for medical professionals, and Appendix B: Studies of Effective Treatment Modalities for Chronic Fatigue and Fibromyalgia, in which I present the results that my research partners and I obtained in our recent study. These will be helpful to your physician.

The book in general, however, is for you, the layperson suffering from chronic fatigue syndrome or fibromyalgia. After giving an overview of the possible causes and patterns of chronic fatigue states in Chapter 1, I home in on the specifics. In Chapter 2, I discuss nutritional problems. In Chapter 3, I focus on hormonal problems. In Chapter 4, I cover immune-system problems and infections, and in Chapter 5, I discuss fibromyalgia. In Chapter 6, getting eight hours of sleep a night and in Chapter 7 how to make your pain go away. Chapters 8 and 9 will teach you about natural remedies. In Chapter 10, I address food allergies, sinus problems, Chiari malformation, and several other possible troublemakers. In Chapter 11, I hope to reassure you that you are not crazy, and that your symptoms are real. And in Chapter 12, I try to help you find a physician who will treat you as a whole person, addressing both the physical and psychospiritual issues inherent in illness. Several appendices offer additional or supporting information.

I think you will find the material presented in this book to be as exciting as my colleagues and I find it. Knowing how problematic brain fog can be, I have tried to keep the text concise and straightforward. However, if you finish the book and find yourself wishing for more information, check Appendix I: Recommended Reading, as well as the Bibliography. Between this book, my website (www.endfatigue.com), my reference sources, and the books and articles I recommend for further reading, you should find the bulk of your most pressing questions answered.

Introduction

I REMEMBER 1975. I WAS IN MY THIRD YEAR OF medical school, doing my pediatrics rotation. I had always excelled, having finished college in three years. Now I was the second youngest in a class of over two hundred medical students, and I was continuing to excel. My approach to life was to move quickly—"full speed ahead." But then a nasty viral illness hit me and made it hard for me to even get out of bed for my pediatrics lecture. I cannot forget walking into an auditorium full of medical students, the professor saying, "Teitelbaum, why are you . . ." As he said "late?" I just about collapsed on the steps.

Although I was barely able to function, I spent the next four weeks working in the electron microscopy and research labs. The work I performed there was considered low key—good tasks for a medical student trying to recuperate. My brain fog made even these duties impossible, and by the end of the month, I was finding it impossible to even get out of bed before noon. I wanted to push forward and try harder. Though it was not what I wanted to hear, one wise professor advised me that this was not a time to push forward but a time to take a leave of absence and regroup. I am still thankful for this teacher's guidance.

My illness seemed to close a door to one chapter of my life and open up other doors to whole new possibilities of self-exploration. Taking off in my '65 Dodge Dart, I had the novel experience of having no agenda, no plans. I was to meet many teachers on my journey. Most important, I was taking time to get to know myself.

With my family's and friends' help and support and my own inner work, I recovered my energy and strength and went on to finish medical school and residency. Though I did well, I continued to intermittently suffer the many diverse symptoms seen in fibromyalgia. My experiences with chronic fatigue syndrome and fibromyalgia left me with an appreciation of the impact of these illnesses. The symptoms that persisted—such as fatigue, achiness, poor sleep, and bowel problems—acted as the arena in which I learned how to help other people overcome these illnesses.

If you have chronic fatigue syndrome (CFS), fibromyalgia syndrome (FMS), myalgic encephalomyelitis (ME), or another disabling chronic fatigue state, you have been through a difficult journey. I remember being told that I was depressed. I *was* depressed. I was unable to function. Most people with chronic fatigue syndrome have to struggle just to get compassion and understanding.

Building on what I have learned since 1975, my research partner, Barbara Bird, and I initially completed an open study (in 1993) of sixty-four patients with disabling chronic fatigue.[1] In 1999, we completed a randomized, double-blind follow-up study, and appreciate the assistance given by National Institutes of Health researchers in developing the study protocol.[2] Mrs. Bird and I have treated thousands of other patients before and after the study. Over 40 percent of our patients have been cured—that is, their symptoms are no longer a major problem—with our treatment, while most of the remainder have shown significant, albeit incomplete, improvement. Only 10 to 15 percent have had no significant improvement.[3] We have found that, on average, patients begin to feel better in about two months.[4]

If you suffer from CFS, FMS, or ME, this book will provide you with the tools and information you need to move beyond fatigue and into wellness. If you are a physician, it will teach you how to help—often dramatically—your patients with chronic exhaustion, including those frustrating cases in which no treatment has thus far been successful.

If you have researched chronic fatigue and immune dysfunction syndrome (CFIDS—also called chronic fatigue syndrome or CFS), you will find some information here that is familiar, but you will also discover much that is new. For instance, Mrs. Bird and I have found that the key to eliminating chronic fatigue is to treat all of the underlying problems simultaneously. Most sufferers of chronic exhaustion have a mix of at least five or six underlying problems (out of dozens of possible problems), which vary from person to person. This occurs because each problem can cause several others. You may have found some relief in the past by treating one, or a few, of these problems; I think you will be happily surprised at what happens when you treat all your underlying problems simultaneously.

Certainly, we still have much more to learn in this area. However, we have now crossed a threshold and can effectively treat the illness. Many patients still obtain significant but incomplete relief. As new information surfaces, more and more people will hopefully join the ranks of those who find their chronic fatigue resolves with the proper treatment!

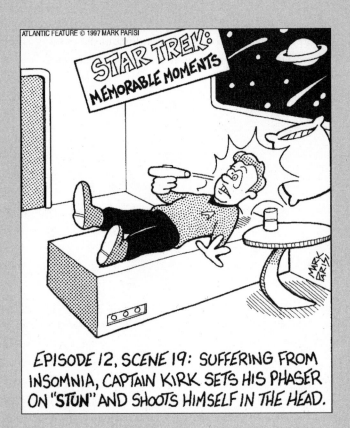

What Is Chronic Fatigue Syndrome?

CHRONIC FATIGUE AND IMMUNE DYSFUNCTION syndrome (abbreviated CFIDS or CFS) is a group of symptoms associated with severe, almost unrelenting fatigue. The predominant symptom is fatigue that causes a persistent and substantial reduction in activity level. Poor sleep; achiness; difficulties with short-term memory, concentration, word finding, word substitution, and orientation (a group of symptoms collectively known as "brain fog"); increased thirst; bowel disorders; recurrent infections; and exhaustion after minimal exertion are some of the more common associated symptoms. A related problem, fibromyalgia syndrome (FMS), also features painful knots at specific points in the muscles. For most people, fibromyalgia and CFIDS/CFS are the same illness. If this sounds like you, I would assume you have CFIDS unless it can be proven otherwise. I use the terms *CFIDS* and *CFS* interchangeably, and *CFIDS/FMS* to refer to the overall process, with muscle pain. *Myalgic encephalomyelitis* (ME) is another term sometimes used to refer to such syndromes.

How Is CFIDS Defined?

The U.S. Centers for Disease Control and Prevention (CDC) has put together an updated list of criteria for the diagnosis of chronic fatigue syndrome (see the inset on page 3). Although the CDC's criteria has helped researchers define groups for studies, its original criteria for chronic fatigue syndrome excluded all but about 5,000 to 20,000 people in the United States.[1] Unfortunately, over 25 million Americans have *severe* fatigue (lasting at least one month) at any given time.[2] Of these, around 6 million people currently suffer from fibromyalgia.[3] Research has shown that people with disabling fatigue who do not fit the CDC criteria have the same immunologic changes and responses to treatment as do those who do fit.[4] My experience, too, suggests that the underlying causes of patients' chronic fatigue and their responses to treatment are not affected by whether they strictly meet the CDC guidelines.[5]

Because of problems with defining CFIDS, I prefer to use the following definition. If you have unexplained fatigue that significantly interferes with your functioning and is associated with any two of the following symptoms:

1. Brain fog;
2. Poor sleep;
3. Diffuse achiness;
4. Increased thirst;
5. Bowel dysfunction; and/or
6. Recurrent and/or persistent infections or flulike feelings,

then you have CFIDS until proven otherwise!

Why Has CFIDS Been Ignored by Doctors?

Unfortunately, although the CDC is a wonderful organization, the bureaucrat and researcher *in charge* of CFIDS research at the CDC in 1999 faced possible indictment for "stealing" the money allocated to CFIDS research and applying it elsewhere. A feeling that the suffering of people with this condition is unimportant seems to be reflected in the CDC's actions. They seem to do their best to underestimate how common CFIDS is and to recommend that little be done about it. To show how bizarre this behavior is, let's look at the numbers.

Fibromyalgia—whose definition was created by the American College of Rheumatology (ACR), not the CDC—is conservatively estimated to af-

---

Updated CDC Criteria for Chronic Fatigue Syndrome

A case of chronic fatigue syndrome is defined by the presence of the following:

1. Clinically evaluated, unexplained, persistent, or relapsing chronic fatigue that is of new or definite onset (has not been lifelong); is not the result of ongoing exertion; is not substantially alleviated by rest; and results in substantial reduction in previous levels of occupational, educational, social, or personal activities.

2. Concurrent occurrence of four or more of the following symptoms, all of which must have persisted or recurred during six or more consecutive months of illness and must not have predated the fatigue:

   A. Self-reported impairment in short-term memory or concentration severe enough to cause substantial reduction in previous levels of occupational, educational, social, or personal activities.
   B. Sore throat.
   C. Tender cervical [neck] or axillary [underarm] lymph nodes.
   D. Muscle pain.
   E. Multijoint pain without joint swelling or redness.
   F. Headaches of a new type, pattern, or severity.
   G. Unrefreshing sleep.
   H. Postexertional malaise lasting more than twenty-four hours.

Adapted from the Annals of Internal Medicine *121 (14 December 1994). Used with permission.*

---

fect 6 million Americans. In our study, sixty-nine of seventy-two patients with fibromyalgia (approximately 95 percent) had CFIDS. In another recent study, by Dr. Dedra Buchwald, 64 percent of her FMS patients also had CFIDS. Because of this, you would expect at least 4 to 5 million cases of CFIDS. In addition, about 10 to 20 percent of CFIDS patients don't have fibromyalgia, so there should be almost 6 million cases of CFIDS. Yet the CDC seems to want to believe that only a few hundred thousand people are affected!

I teased a colleague of mine, Leonard Jason of DePaul University, about this discrepancy. Dr. Jason is the world's foremost epidemiologist for CFIDS. He said that the CDC definition requires (in small print) that you rule out other possible causes of fatigue and adds other criteria that systematically whittle down the number. Yet the big print strongly discourages doctors from looking for these other problems!

Let's break it down further. In Dr. Jason's study, which was published in the prestigious *Archives of Internal Medicine* (the American Medical Association [AMA] internal medicine journal), he found that:

- 11.9 percent of the population currently had "severe fatigue, extreme tiredness or exhaustion" lasting over one month.
- 4.2 percent had these symptoms for over six months.
- 2.2 percent also had no other medical or psychological diagnosis that could cause fatigue (approximately 2 percent of Americans have FMS).
- 0.4 percent is all that was left over after doctors and a psychiatrist looked for any problems that could be used as an excuse to account for fatigue (now or in the past).[6]

These numbers suggest a CFIDS-like *process* may affect at least 2 to 4 percent of the population, and perhaps as many as 12 percent. Dr. Jason is a wonderful, compassionate man. Nonetheless, in the end, by applying the rigid criteria the CDC uses, he still found that over one-half million Americans have CFIDS. The CDC underplays even this.

Why would the CDC do this? As I mentioned, the CDC *overall* is an excellent organization. By downplaying the number of people with CFIDS, Congress underestimates the severity of the problem and allocates research dollars to other projects. Because the doctors at the CDC don't seem to take CFIDS seriously (their mouths say "yes" but their actions clearly say "no, they don't") they get to have the medical research dollars Congress allocates given to their pet projects instead of being "wasted" on CFIDS. Imagine where cancer research would be if the people *in charge* of cancer research thought cancer didn't exist and tried to prevent research from getting funding. If you applied their criteria to cancer—you have to have had it for six months, you have to have no other medical problems and no history of severe depression, and so on—you could make believe cancer doesn't exist, either!

What Causes CFIDS?

People who suffer from CFIDS/FMS usually have a combination of several different problems. The exact combination varies from individual to individual. There are dozens of major underlying factors, with individual people displaying an average of five to six factors each.[7] It is important to look for and treat all of the factors simultaneously. CFIDS/FMS are unusual in that each separate problem can trigger other problems. Because of this, it is rare to have only one single underlying problem by the time a person seeks medical help.

To use an analogy, a person with a chronic fatigue state is like an automobile with a dead battery that short-circuited the starter. If we only charge the battery, the car will not run. If we only repair the starter, the car will not run. However, if we both charge the battery and repair the starter, the car will be fine. In the same way, if we treat all of a CFIDS/FMS patient's problems simultaneously, the person will feel well!

Some Common Patterns of Chronic Fatigue Syndrome

Many common subsets and patterns are seen in severe chronic fatigue states. They include infections (what I call the drop-dead flu), disrupted sleep, and hormonal problems, including what I call the autoimmune triad.

INFECTIONS—THE DROP-DEAD FLU

The most notorious pattern seen in severe chronic fatigue states is one in which a person who is feeling fine suddenly comes down with a brutal flu-like illness that never goes away. The sudden onset of the illness after an infection is a mark of this classic pattern. In most of these CFIDS patients, an underlying viral or other infection is suspected.[8] These infections can suppress the hypothalamus, located in the brain.[9] Hypothalamic dysfunction is common in chronic fatigue states.[10]

What happens when the hypothalamus is injured? The hypothalamus is the body's master gland. It controls most of the other glands, including the adrenal, ovarian, testicular, and thyroid glands. If the hypothalamus is suppressed, the individual will often have a subtle but disabling decrease in the functioning of several of these glands. However, a person can experience fatigue and flulike symptoms from suppression of the adrenal glands alone.

For most people, the suppression of the hypothalamus ends when the flu is over. Dr. William Jefferies, a retired endocrinologist and assistant professor of medicine at Case Western Reserve University, has theorized that people who remain chronically ill after an infection have long-term, sometimes permanent, hypothalamic suppression. He has found that treating such patients with adrenal hormone (in doses that are normal for the body) can safely bring about marked improvement.[11] My research supports his findings.[12]

What happens if the adrenal gland no longer functions properly? In severe cases, people have gone into shock and died from even minor stresses, such as dental work. In most cases, however, the suppression is less severe. Dr. Jefferies discusses adrenal suppression in his excellent 1996 monograph, *Safe Uses of Cortisol.* He explained that the flu causes suppression of adrenocorticotropic hormone (ACTH), which is the hormone that causes the adrenal gland to make adrenal hormone. If the adrenal gland is suppressed—that is, if the adrenal gland does not make sufficient adrenal hormone—a variety of fatigue symptoms result. When Dr. Jefferies gave fatigue and flu patients low doses of adrenal hormone, the flulike symptoms often improved markedly.

Even though a gland is underactive, a blood test can often (I believe mistakenly) suggest that the gland is technically normal, albeit in the low range (more on this in later chapters).[13] This is why patients are often told that their thyroid or adrenal glands are healthy when indeed they are not. Because of this, doctors must know how to correctly interpret blood tests and how to identify subclinical hormonal deficiencies.

The drop-dead flu also causes many people to develop poor immunity, facilitating repeated bladder, respiratory, or sinus infections. I have found that patients who then take repeated courses of antibiotics for any reason often end up with an overgrowth of yeast in the bowel. Bowel parasites and other infections are also common in CFIDS patients.[14] Some of these infections can sneak up on you slowly. Suppressed hypothalamic function from chronic infections can then trigger disordered sleep.

Poor Sleep

Fibromyalgia is basically a sleep disorder associated with shortened, achy muscles that have multiple tender knots. Trying to sleep on the tender knots is like trying to sleep on marbles. In addition, the day/night cycle is confused, leading the brain to be wide awake and thinking, "It's morning!" just about the time one goes to bed. Because of this, people with fibromyalgia have trouble staying in the deep, restorative stages of sleep (stages 3 and 4) that recharge their batteries. Instead, these people stay in the light sleep stages (stages 1, 2, and REM) and often wake up repeatedly during the night. Some of us joke that there's an invisible alarm clock set for 3:00 to 4:00 A.M. that can be heard only by people with fibromyalgia! They finally fall fast asleep just before the alarm clock is set to ring. In essence, fibromyalgia sufferers may not have slept *effectively* for several years. When normal sleep patterns are restored, they feel much better. Please note, however, that most sleeping pills—especially benzodiazepines, such as diazepam (better known by its brand name, Valium), triazolam (Halcion), and flurazepam (Dalmane)—actually worsen deep sleep.

I suspect that poor sleep further suppresses the hypothalamus (more about this in Chapter 3). Poor sleep can then cause immune suppression, with secondary bowel infections.[15] The bowel infections seen in chronic fatigue can cause decreased absorption of nutrients and may prompt increased nutritional needs, which in turn can lead to vitamin and mineral deficiencies. The hormonal and nutritional deficiencies cause the fibromyalgia to persist, and the fatigue cycle thus continues. (For a simplified illustration of this cycle, see Figure 1.1. For a more detailed illustration, see Figure 8.1 on page 149.)

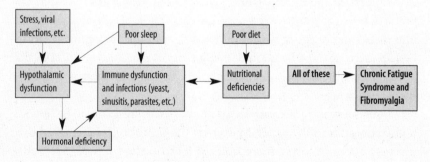

FIGURE 1.1 *The Fatigue Cycle*

Many people enter the fatigue cycle directly through disrupted sleep. Fibromyalgia can be triggered by anything that suppresses the hypothalamus, disrupts sleep, or causes tight muscles. These include a trauma, such as an accident; a parasitic or other infection; chronic emotional or physical stress; hormonal imbalances; and/or recent childbirth. It can also be triggered by a number of other problems, such as an anatomic problem (for example, having legs of different lengths) or temporomandibular joint (TMJ) syndrome, which is characterized by tenderness and clicking in the jaw.

The Autoimmune Triad and Hormonal Deficiencies

Another common pattern seen in severe chronic fatigue states is the *autoimmune triad.* In autoimmune disorders, the body mistakes parts of itself for outside invaders. The autoimmune triad seen in CFIDS patients involves the thyroid and adrenal glands, as well as the cells in the body that assist in the absorption of vitamin B_{12}. When the body attacks these "invaders," the resulting low levels of thyroid and adrenal hormones and vitamin B_{12} trigger fibromyalgia and poor sleep, which then suppresses the hypothalamus gland, setting the fatigue cycle in motion. Multiple other hormonal problems (especially low estrogen in the ten to fifteen years before one is "officially" in menopause—see page 50) can also trigger CFIDS/FMS.

Is the Pattern Important?

Some people fit into one of the patterns just described, but many other patterns also exist. When I ask patients when their problems began, I sometimes get an answer to the exact date—year, month, and day. These patients usually fall into the first category because they had an infection that suppressed the hypothalamus gland. Other people answer, "Oh, the problem began about three to four years ago." These people most often fall into the second category, with disordered sleep as the predominant factor, perhaps accompanied by an underlying yeast or parasitic infection in the bowel. However, they also commonly fall into the third category—hormonal deficiencies.

Sometimes, the exact pattern cannot be determined, and to be honest, it often does not really matter. I now treat the entire process at once so that my patients can recover more quickly. This method has its trade-offs, though. Because I treat all the processes simultaneously, I sometimes cannot tell exactly which treatment is producing the main benefit. However, I feel that treating all the suspected processes at the same time works more efficiently. Then, when the patient is feeling better, I taper off the treatments to see which ones are still needed. The choice of whether to treat multiple problems simultaneously or only one at a time is best made by you and your physician. The educational program on my website (www.endfatigue.com; see Appendix J: Resources) can help you determine which treatments are likely to be needed in your case.

What Chronic Fatigue Syndrome Feels Like

Chronic fatigue syndrome and fibromyalgia occur in varying degrees of severity. Many people have mild to moderate fatigue with achiness and poor sleep. Often, these people attribute the symptoms simply to aging or stress—feeling like they're fifty years old when they're only thirty. Others have fatigue so disabling that they cannot even get out of bed, let alone participate in regular day-to-day activities.

The most common complaints that chronic fatigue and fibromyalgia patients have are:

- *Overwhelming fatigue.* Most people with CFIDS are fatigued most or all of the time. Occasionally, they have periods—that is, short spans of time lasting for several hours or days—during which they feel better. However, what they usually try to do during those good periods is to make up for lost time. They then end up crashing and burning.

  Most CFIDS patients wake up tired. This is especially true of fibromyalgia patients. In addition, exercise often makes the fatigue worse. When CFIDS patients try to exercise, they feel worse that day and usually feel as if they were hit by a truck the next day. This causes further deconditioning and discouragement.
- *Frequent infections.* Many CFIDS patients have recurrent sinus or respiratory infections, sore throats, swollen glands, bladder infections, and/or vaginal, bowel, or skin yeast infections. These are usually best treated without antibiotics (see Treating Infections Without Antibiotics in Chapter 4). Some have a recurrent rash that is resistant to treatment. They often find that the rash goes away for the first time in years when they have their bowel fungal overgrowth treated. Abdomi-

nal gas, cramps, and bloating are also very common, as is alternating diarrhea and constipation. These digestive complaints are attributed to spastic colon and are often triggered by bowel yeast or parasitic infections. Poor food absorption and food sensitivities may also play significant roles in the onset of bowel symptoms.

• *Brain fog.* Brain fog is almost routine. Chronic fatigue patients often suffer from poor short-term memory, difficulty with word finding and word substitution, and, occasionally, brief episodes of disorientation lasting one-half to two minutes that occur despite being in a familiar place. Brain fog is one of the most frustrating symptoms of CFIDS for some patients and is often the scariest. It is also a complaint that routinely resolves with treatment.

• *Achiness.* Chronic diffuse achiness in both muscles and joints is also very common in chronic fatigue patients. For most, this achiness comes from disordered sleep, low thyroid function, yeast infections, and nutritional deficiencies. (The achiness associated with fibromyalgia and how to treat it will be discussed in detail in Chapter 5.)

• *Increased thirst.* When I meet a new patient who has a water bottle in hand, I usually know what his or her main complaint will be. As part of their hormonal problems, people with chronic fatigue have increased urine output and, therefore, increased thirst. A classic description of a CFIDS/FMS patient is that he or she "drinks like a fish and pees like a racehorse." Drinking a lot of water is very important. In fact, many CFIDS patients find that they need to drink two to three times as much liquid as the average person. I recommend filtered water (more about this in later chapters).

• *Allergies.* Fatigue patients often have a history of being sensitive to many foods and medications. They often get away with small doses of medications and respond adversely to normal or large doses. Fortunately, severe environmental sensitivity is much less common. I find that food and other sensitivities usually improve when the adrenal insufficiency and yeast or parasitic overgrowth are treated. Desensitization techniques (such as the Nambudripad allergy elimination technique [NAET] or sublingual provocation and neutralization) can also be very helpful (more about these in Chapter 10).

• *Anxiety and depression.* One-eighth of the people with CFIDS have marked anxiety, with palpitations, sweating, and other signs of panic. The CFIDS, combined with nutritional deficiencies, aggravates the tendency to anxiety and depression. These symptoms, too, often improve with treatment.

- *Weight gain.* Despite no change in diet, people often gain twenty to fifty pounds in the first six to twelve months of their illness. I suspect this occurs because of changes in metabolism (for example, low thyroid function despite "normal" tests, yeast overgrowth, a deficiency of acetyl-L-carnitine [this will be discussed in detail in Chapter 8], and so on).

- *Decreased libido.* When I ask CFIDS patients how their libido is, the majority answer "What libido?" In addition to pain and generally feeling "yucky," hormonal deficiencies also contribute to this. Happily, libido often improves with treatment.

You may have recognized yourself as you read through this list. If you did, please be assured that you are not alone. You are part of a large group of over 50 million people worldwide. Many excellent support groups exist, including the Fibromyalgia Network and the Chronic Fatigue and Immune Dysfunction Syndrome Association of America. These are effective support groups that are actively searching for answers to the CFIDS puzzle. Their addresses, as well as those of some other excellent support groups and additional organizations, may be found in Appendix J: Resources.

Many pieces of the CFIDS puzzle are still missing. The outlook is bright, however, with new research continually providing important clues on how to improve treatment. And for the vast majority of people with CFIDS/FMS/ME-related symptoms, effective treatment is now available!

Important Points

- Chronic fatigue patients usually have a variety of symptoms in addition to fatigue. Common ones are achiness, poor sleep, brain fog, increased thirst, weight gain, low libido, and frequent infections.
- Chronic fatigue usually has a mixture of underlying causes. This is because each problem can trigger other problems. For example, poor sleep and hormonal problems can trigger disordered immunity, which can trigger bowel yeast, parasitic, and other infections, which can trigger fibromyalgia, which can further worsen sleep and hormonal problems.
- New research shows that effective treatment is available for over 85 percent of patients with CFIDS/FMS.

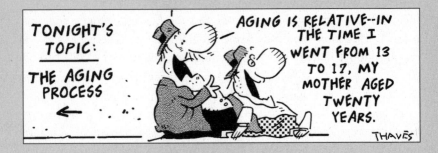

CHAPTER 2

Going After the Easy Things First

OFTEN, PEOPLE COME IN TO MY OFFICE COMPLAINING of longstanding fatigue that is not quite as disabling as the fatigue seen in chronic fatigue syndrome or fibromyalgia. I never cease to be amazed at how often these people improve dramatically by simply cleaning up their diets a little—cutting down on their sugar, caffeine, and alcohol intake; substituting whole grains for white flour; and adding an excellent multivitamin supplement with magnesium to their daily regimens. So let us start with the easy things first.

Sugar and White Flour

The average American's diet includes over 140 pounds of added sugar per year.[1] This added sugar accounts for 18 percent of the average American's caloric intake. Since a healthy diet without added sugar may have only a 5- to 15-percent margin of safety for supplying optimum amounts of vitamins and minerals, the added sugar alone makes the average American diet a disaster.

Sugar also suppresses the immune system, nurtures the growth of yeast in the bowel, and stimulates yeast overgrowth in the bowel. Yeast grows by fermenting sugar, and the yeast say thank-you by making billions of baby yeasties. Physicians working in this field have found that although most sugar is usually absorbed before it gets to the bowels, excess sugar can markedly aggravate yeast overgrowth.[2] (A complete discussion of yeast overgrowth appears in Chapter 4.) Yeast can also aggravate sugar craving. This may mimic hypoglycemia, which is commonly found in people with an underactive adrenal gland. (Hypoglycemia is discussed in Chapter 3.)

I often hear people express skepticism about the importance of nutritional supplements. A typical comment that I hear is, "Five hundred years ago, there were no vitamin tablets, and people seemed to do just fine." Well, 500 years ago, sugar was expensive and not readily available. The King of England might have sprinkled a teaspoon of sugar on his food as a sign of power, but when he wanted sugar and had none left, he had to send someone to the West Indies to get it!

Another dietary disaster is white flour. Vitamins were supposedly discovered by a settler who went on sailing expeditions with Dutch explorers. Soon after the settler helped a group of colonists establish their new home, he found that the colonists were becoming ill. He also noticed that the colony's chickens were looking unusually healthy. Being a curious fellow, this man began feeding the chicken food to the people. Over a period of several weeks, the people became stronger and healthier. Since the settler was also a good businessman, he (incorrectly) named the chicken feed *vital amines,* meaning "vital proteins," and began selling it. The name was later shortened to *vitamins.*

Today, scientists understand what happened to those colonists. Polishing off the brown outer coat, or bran, from rice had become fashionable. The rice bran was then used as chicken feed. The bran, however, contains most of the vitamins and minerals that are present in rice. The colonists therefore quickly became nutritionally deficient, while the chickens flourished.

In the United States, approximately 18 percent of the average person's calories come from white flour. However, white flour, just like white rice, has had the bran removed and therefore is also significantly depleted of vitamins and minerals.[3] Although some foods made of white flour are now fortified with vitamins and minerals to make up for this, *most* of the nutrients that were removed continue to be missing.

As you can see, from just the use of white flour and added sugar, Americans often reduce their vitamin and mineral intake by around 35 percent. Add to this the nutrients that are lost in the canning of vegetables, which can cause vitamin losses of up to 80 percent, and in the processing of other foods.[4] As Dr. S. B. Eaton noted in his study in the prestigious *New England Journal of Medicine,* "Physicians and nutritionists are increasingly convinced that the dietary habits adopted by Western society over the past one hundred years make an important etiologic [causative] contribution to coronary heart diseases [angina], hypertension, diabetes, and some types of cancer.[5] This is the same conclusion that was reached by the authors of *Western Diseases: Their Emergence and Prevention.*[6]

Caffeine and Alcohol

I am constantly astonished at the number of people who complain about being tired who drink more than ten cups of coffee a day. Caffeine is a loan shark for energy and also accentuates hypoglycemic symptoms. Many chronic fatigue patients fall into the trap of drinking ever-increasing amounts of coffee to boost their energy so that they can function. What these people do not realize is that as the day goes on, caffeine takes away more energy than it gives. Coffee drinkers are often caught in a vicious cycle. I advise all my coffee drinkers to stop ingesting coffee completely for two to three months. After this initial period, I tell them that they can add back up to eight ounces of coffee a day if they are feeling better. Black and green teas, in leaf and teabag forms, are high in antioxidants, however, and are much more healthful than coffee.

If you drink more than three cups of coffee a day, you should remove it from your diet gradually. To begin, cut your coffee consumption in half every week until you are down to about one cup a day. For example, if you generally drink four cups of coffee a day, cut your intake to two cups a day the first week, then to one cup a day the second week. The final week, switch to tea, which improves your health, with some caffeine. I usually tell my patients that I do not want to see them until ten days after their last cup of coffee. Caffeine is an addictive drug and removing it from the diet brings withdrawal symptoms—grouchiness, headache, and fatigue. Once the withdrawal symptoms are gone, however, my patients usually feel much better and are very happy that they went through the process. By tapering the coffee as just described, it takes a little longer to feel well, but the withdrawal symptoms are not as severe.

Limit alcohol to one to two drinks a day. One drink equals six ounces of wine, twelve ounces of beer, or one and a half ounces of whiskey. If you drink more than these amounts, you should stop drinking alcohol completely for three months. If you decide to return alcohol to your diet at the end of that time, make two drinks a day your limit. Some people with yeast overgrowth find that even the smallest amount of alcohol makes them feel poorly.

Vitamin and Mineral Supplements

The argument about people not needing vitamin tablets 500 years ago does not apply to the average modern American. One study that was reported in the *American Journal of Clinical Nutrition* showed that fewer than 5 percent of the study participants consumed the recommended daily amounts (RDAs) of all their needed vitamins and minerals.[7] What is frightening is that this study was conducted in Beltsville, Maryland, on U.S. Department of Agriculture (USDA) research center employees.

Despite this, some cynics still like to say that the vitamins go out in your urine, so all you're doing by taking vitamin supplements is making expensive urine. Using this line of reasoning, these cynics can stop drinking water (it just goes out in their urine!). That way, they'll soon stop annoying people who are in the process of getting themselves well!

Why are vitamins and minerals so important? Dr. Janet Travell, White House physician for presidents John F. Kennedy and Lyndon B. Johnson and professor emeritus of internal medicine at George Washington University, cowrote *Myofascial Pain and Dysfunction: The Trigger Point Manual*, which is acknowledged as the authoritative work on muscle problems. In one chapter alone, Dr. Travell and coauthor Dr. David Simons reference 317 studies showing that problems such as hormonal, vitamin, and mineral deficiencies can contribute to muscle disorders.[8]

Numerous other studies have shown that adequate amounts of vitamins and minerals, especially folic acid, zinc (found to be very low in people with FMS), and selenium, are critical for proper immune function— that is, for defense against infections. Vitamin A, beta-carotene, vitamin B_6, vitamin C, vitamin E, iron, and many other nutrients also have been found to be very important in keeping the body's defenses strong.[9]

Multiple Vitamin and Mineral

Every vitamin and nutritional mineral is *very* important in some way to health. The body depends on receiving vitamins and minerals from the diet because it cannot make them itself. Especially important are the B vitamins, zinc, iron, and magnesium. If you are low in vitamins and minerals—whether because you eat junk food and are not taking in the required nutrients or because you are consuming the proper foods but your body is unable to metabolize them correctly—your fibromyalgia simply will not subside. An excellent multivitamin supplement is therefore critical to your improvement.

Taking a multivitamin that supplies at least 25 milligrams each of vitamin B_1 (thiamine), vitamin B_2 (riboflavin), vitamin B_3 (niacin), and vitamin B_6 (pyridoxine), as well as good amounts of folic acid, vitamin B_{12}, and biotin and an adequate representation of minerals can have a dramatic effect on your well-being. An excellent single tablet a day multivitamin is Natrol's My Favorite Multiple—Take One (don't confuse this with My Favorite Multiple, which is a different product). Another recommended multivitamin formula is the From Fatigued To Fantastic Foundation Formula. (See Appendix J: Resources for further information about these products and how to find them.) I recommend these brands because all vitamins are not created equal and many are made very poorly. (My entire share of any profit from my formula goes to charity.)

The main side effect of taking multivitamins is an upset stomach, which occurs in a small percentage of people. If this is a problem for you, try taking the vitamin with a meal or at bedtime, or split it and take one-half or one-third the dose two to three times a day. If the stomach discomfort persists, switch to another brand, such as a Centrum multivitamin supplement in the morning and a B-complex supplement in the afternoon or evening. If you still have problems, experiment until you find a brand of multivitamin that your stomach can tolerate. Please note that any non-time-released supplement containing B vitamins will turn your urine bright yellow. This is normal.

Iron

Iron is important because an iron level that is too high or too low can cause fatigue, poor immune function, cold intolerance, decreased thyroid function, and poor memory.[10] I routinely recommend that all my chronic fatigue patients have their iron level and total iron binding capacity (TIBC) checked. Although not useful by themselves, dividing the iron level by the TIBC gives you a *percent saturation,* which is a useful measure. In addition, I recommend that they have their ferritin blood level checked. These three tests all measure iron status. Some insurance companies balk at paying for all three tests, but the data and my clinical experience strongly support having them all done. Even if a person's iron percent saturation is low but still normal, that person will often feel fatigued, despite not being anemic. The ferritin level, however, will pick up subtle deficiencies. Unfortunately, even minimal inflammation, such as a bladder infection, will falsely elevate the ferritin measurement and make it appear to be falsely normal. This is why all three tests are necessary to determine iron deficiency.

One study reported in the British medical journal *Lancet* showed that infertile females whose ferritin levels were between 20 and 40—a ferritin level over 9 is technically normal—were often able to become pregnant when they took supplemental iron.[11] Other research shows that low-normal iron levels cause poor mental functioning and poor immune function. This suggests that levels considered sufficient to prevent anemia are often inadequate for other body functions. Because of this, anyone whose ferritin level is below 40, *or* whose percent saturation is less than 22 percent, should be considered a prime subject for a trial treatment of iron therapy. However, if you have a high risk of heart disease, such as a strong family history or a high cholesterol count, you should take a multivitamin *without* iron unless your blood tests show that you are low in that mineral. Although iron is important, it is also pro-oxidative (that is, it promotes free-radical activity) and can cause inflammation if the level is too high. This helps remind us that more is not always better!

A surprisingly large number of people display early hemochromatosis on their iron studies. Hemochromatosis is a disease of excess iron. Early in the disease, fatigue is often the only symptom. If caught early, hemochromatosis is remarkably easy to treat. If caught late, however, it is disabling and even life-threatening. This is an additional reason to check the iron level carefully.

VITAMIN B$_{12}$

Vitamin B$_{12}$ is another key nutrient in CFIDS. Technically, the B$_{12}$ level is normal if it is over 208 picograms per deciliter (pg/dL) of blood. However, studies have shown that people can suffer severe and sometimes long-term nerve and brain damage from B$_{12}$ deficiency even if their levels are as high as 300 pg/dL.[12] Why are the "normal" levels set so low? In part, the normal values were initially set according to what prevents anemia. But the brain's and nervous system's needs for vitamin B$_{12}$ are often much higher than those of the bone marrow. Also, as much as I hate to admit it, the medical establishment has greatly enjoyed poking fun at the old-time doctors who gave vitamin B$_{12}$ shots for fatigue. The use of B$_{12}$ shots despite "normal" levels is considered almost a symbol of unscientific, archaic medicine. As noted in an editorial in *The New England Journal of Medicine,* however, current findings suggest that those old-time doctors may have been right.[13] I suspect, though, that the modern medical establishment will be a little slow to eat crow.

I have been told (although I have been unable to confirm it), that a B$_{12}$ level under 400 pg/dL is often considered abnormal in Japan and treated. In addition, a recent study using the respected Framingham database showed that metabolic signs of B$_{12}$ deficiency occur even with levels over 500 pg/dL.[14]

Furthermore, people with Alzheimer's disease have been found to have an average B$_{12}$ level of only 472 picograms per deciliter, compared with people who have confusion from a non-Alzheimer's condition (such as a stroke), whose average B$_{12}$ levels run 887 picograms per deciliter.[15] These and other studies suggest that many people need significantly highter B$_{12}$ levels than what is currently considered normal. More importantly, recent research shows that despite their having low normal B$_{12}$ levels in the blood, CFIDS patients often have *very low* (and sometimes absent) B$_{12}$ levels in their brains![16] This suggests that, because of the metabolic problems present in CFIDS/FMS, you may need quite high B$_{12}$ levels in your blood to get adequate levels past the blood-brain barrier (the membrane that separates the brain from the blood to protect the brain from circulating toxins) and into the brain, where B$_{12}$ is needed. In addition, vitamin B$_{12}$ helps reduce excessive levels of nitric oxide, a neurotransmitter that can be too high in people with CFIDS/FMS and that can easily contribute to symptoms. More and more, research studies are supporting what doctors who effectively treat CFIDS/FMS using B_{12} shots have said for years!

It is no surprise then, when their other problems are also treated, many people respond dramatically to B_{12} injections. If a patient's B_{12} level is under 540 pg/mL, I treat that person with a 1-cc (1,000- to 3,000-microgram) injection one to five times a week for fifteen injections. These shots are very safe and fairly inexpensive. Although most regular pharmacies carry only the 1,000-microgram-per-cc strength, holistic pharmacies (see Appendix J: Resources) can make up injectable vitamin B_{12} that contains 3,000 to 10,000 micrograms per cc. Usually, if a patient is going to benefit from the shots, I see improvement by ten weeks. I usually stop after ten to fifteen shots. If a patient feels worse when the injections are stopped, I resume giving the shots, usually every one to five weeks (but as often as three to four times a week in some cases) for an extended period of time. Many people, however, can maintain their B_{12} level after fifteen injections by taking a good multivitamin supplement.

Why is a low B_{12} level such a common problem in CFIDS patients? Several possibilities exist. Among them are the following:

- Vitamin B_{12} is important for the repair of nerve injuries. Evidence suggests that brain dysfunction occurs in CFIDS. In repairing this injury, the body may overutilize vitamin B_{12} and deplete its stores.
- If an autoimmune process impairs the thyroid or adrenal gland, it may also attack the area responsible for our ability to absorb vitamin B_{12}. (For a discussion of autoimmunity, see page 29.)
- Overgrowth of yeast or parasites in the bowel or problems with absorption may prevent the proper absorption of vitamin B_{12}.
- Vitamin B_{12} has trouble getting across the blood-brain barrier.[17]
- Vitamin B_{12} may be important for, and used up in, detoxification.

Whatever the cause, I have found that treating patients with vitamin B_{12}, even if their levels are technically normal, often results in marked improvement.

MAGNESIUM

In addition to the multivitamin supplement and B_{12} shots, I also urge my CFIDS patients to take a magnesium supplement. Magnesium is involved in hundreds of different body functions, but is routinely low in the American diet as a result of food processing. The average American diet supplies less than 300 milligrams of magnesium per day, while the average Asian diet supplies over 600 milligrams per day.[18] I generally recommend taking 1,800 milligrams of malic acid and 450 milligrams of magnesium glycinate a day for eight months, and then cutting back to one-third this dose. If diarrhea and cramps are not a problem, you can take up to twice this amount. If your magnesium level is low, your muscles will stay in spasm and your fibromyalgia will not resolve. This is one of the reasons that taking magnesium is so critical. In addition, magnesium is important for the muscles' and body's strength and energy.[19] Most of your magnesium is inside your cells and the blood test only measures the magnesium in your blood—making blood tests an unreliable measure. I suspect that magnesium has trouble getting into the cells in people with CFIDS/FMS. When CFIDS/FMS is properly treated, the magnesium may then be better able to get inside the cells. The cells then soak it in like a thirsty sponge and your blood level may even drop—despite taking large amounts of oral and even intravenous magnesium. So keep in mind that magnesium blood tests do not drop below normal until *severe* magnesium depletion occurs and *everyone* with CFIDS/FMS, fatigue, or muscle achiness should take magnesium.[20] An exception is if you have kidney failure with a blood creatinine level over 1.6 milligrams per deciliter (mg/dL)—very rare in CFIDS/FMS.

If you get uncomfortable diarrhea from the magnesium, cut the dosage back and then slowly increase the dose as is comfortable. If your creatinine is 1.5 to 1.6 mg/dL, take just 150 milligrams of magnesium a day for two to three months and discuss your dosage and regimen with your physician.

Magnesium absorption is very difficult, which is why I like to use the glycinate forms. The forms I recommend are found in Fibrocare from To Your Health and in the From Fatigued To Fantastic powder formula. Plain magnesium oxide is also available and is the most inexpensive form of magnesium. Your body may not absorb it well, however, resulting in gas and diarrhea. If you choose to take magnesium oxide, take 500 milligrams per day.

Although I strongly recommend taking nutritional supplements to ensure obtaining the necessary nutrients, I also want to stress that eating a good healthy diet is important. Eat a lot of whole grains, fresh fruits (whole fruit, not fruit juice), and fresh vegetables. Many raw vegetables have enzymes that help boost energy levels. You do not have to cut out all foods that might be bad or eat a diet that is impossible to follow. All you need to do is eat a diet that is reasonably healthy and low in caffeine and added sugar. The more unprocessed your diet is, the healthier you will be. Your body will tell you what's good for you by making you *feel good!*

IMPORTANT POINTS

- Remove sugar and other sweeteners from your diet. Stevia, a sweet-tasting herb, and Sweet Balance, a product derived from the lo-han fruit, can be used as substitutes. They taste good and are healthy.
- Use whole-grain flour instead of white flour whenever possible.
- Remove caffeine from your diet.
- Limit alcohol consumption to one or two drinks daily.
- Treat nutritional deficiencies with a daily multivitamin that has as least 25 milligrams each of vitamins B_1, B_2, B_3, and B_6, as well as all the essential minerals. It is also important to take magnesium glycinate with malic acid.
- Treat a suboptimal iron level with an iron supplement. A high iron level also needs to be treated properly.
- Vitamin B_{12} injections can be *very* helpful.
- In addition to taking supplements, eat a healthy diet that includes lots of fresh fruits and vegetables and a minimum of processed foods.

CHAPTER 3

Hormones—The Body's Master Control System

YOUR BODY'S METABOLISM IS CONTROLLED BY A series of glands that create messengers called hormones. These hormones are controlled by feedback mechanisms that are constantly interacting with one another in an elaborate dance. This dance is initiated by the hypothalamus, an ancient structure that is located deep inside the brain. The hypothalamus is the body's master gland and acts like the conductor in an orchestra. It sends hormones to its next-door neighbor, the pituitary gland, which in turn controls the thyroid gland, the adrenal glands, and the ovaries in females and testicles in males. The hypothalamus also monitors the levels of the hormones that all these glands make and tells the glands whether to make more or less.

Many factors determine how much hormone the hypothalamus directs each gland to make. A very mysterious gland in the brain called the pineal gland makes melatonin (and possibly also other hormones, as yet unknown). This gland also likely regulates your body's circadian rhythm—that is, your day/night cycles. Many functions in the body are rhythmic. The adrenal gland, for example, makes most of its cortisol hormones during the day. If it makes too much at night, the person has trouble sleeping. Evidence suggests that in people with chronic fatigue, the adrenal glands make too much cortisol at night and not enough during the day. Stress, such as an infection, also causes the hypothalamus to direct the adrenals to make more cortisol. These are just a few of the many factors that regulate hormone production.

Functions of the Different Glands

As just noted, the pineal, hypothalamus, and pituitary glands, located deep within the brain, work together to direct and balance the metabolic system (the body's energy) and the immune system (the body's defense systems), as well as the the autonomic [sympathetic-parasympathetic] nervous system (the part of the nervous system that controls blood flow to the skin, muscles, and organs). Current evidence suggests that a major portion of the symptoms of CFIDS and fibromyalgia are manifestations of a poorly functioning hypothalamus.

What roles do the other glands play? The thyroid gland is the body's gas pedal. It slows or speeds up the metabolism. If it is underactive—that is, if it produces too little thyroid hormone—as is common in CFIDS/FMS, you can have fatigue, achiness, weight gain, poor mental functioning, and intolerance to cold.

The adrenal glands are really several glands in one. They help direct the body's defense systems plus assist the body in dealing with stressful situations. If they are underactive, the result is fatigue, recurrent or persistent infections, hypoglycemia, allergies or environmental sensitivities, low blood pressure, dizziness, sugar craving, and poor ability to cope with stress.

The ovaries in females and the testicles in males support and cycle the reproductive system. The ovaries regulate menstruation in women, and both the ovaries and testicles contribute to libido (sexual desire). The male and female states of mind are powerfully influenced by the hormones produced by these glands. Although testosterone is known as a "male hormone," it is also important in females. If either testosterone or the female hormone, estrogen, is low, the person may feel tired, depressed, weak, or moody. He or she may also feel a loss of libido and suffer from disordered sexual function and hot flashes.

Suppression of the hormonal system plays a dramatic role in CFIDS and fibromyalgia. This often occurs despite your hormonal blood tests being normal! This chapter will present an overview of how to handle this problem.

Hypothalamic Dysfunction

There is an old story of the blind men who stumbled upon an elephant. One felt its trunk and believed it was a snake. Another felt its leg and thought it was a tree trunk. Yet another, missing the elephant entirely, was certain nothing was there and told his friends they must be crazy. This seems to be the current state of affairs in our understanding of CFIDS/FMS.

Even so, we are lucky to be at a point where we have as many pieces of the puzzle as we do. Let's examine what we do know, beginning with two assumptions that I believe to be true:

1. CFIDS/FMS are part of the same process in most cases.
2. CFIDS/FMS represent a common endpoint of a large number of possible underlying triggers—that is, many different things can trigger the syndrome. Once triggered, the process is similar and self-perpetuating, regardless of what the triggers were and whether or not the triggers are now gone. For example, an auto accident or viral syndrome can both trigger CFIDS/FMS in different people.

Furthermore, we know that several processes are common in people with CFIDS/FMS:

- Disordered sleep.
- Multiple hormonal dysfunctions.
- Immune dysfunction.
- Autonomic nervous system dysfunction, with neurally mediated hypotension (NMH), a problem with blood pressure regulation that results in weakness and dizziness when standing.
- Low body temperature.

Things simplify a bit when one realizes that all of the above processes are controlled by the hypothalamus. Let's look at each of them in turn.

DISORDERED SLEEP

When we look at sleep deprivation research, several things stand out. Among other things, sleep deprivation can cause:

- Immune dysfunction, with multiple opportunistic infections.
- Decreased metabolic activity, specifically in the hypothalamus, limbic system, and thalamus. This (as well as low estrogen levels) could account for the decreases in blood flow to the brain.
- Suppression of thyroid hormones.
- Autonomic and temperature regulation dysfunction. When given the choice, sleep-deprived test animals will often choose a higher room temperature. Higher nighttime room temperatures may further worsen sleep quality.
- Changes in phosphate metabolism. Dr. R. Paul St. Amand, FMS researcher and author, postulates that a defect of phosphate metabolism is important in FMS and has found that guaifenesin, an expectorant that is a common ingredient in over-the-counter cough medicines, and other agents that promote the excretion of uric acid can improve symptoms. It is possible that the sleep disorder triggers the phosphate defect. Although a controlled study by Dr. Robert Bennett of the University of Oregon, a superb FMS researcher, did not find guaifenesin to be beneficial, Dr. St. Amand feels that that study had critical design flaws. There have been enough reports of benefit from patients who found no relief from other treatments to encourage me to study guaifenesin further, despite the negative study. I rarely prescribe guaifenesin myself, though.
- Allodynia, a condition in which normally comfortable touch causes discomfort. It is postulated that in FMS, this is caused by elevated levels of a compound known as substance P, a neurotransmitter involved in the sensation of pain, secondary to low brain levels of another neurotransmitter, serotonin. Low estrogen also can cause low serotonin, as well as low levels of still another neurotransmitter, acetylcholine. If sleep deprivation causes allodynia, might it also cause increased levels of substance P and a decrease in serotonin? Evidence suggests that low acetylcholine function can contribute to CFIDS/FMS, and a recent study found that treating this with a type of drug called an acetylcholinesterase inhibitor, which results in increased acetylcholine, resulted in some improvement in CFIDS symptoms.

Hormonal Dysfunction

The hypothalamus is the master gland, controlling the activity of most other glands in the body. Autoimmune injury can also damage glands. The effects of hypothalamic dysfunction on the body's hormone levels can include:

- Low thyroid hormone. This can cause decreased metabolism, with weight gain and low body temperature, which can cause poor enzyme and metabolic function.
- Low vasopressin (antidiuretic hormone). This causes decreased ability to hold onto fluid, resulting in frequent urination and increased thirst. Dehydration then occurs, despite increased water intake. Because vasopressin is also a stimulus for adrenocorticotropic hormone (ACTH) and adrenal function, low vasopressin could also result in decreased adrenal function. Both dehydration and low cortisol (a hormone secreted by the adrenals) can increase the susceptibility to NMH.
- Low growth hormone. This also causes low levels of dehydroepiandrosterone (DHEA), another hormone produced by the adrenal glands. DHEA is used by the body to make other hormones, including estrogen and testosterone, and is tied to energy levels and a general feeling of well-being.
- Decreased cortisol. Low levels of this "stress hormone" causes immune dysfunction and hypotension and the tendency to "crash" in stressful situations.
- Low ovarian and testicular function. Low estrogen can contribute to the decreased blood flow to specific areas in the brain that is seen in CFIDS/FMS. Low testosterone (in both males and females) can cause immune dysfunction. Although total testosterone levels are often normal, I have found that the levels of active (free, or unbound, serum) testosterone are low in the majority of people with CFIDS/FMS. In men, bringing free testosterone levels back to mid- to high-normal (with testosterone injections or creams) often dramatically improved symptoms after two months.
- Elevated prolactin. Prolactin is a hormone whose principal action is to stimulate and maintain milk production after childbirth. The hypothalamus normally suppresses prolactin production. It is not clear what role (if any) elevated prolactin plays in CFIDS. However, lower-

ing an elevated prolactin may improve symptoms. Excessive melatonin intake can also cause elevated prolactin levels.

- Low oxytocin. Oxytocin is a hypothalamic neurotransmitter. Many
CFIDS/FMS patients improve with oxytocin therapy. At this point,
though, it is not clear what, besides low estrogen and amino acid (protein) deficiencies, causes the decreased levels of multiple neurotransmitters.

IMMUNE DYSFUNCTION

Although the causes of immune dysfunction in CFIDS/FMS are not clear,
hypothalamic dysfunction and poor sleep likely play a role. The implications are that CFIDS patients also seem to have opportunistic infections
(that is, infections caused by organisms that usually do not cause illness in
most people) and other recurrent infections. These infections can cause
CFIDS/FMS to persist. Some common types of infections that affect
people with CFIDS/FMS are:

- Chronic sinusitis. This can be bacterial or fungal.
- Chronic prostatitis. This is common in men with CFIDS. It is often
subtle, however.
- Bowel infections. These are a major player in CFIDS/FMS. Parasitic,
fungal, and bacterial overgrowths are common, and often account for
irritable bowel syndrome. They can cause CFIDS/FMS and contribute to the nutritional deficiencies by causing malabsorption and a
"leaky gut." These problems in turn can lead to food sensitivities and
liver overload (the liver may have to detoxify many large molecules
that should not have been absorbed intact or that normally would
have been broken down before absorption). Liver overload, combined
with immune system overactivation and decreased adrenal function,
can contribute to the food, chemical/environmental, and medication
sensitivites. This can occur when the liver is overwhelmed and more
slowly metabolizes or detoxifies these substances.
- Infections caused by rickettsia, mycoplasma, chlamydia, and other unusual organisms. Several organisms that are difficult to test for may
both trigger and perpetuate CFIDS/FMS. Doxycycline, a tetracycline

antibiotic (also sold under the brand names Doryx, Monodox, Vibramycin, and Vibra-Tabs), or ciprofloxacin (Cipro), another antibiotic, given for anywhere from six months to years at a time may eradicate these, but may cause yeast overgrowth, necessitating the use of an antifungal medication.

- Viral infections. Some viruses can cause hypothalamic suppression. Although in most people this resolves when the virus goes away, if you have CFIDS/FMS, it may not. Because many patients get well without antiviral treatments, I suspect the virus is long gone by several months after the illness begins, or is eliminated when the immune suppression is treated and resolves. Post-polio syndrome, herpesvirus type 6 (HHV-6), cytomegalovirus (CMV), and the Epstein-Barr virus are four of many suspected culprits.

AUTONOMIC DYSFUNCTION

The autonomic (sympathetic/parasympathetic) nervous system, the part of the nervous system that controls such basic bodily processes as circulation and breathing (among others) is controlled by the hypothalamus. Improper functioning of the autonomic nervous system can cause a variety of problems, among them:

- Neurally mediated hypotension (NMH). This can cause dizziness and weakness, especially when standing.
- Night and day sweats. The night sweats can disrupt sleep.
- Nasal congestion, with fatigue and an increased risk of chronic sinusitis.

ALTERED TEMPERATURE REGULATION

A low body temperature causes the body's energy and enzyme systems to work inefficiently (enzyme function is very temperature-sensitive). If the body temperature is raised back to 98.6°F (using sustained-release thyroid hormone), people often feel much better. Stress, including infection, or starvation (that is, dieting) may trigger persistently low levels of triiodothyronine (T_3), the active form of thyroid hormone, and cause low body temperature. Unfortunately, since T_3 is mostly made inside the cells, low T_3 levels do not show up on standard blood tests for thyroid function. Altered temperature regulation may also further contribute to impaired sleep.

THE GOOD NEWS

As you can see, hypothalamic dysfunction can cause a cascade of problems that can account for many, if not most, of the abnormal findings seen in CFIDS/FMS. These processes can then perpetuate hypothalamic suppression. They also explain the multitude of symptoms seen in these illnesses.

The good news is that everything I have discussed above is treatable. The trick is to sort out which problems are most active in each individual and to treat them all. We certainly have much more to learn (I really do not think I have defined "the whole elephant" yet!). As we continue to integrate what we learn, we may begin to see the whole picture.

Adrenal Insufficiency

The adrenal glands, which sit on top of the kidneys, are actually two different glands in one. The center of the gland makes adrenaline (epinephrine) and is under the control of the autonomic nervous system. Although it is known that this part of the nervous system is also on the fritz in chronic fatigue patients—contributing to such symptoms as hot and cold sweats, cold sweaty hands, neurally mediated hypotension, and panic attacks—it is not understood if or how this ties into the adrenal's ability to make adrenaline in CFIDS/FMS. More likely, adrenaline deficiency is a central brain problem.

The outer part of the adrenal gland, the cortex, also makes many important hormones. These include:

- Cortisol. The adrenal glands increase their production of cortisol in response to stress. Cortisol raises the blood sugar and blood pressure levels and moderates immune function, in addition to playing numerous other roles. If the cortisol level is low, the person has fatigue, low blood pressure, hypoglycemia, poor immune function, an increased tendency to allergies and environmental sensitivity, and an inability to deal with stress.

- Dehydroepiandrosterone sulfate (DHEA-S). Although its mechanism of action is not clear, DHEA is the most abundant hormone produced by the adrenal cortex. If it is low, you will feel poorly. Patients often feel dramatically better when their DHEA-S levels are brought to the mid-normal range for a twenty-nine-year-old. DHEA-S levels normally decline with age, prompting many people to feel that this deficiency causes people to age and die to make room for newborns. DHEA-S levels appear to drop prematurely in chronic fatigue patients.
- Aldosterone. This hormone helps to keep salt and water balanced in the body.
- Estrogen and testosterone. These hormones are produced in small but significant amounts by the adrenals as well as by the ovaries and testicles.

CAUSES OF ADRENAL INSUFFICIENCY

About two-thirds of chronic fatigue patients appear to have underactive adrenal glands.[1] One reason may be that the hypothalamus does not make enough corticotropin-releasing hormone (CRH), which is the brain's way of telling the adrenals that more cortisol is needed. I suspect that many people also have adrenal burnout. Dr. Hans Selye, one of the first doctors to research stress reactions, found that if an animal becomes severely overstressed, its adrenal glands bleed and develop signs of adrenal destruction before the animal finally dies from the stress.

If you think back to your biology classes in high school, you may remember something called the *fight-or-flight response.* This is a physical reaction that occurs during times of stress. During the Stone Age, when a caveman met an animal that wanted to eat him, the caveman's adrenal glands activated multiple systems in his body that prompted him to either fight or run. This reaction helped the caveman survive. In those days, however, people probably had a couple of weeks or months to recover before facing the next major stress.

In today's society, people often experience stress reactions every few minutes. For example, when driving to work, a woman is delayed because of heavy traffic. While sitting behind the wheel, she frets about the consequences of her walking into the office late. Every time she hits a red light or pulls up behind a car that has slowed down, her adrenal glands' fight-or-flight reaction goes off again. When she finally arrives at work, she finds her boss waiting for her, which triggers the reaction once more. During the day, the woman may also have to deal with stresses such as angry customers or difficult coworkers. Her husband or children may phone, forcing her to deal with family stresses. If the woman is ill—suffering from CFS, for example—she has another major stress. The different problems associated with CFS, such as sinus infections and pain, put more stress on her adrenal glands.

I suspect that many people suffer exhaustion of their adrenal glands but without the adrenal gland destruction that Hans Selye saw in his experimental animals. With the kinds of stresses common in modern society, a person's adrenal test may show hormonal levels that are actually higher than usual, since the adrenal gland tends to overcompensate to deal with stress. Over time, this may exhaust the adrenal reserve—that is, the adrenal's ability to increase hormone production in response to stress. In endocrinologist Dr. William Jefferies's experience (and in mine as well), people with either low hormone production or a low reserve often respond dramatically to treatment with a low dose of adrenal hormone.[2]

Dr. Jefferies's opinion is that everyone who has unexplained, disabling chronic fatigue should be given a low-dose trial of adrenal hormone.[3] Although Dr. Jefferies may well be on the mark, I tend to use this treatment first only on patients who fail morning cortisol and/or cortrosyn stimulation tests, which test adrenal function. However, the test can be interpreted in many different ways, and I tend to be *much* more liberal than most when interpreting the results.

Symptoms of Adrenal Insufficiency

If your adrenal glands are underactive, what might you be experiencing? Low adrenal function can cause, among other symptoms:

- Fatigue.
- Recurrent infections.
- Difficulty shaking off infections.
- Poor response and "crashing" during stress.
- Achiness.

- Hypoglycemia.
- Low blood pressure and dizziness upon first standing.

Hypoglycemia deserves special mention. Many people sometimes become shaky and nervous, then dizzy, irritable, and fatigued. These people often feel better after they eat sweets, which improve their energy and mood for a short period of time. Because of this, these people often crave sugar, not realizing that it makes their blood sugar level initially shoot back up to normal, which is what makes them feel better, but then makes it continue shooting up beyond normal. The body responds to this by driving the sugar level back down below normal again. The effect, energywise, is like a roller coaster.

Dr. Jefferies has noted—and again, my experience confirms his finding—that most people with hypoglycemia have underactive adrenal glands. This makes sense because the adrenal glands' responsibilities include maintaining blood sugar at an adequate level. Sugar is the only fuel that the brain can use. When a person's blood sugar level drops, he or she feels poorly.

Treating Adrenal Insufficiency

People with hypoglycemia can treat low blood sugar symptoms by cutting sugar and caffeine out of their diets; having frequent, small meals; and increasing their intake of complex carbohydrates such as whole grains and vegetables. Fruit—not fruit juices, which contain concentrated sugar—can be eaten in moderation, about one to two pieces a day, depending on the type of fruit. Taking 250 micrograms of glucose tolerance factor (GTF) chromium twice a day for six months often helps smooth out hypoglycemic symptoms.[4]

More directly, treating the underactive adrenal problem with low doses of adrenal hormone usually banishes the symptoms of low blood sugar. I prefer using prescription hydrocortisone such as Cortef instead of the adrenal glandulars available at health food stores. The adrenal content of over-the-counter adrenal glandulars is unknown and varies from batch to batch. Toxicity, or overdosing, is too easy. If you can't get Cortef, or prefer to try a natural approach first, you can try using licorice, vitamin C, ginseng, and echinacea to improve adrenal function, as follows:

- Take 2 to 3 grams (2,000 to 3,000 milligrams) of licorice root (*not* de-glycyrrhizinated licorice [DGL]) twice a day for six to eight weeks. You may then taper off over a period of ten to fourteen days. Licorice can raise blood pressure or cause an overly high cortisol level if taken on an ongoing basis. It is best used short-term as a "jump-start" in raising cortisol levels.
- After four to six weeks on licorice root, add 100 milligrams of Asian ginseng twice a day. This is safer than licorice. If it helps, you can take it for an extended period (one to two years) in cycles of six weeks on and one to two weeks off.
- Take 325 to 650 milligrams of encapsulated freeze-dried echinacea plant *or* 1,000 to 2,000 milligrams of dried echinacea root three times a day. Take it in cycles of six weeks on and two weeks off—if taken continuously, it stops working.
- Take 500 to 2,000 milligrams of vitamin C each day.

For further information on the herbs recommended above, read on.

Licorice

Licorice acts as an adrenal stimulant and antacid. It contains glycyrrhizin, a compound that raises the body's levels of the adrenal hormone cortisol. This occurs because licorice slows the breakdown of cortisol produced by the body. As adrenal function is often suboptimal in CFIDS/FMS, licorice can be helpful. Licorice also protects against stomach ulcers, whether in its ordinary form or in the form of deglycyrrhizinated licorice (DGL), a type of licorice extract from which the glycyrrhizin has been removed. In several head-on studies against pharmaceutical antacids and acid inhibitors such as cimetidine (Tagamet), DGL was found to be at least as effective against stomach and duodenal ulcers. Moreover, antacids and acid inhibitors may also worsen digestion; prevent proper absorption of proteins, vitamins, and minerals; and allow infection with parasites, fungi, bacteria, and viruses that would otherwise be killed by the stomach's acid. They also prevent absorption of itraconazole (Sporanox), an anti-yeast medication. In contrast, DGL increases the stomach lining's natural protection against stomach acid and decreased aspirin-induced stomach bleeding by 20 percent. DGL and cimetidine *combined* had an even more pronounced effect in preventing aspirin-induced stomach bleeding. Chewable tablets containing 380 milligrams of DGL, made by Enzymatic Therapies, are available in health food stores. Use the sweetened form (the other tastes awful). For best results, chew two tablets three times a day. When the stomach feels better, the dose can be decreased to one to two tablets twice a day. If active stomach ulcers are severe, four tablets three times a day can be used for short periods. For people with CFIDS/FMS, however, it often makes sense to use regular licorice, as DGL does *not* help the adrenal glands.

Ginseng

Asian ginseng (*Panax ginseng*) is the most famous of all Asian medicinal plants. Because the chemical nature varies widely depending on where the plant is grown (with high activity of a compound designated *ginsenoside-RG-1* in Asian plants and high activity of another compound, *ginsenoside-RB-1* in American plants), it is important to know where it comes from. Asian ginseng has the properties we want in CFIDS/FMS, while American ginseng (*Panax quinqefolium*) may worsen symptoms. For example, Asian ginseng enhances energy, raises blood pressure, and improves adrenal function, while American ginseng lowers blood pressure and is a brain depressant. Asian ginseng has such a wide mix of health benefits that its name, *Panax,* comes from the Greek roots of *pan* (meaning "all") and *akos* (meaning "cure")—that is, "cure-all." In CFIDS/FMS, we are interested in its properties of increasing energy and improving adrenal function. Siberian ginseng (*Eleutherococcus senticosus*) has properties midway between American and Asian.

In one study of 232 patients with "functional fatigue," those taking 80 milligrams of ginseng a day for six weeks (using the Ginsana brand) experienced less fatigue than the placebo group. Concentration also improved.[5]

Ginseng has been shown to reduce fatigue and improve exercise capacity. For most purposes, the usual dose of standardized *Panax ginseng* extract, containing 5 to 7 percent ginsenosides, is about 100 milligrams twice a day. Asian and Siberian ginseng (as well as echinacea and licorice) also support adrenal function. Other studies also suggest that Asian (*Panax*) ginseng may protect nerve cells and decrease cancer risk.

Remember, the potency of different forms of ginseng is quite variable. To treat symptoms of underactive adrenal glands, such as hypoglycemia and low blood pressure, use 100 milligrams of Asian ginseng (*Panax ginseng*) twice a day. Or you can take Siberian ginseng (*Eleutherococcus senticosus*), in dosages of 2,000 to 3,000 milligrams of dry powdered root, 300 to 400 milligrams of standardized concentrated extract, *or* 10 cc (2 teaspoons) of alcohol-based extract daily. When using either form of ginseng, take it for six weeks and then skip taking it for one to two weeks before resuming it. Continue this on-off cycle for one to two years or until you feel your ability to handle stress and infections has improved. Adding 500 to 2,000 milligrams of vitamin C a day will also support the adrenal glands. Ginseng is quite safe and well tolerated. Unlike licorice, it does not pose the risk of raising adrenal hormone levels too much.

Echinacea

Echinacea, also known as purple coneflower, is a member of the sunflower family and is indigenous to the rich prairie soils of midwest North America. It was the most commonly used herb in Native American healing traditions and has been the subject of over 350 studies.[6]

Echinacea is very useful as a general immune activator, stimulating the body's white blood cells (for example, natural killer cells and macrophages), which destroy viruses, bacteria, parasites, and yeast. Studies suggest that it can help the body fight off many different infections, including the flu, herpes, common cold viruses, staph and other bacterial infections (including sinusitis, bronchitis, childhood ear infections, and prostatitis) and *Candida* (yeast) infections. In one study of women with recurrent vaginal *Candida,* 60 percent of those treated with topical creams had recurrences six months later, as opposed to only 15 percent who also took echinacea!

Echinacea also has other uses. Very importantly, it can stimulate the adrenal glands.[7] Because the adrenals need a lot of vitamin C, consider taking 500 to 2,000 milligrams of vitamin C a day with the echinacea (adrenal vitamin C levels will otherwise drop while taking the echinacea, as the adrenals "wake up").

Echinacea also strongly protects cancer patients against the drop in white blood cell counts that occur during radiation therapy. These studies suggest that it is a good idea for any cancer patient on radiation or chemotherapy to consider adding echinacea to their regimen.[8]

Uncontrolled trials have shown that topical echinacea speeds wound healing, including the healing of abscesses, eczema, burns, herpes, and varicose ulcers. Although different species and parts of the echinacea plant each has its pros and cons, it is important to use a good brand. The importance of this is reflected in the estimate that over 50 percent of the echinacea sold in the United States in this century was not echinacea at all, but was (the unrelated) Missouri snakeroot! Check the label to document that the brand you use is actually echinacea. One way to do this is to use a standardized fresh-pressed juice that is noted on the bottle to have at least 2.4 percent beta-1,2-fructofuranosides. Proper dosing is important as there tends to be an "all or nothing" effect—that is, too low a dose has *no* effect.

Overall, echinacea is best used to treat rather than to prevent infections. If you have an impaired immune system, though, as do CFIDS/FMS patients with recurrent or persistent yeast or other (for example, respiratory) infections do, long-term use may be helpful. It is *important* to stop the echinacea for seven to ten days every six to eight weeks or it will stop being effective. A set of dosing recommendations made by Michael Murray, N.D., an excellent and very knowledgeable expert on herbal remedies, is as follows.

For acute infections use one of the following:

- 2 to 3 cc (½ to ¾ teaspoon) of juice of the aerial (above ground) portion of *Echinacea purpurea* stabilized in 22 percent ethanol (this is 44-proof alcohol) with a minimum of 2.4 percent beta-1,2-fructofuranosides (it should say this on the bottle) three times a day, *or*
- 1,000 to 2,000 milligrams (1 to 2 grams) of dried root (or as tea), three times a day, *or*
- 325 to 650 milligrams of encapsulated freeze-dried plant three times a day, *or*
- 3 to 4 cc (¾ to 1 teaspoon) of 1:5 tincture three times a day.

Echinacea is quite safe and nontoxic and some experts will even use it during pregnancy. Because it stimulates the activity of the immune system, it makes sense *not* to use it if you have an autoimmune disease such as lupus or multiple sclerosis, or if you have AIDS or are HIV-positive.

Toxicity of Cortisone

Adrenal hormones are essential for life. Without them, a person dies. But, as with any hormone, too much can be dangerous. In the early studies using adrenal hormones, the researchers had no idea what dose was normal and what was toxic. When they gave injections of the hormone to patients, the patients' arthritis went away and they felt better. However, when they gave patients many times more than the normal amount, the patients became toxic and died. Because of this, the researchers became frightened and avoided using adrenal hormones whenever possible. Medical students were taught to avoid adrenal hormones unless no other treatment choices existed.

The use of adrenal hormones needs to be put into perspective, however. Imagine if the early thyroid researchers had given their patients fifty times the usual dose of thyroid hormone. Thyroid patients would have routinely died of heart attacks. The thyroid researchers, though, were fortunate enough to stumble upon the body's healthy dose early on and to skip these negative outcomes. If they had not, people today would not be treated for an underactive thyroid until they displayed symptoms of very advanced thyroid disease (myxedema) and were nearly comatose. Medical science is just beginning to learn that a person can feel horrible and function poorly even with a minimal to moderate hormone deficiency. Waiting for the person to go "off the deep end" of the test's normal scale is not healthy!

Dr. Jefferies has found that as long as the adrenal hormone level is kept within the normal range, the main toxicity that a patient might experience is a slight upset stomach, due to the body not being used to having the hormone come in through the stomach.[9] Taking the hormone with food usually helps. In addition, some patients gain a few pounds. This is because a low adrenal level can cause a person's weight to drop below the body's normal "set point," even if that set point is high because of CFIDS/FMS. However, any weight gain often is more than offset by the weight loss resulting from being able to exercise once again.

Many physicians do not like to prescribe even low doses of adrenal hormone. If your physician is uncomfortable with Cortef, invite him or her to read Dr. Jefferies' material on the safety of low-dose cortisone as well as our recent study.[10] A study by R. McKenzie and colleagues at the N.I.H. Institute of Allergy and Infectious Diseases showed that what they called "low-dose" Cortef (25 to 35 milligrams a day) moderately helped CFIDS patients but caused some patients' adrenal glands to "go to sleep."[11] As noted in my letter to the editor printed in the *Journal of the American Medical Association,* their dose was two to three times as high as most CFIDS patients need and dramatically worsened the sleep disorder.[12] Another study using 10 milligrams of Cortef a day in CFIDS and our studies of CFIDS/FMS patients showed significant benefit without significant toxicity using lower doses.[13] Most patients only need 5 to 12½ milligrams a day, equivalent to 1 to 3 milligrams a day of prednisone—a dose so low that most doctors have never prescribed it! Cortef is better than prednisone, though, for people with CFIDS/FMS. After feeling well for six to eighteen months, most people are able to begin slowly decreasing their adrenal hormone dosage, eventually discontinuing the treatment entirely.

Recently, studies have been published about bone loss with low-dose adrenal hormones, but even these studies do not use the very low doses that we use.[14] Nonetheless, it is reasonable to take estrogen, if you are a menopausal or estrogen-deficient female (see page 50). Also take 600 to 1,000 milligrams of calcium a day, as well as 400 international units (IU) of vitamin D (your multivitamin may already contain this amount). You can also get your calcium by adding two cups of yogurt with live and active yogurt cultures to your daily diet.

If your symptoms started suddenly after a viral infection, if you suffer from hypoglycemia, or if you have recurrent infections that take a long time to resolve, you probably have underactive adrenal glands. About two-thirds of my severe chronic fatigue patients have underactive or marginally functioning adrenal glands or a decreased adrenal reserve.[15]

Although I prefer natural products to pharmaceuticals, in this situation I am most comfortable with standardized hormones. If the amount of hormone given is within the body's normal range, the body can decide for itself how much of the hormone it wants to use. Using natural remedies with the Cortef though, may help you to need a lower dose (or none at all) and help you to be able to stop the cortisol sooner.

Another important function of the adrenal gland is maintaining blood volume and pressure. Low blood pressure, blood volume, and dehydration are common in CFS patients. Recent research has suggested that a low dose of another prescription adrenal hormone, fludrocortisone (sold under the brand name Florinef) can help in 14 percent of CFIDS patients (versus 10 percent of placebo patients). The researchers suspect that in CFIDS, blood pressure may drop precipitously at times and trigger symptoms that can last for weeks.[16] Florinef, which helps the body retain water, can prevent this. Florinef is most likely to help people under eighteen years old, and I rarely use prescribe it for people over twenty-two years old. Begin with one-quarter of a 0.1-milligram tablet per day and increase by a quarter-tablet every four to seven days until you reach one whole tablet. Note that you may not see any effects for three to six weeks. I have found detroamphetamine (Dexedrine) and the antidepressant fluoxetine (Prozac) to be *much* more helpful than Florinef for CFIDS/FMS and for neurally mediated hypotension (NMH).[17] Drinking plenty of water and getting enough

Getting Kids and Young Adults Well—
Information for Patients Under Age Sixteen

If you're under age sixteen, you most likely have neurally mediated hypotension (NMH)—sort of like low blood pressure—and an allergy to milk proteins.[18] Some doctors do a type of test called the tilt table test to diagnose NMH, but I treat NMH without doing the test first. It's not a bad idea to have it done, but it is expensive and uncomfortable.

To treat NMH, your doctor can prescribe the medications fluoxetine (Prozac), ephedrine (*not* pseudoephedrine, or Sudafed), fludrocortisone (Florinef, which is modestly effective), and/or methylphenidate (Ritalin) or dextroamphetamine (Dexedrine).[19] In addition, the following things can be helpful:

- Avoid sugar. Stevia is a healthy sweetener you can use instead. (See page 22.)
- Take an excellent multivitamin. (See page 17.)
- *Dramatically* increase your intake of salt and water. Aim for 8 to 15 grams of salt and 1 gallon of water each day.
- If you have stomach or bowel symptoms, cut out all milk products and any foods containing casein or caseinate (milk protein) as ingredients.
- If you have taken a lot of antibiotics and/or steroid medications (cortisone, Prednisone, or others) ask your doctor to consider treating you with the antifungals nystatin, for five months, and fluconazole (Diflucan), for twelve weeks after that, to get rid of possible yeast overgrowth. (See page 62.)
- If you run frequent fevers (temperatures over 98.8°F), you likely have a hidden infection. Get a parasite test done. It is important that this be done by a laboratory that specializes in this type of testing, such as the Parasitology Center or the Great Smokies Diagnostic Laboratory (see Appendix J: Resources). If the parasite test is negative, ask your doctor to consider giving you a course of the antibiotic ciprofloxacin (Cipro) for twelve weeks. If you are under sixteen years old, your pediatrician can let you know if you can substitute doxycycline without staining your teeth. If you feel better and/or the fevers go away, keep repeating six-week to six-month courses of antibiotic treatment until the fevers stay gone. You should also take nystatin while on the antibiotic. If you're not better after twelve weeks of Cipro or doxycycline, you might want to try taking the antiviral famciclovir (Famvir) in high doses for six months. If these medicines help you feel better, stay on them for as long as you need them. If you're not better, then refer to the rest of the program outlined in this book. Chapter 4 will offer more detailed information on treating infections.

Fortunately, these simple suggestions help most kids get better!

salt and potassium are also helpful. (More information about NMH can be found in the inset on page 40, Getting Kids and Young Adults Well—Information for Patients Under Age Sixteen.)

Dehydroepiandrosterone (DHEA)

The adrenal gland makes many hormones in addition to hydrocortisone. One of these is DHEA. DHEA is often *very* low in CFIDS patients. Although DHEA's function is not yet fully understood, it appears to be important for good health, which makes a low DHEA level worth treating.[20] Some studies suggest that the higher a person's DHEA level is, the longer that person will live and the healthier he or she will be. I'm concerned that pushing the blood level *above* the upper limit of normal may increase the risk of breast cancer. For many patients, when a low DHEA level is treated, the result is a dramatic boost in energy.

If your DHEA-S (*not* DHEA) level is low (under 120 micrograms per deciliter [mg/dL] of blood for females or 325 mcg/dL for males), I recommend beginning treatment with 5 to 25 milligrams of DHEA per day and slowly working up to what feels like an optimal level to you. For women, I suggest keeping the DHEA-S level at around 150 to 180 mcg/dL, which is the middle of the normal range for a twenty-nine-year-old female. For men, I keep the DHEA-S level between 350 and 500 mcg/dL, which is the normal range for a twenty-nine-year-old male. The low ends of the normal ranges are normal only for people over eighty. If you have side effects, such as facial hair or acne, which are uncommon, check your blood level of DHEA-S and decrease your dose. A very good form of DHEA (some are not) is available without a prescription from General Nutrition Centers. I would use their timed-release tablets.

Hypothyroidism

The thyroid gland, located in the neck area, is the body's gas pedal. It regulates the body's metabolic speed. If the thyroid gland produces insufficient amounts of thyroid hormones, metabolism decreases and the person gains weight. It is common, in fact, for CFIDS patients to put on twenty to fifty pounds during the first year of their disease. Other symptoms of hypothyroidism include intolerance to cold, fatigue, achiness, confusion, and constipation.

The thyroid makes two primary hormones. They are:

- *Thyroxine* (T_4). T_4 is the storage form of thyroid hormone. The body uses it to make triiodothyronine (T_3), the active form of thyroid hormone. Most synthetic thyroid medications, such as Synthroid and Levothroid, are pure T_4. These synthetics are fine if your body has the ability to properly turn them into T_3. Unfortunately, many patients find that their bodies do not have this ability.
- *Triiodothyronine* (T_3). T_3 is the active form of thyroid hormone. Although in some life-threatening illnesses the body appropriately makes less T_3, experience suggests that at times it may not be able to turn T_4 into T_3 when necessary. Most doctors never check T_3 levels. Because T_3 readings tell only the level in the blood (and not in the cells where the T_4 is converted to T_3) and also measures inactive forms of T_3 (for example, "reverse T_3"), blood tests can miss most cases of T_3 thyroid deficiency. Nonetheless, it still is worthwhile to check total or free T_3 levels and directly monitor T_3 function. As just mentioned, the synthetic thyroid medications do not contain T_3. However, natural thyroid hormone preparations, such as Armour Thyroid, do.

THE PROBLEM WITH THYROID TESTS

Many years ago, while I was in medical school, physicians were taught to diagnose hypothyroidism, or low thyroid function, by using the newly discovered method of measuring the metabolic rate while the patient ran on a treadmill. Doctors thought that this was a wonderful new test and that they finally had a way to identify patients with underactive thyroids. We congratulated ourselves on being so clever. But then a new test came out. The new test measured protein-bound iodide (PBI). When doctors began using the PBI test, we realized, "Oh, we missed diagnosing so many people with a low thyroid, but this new test will now pick up everybody who has a problem." We patted ourselves on the back and told all our newly discovered thyroid patients that it turned out that they were not crazy—they just had a low thyroid. Doctors were comfortable that we could now determine with certainty when someone had a thyroid problem.

Then the T_4-level thyroid test was developed and we said, "Oh, that silly old PBI test. It missed so many people with a low thyroid, but this new test will find everyone." Then the T_7 test, which adjusts for protein binding of thyroid hormone, came out, and then the thyroid-stimulating hormone (TSH) test. Modern medicine is now into the fifth generation of TSH tests. To make matters more difficult, if the thyroid is underactive because the hypothalamus is suppressed, the TSH test may appear to be normal, or even suggest an overactive thyroid. With each new test, doctors realize they missed many people with underactive thyroids. Fortunately some doctors are finally starting to catch on.

In two studies done by Dr. G.R. Skinner and his associates in the United Kingdom, patients who were felt to have hypothyroidism (an underactive thyroid) because of their symptoms had their blood levels of thyroid hormone checked. The vast majority of them had technically normal thyroid blood tests. This data was published in the *British Medical Journal*.[21] Since that time, Dr. Skinner has done another study in which the patients with normal blood tests who had symptoms of an underactive thyroid—those who your doctor would likely say had a normal thyroid and would not need treatment—were treated with thyroid hormone. A remarkable thing happened when this was done (well, maybe we're not surprised!). The large majority of patients, despite being considered to have a normal thyroid, had their symptoms improve upon taking thyroid hormone (Synthroid), at an average dosage of 100 to 120 micrograms a day.[22]

These two studies, plus another one showing that thyroid blood tests are only low in about 3 percent of patients whose doctors sent blood tests in (and this is at an HMO—where the doctor really suspected that the patient had thyroid problems!), confirm what we have been saying all along.[23] Our current thyroid testing will miss *most* patients with an underactive thyroid. Once again, doctors of decades ago were on target when they knew that one has to treat the patient and not the blood test! (For a more complete discussion of the interpretation of thyroid tests, see Appendix A: For Physicians.)

If you suffer from chronic fatigue plus have achy muscles and joints, heavy periods, constipation, easy weight gain, cold intolerance, dry skin, thin hair, a change in your ankle reflexes called a delayed relaxation of the deep tendon reflex (DTR), *or* a body temperature that tends to be on the low side of normal, you should consider asking your doctor to prescribe a low dose of thyroid hormone. If your doctor won't prescribe it, you may wish to consult one who is open to the idea (for organizations that can help you locate a physician specializing in the treatment of chronic fatigue, see Appendix J: Resources, or visit my website for a list of over 700 health professionals). Before seeing a new doctor, call and ask if he or she sometimes treats people with thyroid hormone if their symptoms show they need it but the blood tests are normal. As long as you do not have underlying angina and you follow up with a blood test to make sure that your thyroid levels are in a safe range (going *above* the *upper limit* of normal may aggravate osteoporosis, a problem already common in CFIDS/FMS) a trial of low-dose thyroid hormone treatment is usually safe and may be dramatically beneficial.

If your symptoms suggest low thyroid function, some physicians recommend checking your axilla (armpit) temperature each morning when you first wake up. Before you get out of bed, put a thermometer under your arm and lie quietly for ten minutes. If your temperature is routinely under 97.4°F, consider a trial of thyroid hormone regardless of what your blood tests show. I prefer to check an oral temperature between 11:00 A.M. and 7:00 P.M. and to treat if it's regularly under 98.1°F.

Some patients have found desiccated thyroid (Armour Thyroid) to be helpful and the synthetic thyroid (Synthroid) not to be. Some have found the opposite. I have found—either through blood testing or according to symptoms—that over 47 percent of my chronic fatigue patients have a low thyroid and that 83 percent of these patients have improved by taking a low dose of thyroid hormone.[24] If you have fibromyalgia and an underactive thyroid that is not treated (even if your blood tests come back normal), your fibromyalgia simply will not resolve. Many physicians who are experts on chronic pain agree.[25]

TREATING AN UNDERACTIVE THYROID

We are constantly learning powerful new tricks for treating hypothyroidism and there are many reasonable treatment approaches. Our treatment protocol information checklist (see Appendix E) gives the "nuts and bolts" of some approaches.

Thyroid Hormone

Most doctors prescribe T_4 (Synthroid) to treat an underactive thyroid. T_4, though, is fairly inactive until the body converts it into T_3, or activated thyroid hormone. If the problem is only with the thyroid gland itself, prescribing Synthroid will work just fine. However, if the body has trouble turning inactive T_4 into active T_3, taking Synthroid can make the problem worse. Because of this problem, many physicians prefer to use Armour Thyroid, which is a mix of T_4 and T_3.

Why might the body have trouble making active T_3 from inactive T_4? During periods when the body wants to conserve energy (for example, during times of infection or famine—which is how the body views an overly restricted diet), the body slows down metabolism. It does this by decreasing the production of active T_3 from T_4, which is turned into inactive "reverse T_3," instead. By a mechanism discussed in Dr. E. Denis Wilson's book, *Wilson's Syndrome—The Miracle of Feeling Well,* (Cornerstone, 1991) the body may get "stuck," and becomes unable to make adequate T_3.

I prefer to start with a trial of Armour thyroid. I begin with ¼ grain (15 milligrams) a day and increase it to ½ grain (30 milligrams) a day in one week. Then, I increase it by ¼ to ½ grain each two to six weeks until the patient finds a dose that *feels* best. If you are shaky, hyper, or have a racing heart (for example, a pulse over 90 beats per minute), lower the dose. I check a *total T_3* (this exact test—*not* a T_3 RU) and free T_4 (thyroid blood tests) about one month after the 1, 2, and 2½ grain levels are reached. *Do not* check a TSH test. It will be low (because of the hypothalamic dysfunction) and your doctor will incorrectly think you're on too much thyroid—even if your blood hormone levels are low normal. This will make you and your doctor crazy! Adjust the thyroid slowly to the dose that *feels* the best, while making certain to *remain within normal range for blood thyroid hormone levels.* When on a stable dose, consider checking the thyroid blood levels every three to six months. You will know if the treatment is working within two to six weeks on a given dose. Although most patients can stop taking thyroid hormone after twelve to twenty-four months, you can stay on Armour Thyroid or Synthroid for as long as it is needed.

One can also try prescribing Synthroid (T_4). One hundred micrograms (0.1 milligrams) of Synthroid "equals" 1 grain of Armour Thyroid. Often, one hormone treatment works when the other does not. Adjust the dose as above.

Another approach is to use a modification of Dr. Wilson's technique. In brief, after tapering off any thyroid hormone (if you are able to), you take *sustained-release* T_3 (T_3SR, *not* short-acting T_3 [Cytomel]) at a dosage of 7½ micrograms twice a day. Increase the dosage by 7½ micrograms a day (for example, to 15 micrograms twice a day, then 22½ micrograms twice a day, and so on) every one to six weeks until your body temperature is 98.6°F or until you feel well. When this occurs, stay at that dose for two weeks. If your body temperature drops before the two weeks are over or if you feel poorly again, continue to raise the dose. I do not routinely recommend going above 45 or 52½ micrograms twice a day. After three months of feeling well, or maintaining a temperature of 98.6°F, or being at 45 micrograms twice a day, decrease the dosage by 7½ micrograms every one to two days, as you are able. This approach helps only a minority of patients, but the effect is often dramatic when it does work. I usually prescribe sustained-release T_3 when other treatments have failed.

Another approach, used by the research center of Jon Lowe, D.C., in Texas, is to use the T_3SR only in the morning. He feels that FMS patients have "thyroid resistance"—that is, it takes a much higher level of thyroid to obtain the normal effect. Even though the body may only make about 25 to 30 micrograms of T_3 a day, his studies found it took an average of 125 mcg a day to make FMS patients feel healthy.[26]

Try taking the full dose of thyroid in the morning or half the dose twice a day to see which feels best. Do not take thyroid hormone within several hours of iron, and perhaps calcium, or you won't absorb the thyroid.[27] Take thyroid on an empty stomach (for example, first thing in the morning).

If a dose of sustained-release T_3 feels optimal, but the effect cannot be maintained when you taper off, stay on the lowest optimal dose. Check the total T_3 and free T_4 thyroid blood tests after four to six weeks on the dose to make certain that the normal range is maintained.

All thyroid treatments must be prescribed and monitored by a physician. Holistic physicians are more likely to be familiar with (and open to trying) these new treatment approaches. Unfortunately, many doctors are (I believe incorrectly) trained to stop increasing the dosage of thyroid hormone once an individual's thyroid tests are in the "normal" range—even if the dose is inadequate for that person. Synthetic T_4 (Synthroid) is available at any pharmacy. Sustained-release T_3 can be obtained from many compounding pharmacies. I use Cape Apothecary (see Appendix J: Resources). When you settle on an optimal dose, a compounding pharmacy can then make a single capsule of that dosage to be taken one or two times a day. This is less expensive because T_3 capsules cost about the same for 7½- and 60-microgram strengths.

Using an ovulation thermometer (available at most pharmacies) will make it easier to check your body temperature accurately. If you are using sustained-release T_3, check your temperature one to three times a day, between 11:00 A.M. and 7:00 P.M., while the dose of thyroid hormone is being adjusted. If you are taking Armour thyroid or Synthroid, check your temperature one to two times a week during the adjustment periods. Aim for an ideal temperature of 98.6°F.

Potential Side Effects

If someone has blockages in the arteries that feed the heart and is on the verge of a heart attack, taking thyroid hormone can trigger a heart attack or angina, just like exercise could. Thyroid treatment can trigger heart palpitations as well. These are often benign, but if chest pain or palpitations occur, though, stop the thyroid and call your doctor at once. Because of this concern, I often recommend that patients at significant risks of angina—people who smoke, have high blood pressure, are over forty-five years old, have cholesterol levels over 260, and a family history of heart attacks in individuals under sixty-five years old—have an exercise treadmill test done before treatment, even if they can't complete the test.

To put the risk in perspective, in the many hundreds of patients that I have put on thyroid, I don't remember any having a heart attack or dangerous problems from taking it. In the long run, I suspect thyroid treatment is more likely to decrease one's risk of heart disease by lowering cholesterol.

The other main concern is that *excess* thyroid hormone can cause osteoporosis (bone thinning). In my research, I have seen *no* studies showing any increase in osteoporosis in premenopausal women if one keeps the T_3 and T_4 thyroid blood levels in the normal range. I do not consider TSH to be a reliable monitor of thyroid levels in CFIDS/FMS because of hypothalamic dysfunction. We don't know for sure if keeping the T_3 level above normal in FMS patients with thyroid resistance worsens the osteoporosis already commonly seen in CFIDS/FMS, but this has not been a problem. If you need to keep T_3 or T_4 above the upper limit of normal, you should have a DEXA (osteoporosis) scan each six to twelve months. If this is showing osteoporosis, lower the thyroid dose. If this is not possible, consider other osteoporosis prevention measures with your physician.

Low Estrogen and Testosterone

Many people going through midlife develop fatigue, poor libido, or depression. This includes men and women alike. Researchers have found that if the estrogen level in females or testosterone level in males or females is low, a trial replacement of these hormones can bring about dramatic improvement and is therefore worth considering. An underactive adrenal gland can aggravate this problem. Although the ovaries make most of a woman's estrogen and the testicles make most of a man's testosterone, the adrenals make significant amounts of both.

Low Testosterone—Not Only a Male Problem!

Low testosterone is a *major* problem in 70 percent of my male patients with CFIDS/FMS. After six to eight weeks, the effect of treatment is often marked. It is important (again, in both men and women) to check the *free,* or *unbound,* blood testosterone level. This measures the *active* form of the hormone. A serum (or total) testosterone level measures only the *inactive* storage form of the hormone. Inactive (total) testosterone levels are often normal while the active (free) testosterone levels are low or barely normal in most male CFIDS/FMS patients. Low testosterone is associated with many problems, including fatigue, poor stamina, muscle wasting, and poor libido. Although testosterone levels are normally much lower in females, deficiencies in women cause these same problems. Testosterone is critical in females, as well as males, and I find low free testosterone levels in many female CFIDS/FMS patients as well.

Again, it is important to check the *free* (not just total) testosterone. Most laboratories can test free testosterone only if they also do the total testosterone—this is a normal procedure. Be sure that the normal ranges for the lab results are broken down by ten-year age groups (thirty-one to forty years old, forty-one to fifty years old, and so on). It is meaningless to have a normal range that includes eighty-year-olds if you're twenty-eight. If your result is below normal, or even in the lowest 25 percent of the normal range, I would consider a trial of testosterone therapy.

Treating Low Testosterone

For men, the standard dose is about 100 to 125 milligrams intramuscularly (by injection) every seven to ten days. It can also be given as 200 milligrams every two weeks, but this can result in peak levels right after the shot that are too high, and levels that go too low for a few days before the next shot. Adding testosterone patches on day nine to fourteen (when getting injections every fourteen days) can avoid the levels going too low. I feel that getting shots weekly is preferable, though. I usually give ½ or 6⁄10 cc of Delatestryl, which contains 200 milligrams of testosterone per cc. Unfortunately, the skin patches are not adequate for the job. I often switch to testosterone cream (100 milligrams per gram in pluronic-lecithin-organogel (PLO gel) from a compounding pharmacy after a man has been on the shots for eight weeks so he can tell what the optimum effect is. Most men need 25 to 100 milligrams rubbed onto thin-skinned areas (for example, your inner upper arms from the elbow to two inches below your armpit) one to two times a day. The problem (for men) with taking tablets, instead of the shots or cream, is that oral testosterone goes to the liver first. The higher dose required by men (as opposed to women) can raise cholesterol levels. I'm beginning to suspect that avoiding other possible side effects by using the hormone cream twice daily (instead of getting high and low levels by taking the shot every week or two) is better. The cost can be markedly decreased by getting the cream as 100 milligrams of testosterone per gram of cream. A plastic plunger that screws onto the top of the tube will measure the grams of cream. A new testosterone gel (Androgel, available in 25- and 50-milligram packets) may also work. Although much more expensive—approximately five dollars a packet—it may be cheaper if your insurance covers prescriptions.

For women, testosterone treatment is easier. Oral natural micronized testosterone (and natural estrogen and progesterone) are available through most compounding pharmacies. (For names of some compounding pharmacies that do mail-order prescriptions, see Appendix J: Resources.) The usual dose is 1.5 to 4 milligrams one to two times a day by mouth or in cream form. If you take the capsules and also need estrogen or progesterone (see below), they can be combined in the same capsule, at a lower cost. I usually begin by prescribing 2 milligrams one to two times a day for six weeks to see the effect, then raise or lower the dosage if needed. With this dosing, most women feel more energy and have thicker hair, younger skin, and improved libido.

I check *free* testosterone blood levels six to eight weeks after starting therapy (in men, just before their eight-week shot) and adjust the dosing accordingly. Blood levels are not reliable, however, if you are taking synthetic methyltestosterone instead of natural testosterone. Check the test one and a half to three hours after taking the tablets or applying the cream, or one day before your injection.

Potential Side Effects

In women, if acne, intense dreams, or darkening of facial hair occurs, the dose is too high and should be decreased. These effects, which can also occur with DHEA supplementation, are usually reversible. These side effects can also be caused by an estrogen level that is too low relative to your testosterone, and may be avoided by supplementing both together. For women, it may be best to use estrogen for four to eight weeks before starting testosterone. This often decreases side effects.

In men, acne suggests the dose is too high. It is important to monitor levels because (as in body builders who abuse testosterone by taking many times the recommended dose) elevated levels can cause elevated blood counts, liver inflammation, a decreased sperm count with resulting infertility (also usually reversible), and elevated cholesterols with increased risk of heart disease. Because of this, in *men,* a complete blood count (CBC), cholesterol test, and liver enzymes test should be done from time to time. Testosterone supplementation can also cause elevated thyroid hormone levels in those taking thyroid supplements. If you are on thyroid supplements, I would recheck thyroid hormone levels after six to twelve weeks or sooner if you get a racing heart or anxious/hyper feelings.

Interestingly, in men, most studies show that bringing low testosterone up to the normal level *decreases* angina and leg artery blockages, improves cholesterol, and may decrease diabetic tendencies! It is not clear if taking testosterone increases the risk of prostate enlargement or cancer beyond that of any other healthy male. While I don't feel being testosterone deficient is a good way to prevent these illnesses, if you are a man over forty-four who is taking testosterone, it is reasonable to do a prostate exam and prostate-specific antigen (PSA) test yearly. For many men, improvements in stamina, energy, and overall sense of wellness have been dramatic, and treating the low testosterone has been critical.

LOW ESTROGEN AND PROGESTERONE

Although not likely to be a problem with men, deficiencies of estrogen and/or progesterone can be major problems in women with CFIDS/FMS. In a wonderful book by Dr. Elizabeth Lee Vliet, *Screaming To Be Heard: Hormonal Connections Women Suspect . . . and Doctors Ignore* (M. Evans and Company, 2000), the role of estrogen deficiency in causing fatigue, brain fog, disordered sleep, fibromyalgia, poor libido, PMS, low levels of serotonin and other neurotransmitters, interstitial cystitis, as well as other problems is reviewed in detail. She notes, appropriately, that the perimenopausal period (the period as you approach menopause) has a gradual onset, and symptoms of estrogen deficiency can occur well before your blood tests and periods become abnormal. As noted above, hypothalamic dysfunction can cause estrogen deficiency as well.

By checking the blood levels and noting if symptoms are cyclic through the month (that is, worse during ovulation, which occurs about fifteen days after the first day of your period, and especially premenstrually), one can tell if a trial of *natural* estrogen supplementation is warranted. For example, panic attacks, migraines, and palpitations that occur for one to two days around ovulation or around your period often are triggered by dropping estrogen levels. Because of this, it can be very helpful to keep a symptom log relative to your periods.

Part of the difficulty in checking estradiol (the most active form of estrogen) and progesterone levels is that the normal range fluctuates widely during your cycle. Dr. Vliet feels that at menopause, estradiol levels should be kept over 100 picograms per milliliter (pg/mL) of blood, and that symptoms are likely if levels are under 50 pg/ml (normal peak levels are over 200 pg/ml at ovulation). If levels of follicle-stimulating hormone (FSH) or luteinizing hormone (LH), two other hormones involved in regulating the menstrual cycle, are high *or* low-normal and/or your symptoms cycle with your periods, a trial of estrogen is helpful.

Treating Low Estrogen and Progesterone

In my experience, and that of Dr. Vliet, many of the symptoms noted above can improve dramatically with estrogen replacement. Dr. Vliet notes that 17-beta-estradiol is the major active form of estrogen naturally found in the human female. For menopausal women, this can be found in Estrace tablets or Climara or Estraderm patches. Some physicians prefer natural biestrogen from a compounding pharmacy. This contains estradiol plus estriol, a weaker form of estrogen that is present at low levels except if you're pregnant.

Unless you have had a hysterectomy, if you take supplemental estrogen, you *must* also take progesterone. I prefer natural progesterone—for example, 200 milligrams of Prometrium a day for the first ten days of each month, or 100 milligrams every day. Taking both estrogen and progesterone every day will often result in your periods going away after six to nine months, and most women over forty-eight or so prefer this approach.

If you're under thirty-eight years of age, or have significant PMS symptoms, monophasic birth control pills (BCPs) that are *low* in progesterone, such as Ovcon-35, Modicon or Brevicon, can be very helpful, and are better for women with CFIDS/FMS and PMS than the newer triphasic BCPs. If you don't have PMS and you find anxiety—*not* mood shifts and easy crying—is a major problem throughout your cycle, a BCP with a bit more progesterone may be worth trying. Most women find Ovcon-35 to be too strong, so I usually use Ortho-Novum 1/35 or 1/50s. I prefer to use natural biestrogen and progesterone. Compounding pharmacists can help you and your physician tailor the optimum dosing and timing for *you*. (For names of some compounding pharmacies that do mail-order prescriptions, see Appendix J: Resources.)

Premarin is the brand of estrogen most commonly prescribed for menopausal women. It contains a form of the hormone that comes from pregnant horse urine (*pre* = "pregnant," *mar* = "mare," *in* = "urine"). I think it's great for horses, but I rarely prescribe it for human females anymore.

Potential Side Effects

Although estrogen can cause a slightly increased risk of breast cancer (seen mostly in studies using the conjugated, or more powerful, horse estrogen), I feel that estrogen's benefits of improving well-being, while significantly decreasing the likelihood of developing osteoporosis, and possibly heart disease, generally outweigh this risk. You should not smoke while taking estrogen as this increases the risk of blood clots and strokes. Caution should also be used if your mother or sister have had breast cancer.

As we learned above, low estrogen can cause disordered sleep; low levels of serotonin, dopamine, norepinephrine, and acetylcholine, neurotransmitters that appear to be low in CFIDS/FMS; cyclic panic and palpitations; decreased libido; and other symptoms often seen in CFIDS/FMS. Low progesterone can cause low levels of gamma-aminobutyric acid (GABA), another neurotransmitter, and this can cause anxiety. Low testosterone can cause low libido, fatigue, poor stamina and many other problems. Fortunately, all of these are treatable. Women should note that it is normal for menstruation to become irregular for the first several months of treatment. This occurs even in women who do not take hormonal treatment, and it resolves on its own.

Low Oxytocin

Dr. Jay Goldstein, a physician who does a lot of work with CFIDS patients, has found that many patients improve through the use of oxytocin. Oxytocin is a hormone produced by the hypothalamus. It is recognized primarily for its function in labor and lactation (milk production), but it also appears to be important in the day-to-day performance of the hypothalamus, the master gland of the body. It is also an important neurotransmitter in the brain.[28] Dr. Goldstein's theory is supported by recent research showing that oxytocin levels are decreased in FMS. Unfortunately, the test for oxytocin is only available in research labs. Fortunately, it's easy to tell if oxytocin will help by simply taking one injection. If it doesn't help, consider first bringing your DHEA-S level up to midrange for three months (see page 41) and consider taking 1,500 milligrams each of choline and inositol every day for several weeks before retrying the oxytocin. People who are pale and have cold extremities seem most likely to benefit from oxytocin treatment. The usual dose is 10 international units (1 cc by intramuscular injection) per day. If the oxytocin treatment is going to help, it should do so in thirty to sixty minutes.

Growth Hormone, Vasopressin, and Prolactin

Clinical experience has shown that some patients with diffuse hypothalamic or pituitary disease do not respond to treatment, even when their adrenal hormone, thyroid hormone, oxytocin, estrogen, and testosterone are replaced. Current research suggests that inadequate levels of growth hormone (GH) may be an important factor for these patients.[29] GH is synthesized and stored in the pituitary gland and assists in protein synthesis in the body and bone growth in the limbs. It is also responsible for stimulating DHEA production. Excellent studies recently completed by Drs. Robert Bennett and Peter Behan, noted CFIDS/FMS researchers, show that people with CFIDS have significantly diminished GH levels. Other studies have shown that low GH levels can be associated with significant fatigue and CFIDS-like symptoms. GH is produced during the deep stages of sleep (stages 3 and 4) that are missing in CFIDS/FMS.[30] Getting this deep, restorative sleep may well be the best way to raise GH. GH is important, and FMS symptoms have been shown to improve with GH treatment. In the future, growth hormone may help those few CFIDS patients who do not improve with the current treatment approach. However, treatment with growth hormone is expensive, averaging around $15,000 per year. Fortunately, though, there is a good chance that much of the benefit of GH treatment can be obtained by treating your sleep and by taking DHEA. In addition, natural GH secretagogues (that is, glandulars, amino acids, and nutrients that increase GH secretion) are available and have been found to be helpful in FMS. One such product is SomatoPlex from VesPro, which costs approximately ninety-five dollars a month. Colostrum may also help because it contains IGF-1, a hormone that does a lot of growth hormone's work, but it takes four to five months to be effective.

People who are lightheaded or drink more water than normal—that is, most CFIDS/FMS patients—may be low in vasopressin.[31] This can cause low blood pressure and secondary fatigue. Vasopressin, which is also known as the antidiuretic hormone (ADH), is secreted by the pituitary gland and keeps the body from losing too much water by increasing the amount that is reabsorbed by the kidneys. The simplest treatment for a low vasopressin level is to use plenty of salt and drink plenty of water. A small percentage of patients find that taking 0.1 milligram of fludrocortisone (Florinef), another adrenal-like hormone, along with potassium every day, dramatically improves their symptoms. It is worth a six- to eight-week trial. This is especially important in younger people with CFIDS/NMH (see page 40). The use of prescription adrenocorticoids such as Florinef for fatigue states, however, is still considered controversial. However, they are routinely used for other conditions and are considered fairly safe. Recent research at Johns Hopkins Hospital has shown that Florinef helps neurally mediated hypotension (NMH), which is common in CFIDS. An National Institutes of Health (NIH) study, however, found it helped only 14 percent of CFIDS patients.[32] Desmopressin, a synthetic derivative of vasopressin that is available as a nasal spray, is even less helpful. We've found other agents that treat NMH (fluoxetine [Prozac], sertraline [Zoloft], dextroamphetamine [Adderall, Dexedrine], or ephedrine) to be much more effective than Florinef for people with CFIDS.[33] Do not combine ephedrine with ephedra (ma huang), which is often found in weight-loss products, or with pseudoephedrine (Sudafed). These are all essentially the same (except that Sudafed won't help NMH). Too high a dose can be very toxic and has been fatal.

Prolactin levels are sometimes mildly elevated in CFIDS patients. Prolactin is synthesized and stored in the pituitary gland, and is best known for stimulating milk production after childbirth. A mildly elevated prolactin level usually has no effect and may simply reflect hypothalamic injury. The hypothalamus suppresses, instead of stimulates, prolactin production. To make sure that no (benign) pituitary tumor exists, however, I may order a magnetic resonance imaging (MRI) scan in patients who still have elevated prolactin levels after four months of treatment. The MRI generally shows that everything is normal. Some medications, such as risperidone (Risperdal) can also elevate prolactin levels.

Some physicians have also reported diabetes mellitus in the later stages of CFIDS, although I have not seen this problem in my patients. Dr. Jefferies, interestingly, has found that diabetes often improves through treatment with low-dose cortisol.

As you can see, many problems can occur when the body's glands do not function properly. The good news is that most of these problems can be treated. In my experience, this has often resulted in dramatic improvement. It is important, though, to treat the *whole* person, not simply the hormonal problem.

Important Points

- Underactive adrenals are common in CFIDS. Treat low or borderline adrenal function with *low-dose* Cortef and/or DHEA (adrenal hormones). If you take Cortef, consider also taking supplemental calcium and vitamin D, or yogurt. If your blood pressure is low, try Florinef, Prozac, Dexedrine, or ephedrine; increase your water intake; and make sure you consume enough salt.
- Hypothyroidism is also very common in CFIDS. Treat symptoms of low or borderline thyroid function with Synthroid, Armour Thyroid, or sustained-release T_3—even if your blood tests are normal!
- If you are a woman with an estrogen deficiency or a person of either sex with a testosterone deficiency, consider a trial replacement of these hormones.
- Treat an oxytocin deficiency with oxytocin injections.

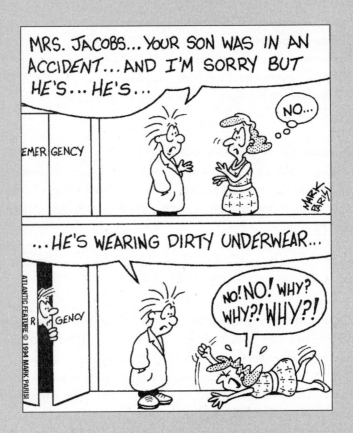

CHAPTER 4

When Your Defenses Are Down—
Those Persistent Infections

MEDICAL SCIENCE HAS KNOWN FOR QUITE SOME time that chronic fatigue syndrome is associated with changes in the body's immune system. In fact, the acronym *CFIDS* stands for chronic fatigue *and immune dysfunction* syndrome. People with CFIDS can have several different and unusual infections at one time. Many of these infections need to be treated directly. Other infections will go away on their own as your immune (defense) system comes back "on line" as a result of using the effective treatment protocol detailed in this book. In this chapter, we will look at some of the more common yet not-usually-thought-of (at least in "regular" medicine), infections.

What kinds of infections are people with CFIDS most at risk for? Although CFIDS that comes on suddenly often seems to be triggered by viral infections—for example, infection with the Epstein-Barr virus (EBV), human herpesvirus type 6 (HHV-6), or cytomegalovirus (CMV)—those infections, I suspect, are "simmering" or no longer active in many cases. However, the body acts as if they are active. This may result in elevated levels of interferon. I suspect this was what triggered my CFIDS.

The body produces interferon to fight viral infections. When a person with cancer or hepatitis is injected with interferon, he or she becomes achy, fatigued and brain-fogged.[1] Underactive adrenal glands can also cause interferon levels to become elevated.[2] Because of this elevation, it is more accurate to say that the body's immune system is not functioning properly than to say that it is underactive. Indeed, in many ways, the immune system may be in overdrive and soon exhaust itself. The immune system malfunctions in many other ways, too, among them decreasing the effectiveness of the body's natural killer cells, which are an important defense mechanism.[3]

Many other recurrent or unusual infections can also occur because of a malfunctioning immune system. Chronic sinus, bladder, prostate, and respiratory infections are common and are often treated with repeated courses of antibiotics. The large amount of antibiotics introduced into the system can lead to a secondary yeast overgrowth, as antibiotics change the natural balance between the bowel's healthy bacteria and yeast. The original immune dysfunction also contributes to the yeast overgrowth. Although the theory is controversial, many physicians believe that chronic overgrowth of yeast due to overuse of antibiotics is a potential and strong trigger for chronic fatigue, fibromyalgia, and further immune dysfunction. What makes the theory controversial is that no definitive tests exist to distinguish fungal overgrowth from normal fungal levels. Also, many of the symptoms ascribed to yeast overgrowth can also come from the many other problems present in chronic fatigue syndrome and fibromyalgia. On the other hand, most doctors who try treating yeast in at least three or four CFIDS patients see how well it works and keep using it.

People with CFIDS also frequently have bowel parasite infections. Bowel parasites can cause severe allergic or sensitivity reactions, which in turn can trigger fibromyalgia and fatigue. Often, a patient will finally recover from longstanding and disabling fatigue within a week or two after beginning treatment for bowel parasites.

Many other CFIDS/FMS patients are left with disabling fatigue after a bout with viral infections such as polio, HHV-6, CMV, or EBV infections. This fatigue also usually responds to the treatments discussed in this book. In addition, infections with unusual organisms such as rickettsia (for example, Lyme disease), chlamydia, and mycoplasma may also be problematic.

Yeast Overgrowth

Everyone's immune system has strong spots as well as weak spots. Some people never get colds but have frequent bouts of athlete's foot or other skin fungal infections. Others never get fungal infections but tend to get colds. Many people seem to have a diminished ability to fight off fungal infections.

Fungi are very complex organisms. Fungal overgrowth may suppress the body's immune system. The body may also develop allergic reactions to components of the yeast.

This allergic reaction was suggested in a study that connected the fungal organism *Candida albicans* with allergic skin dermatitis (eczema). This study was published in *Clinical Experimental Allergy* in 1993.[4] It found that there is a significant correlation between the body having antibodies to *Candida albicans* and allergic dermatitis or eczema. In addition, we have found that unexplained rashes that have lasted for many years often clear up with antifungal treatment. Many physicians feel that yeast overgrowth causes a generalized suppression of the immune system. In other words, once the yeast gets the upper hand, it sets up a cycle that further suppresses the body's defenses.[5] Interestingly, a recent Mayo Clinic study showed that most cases of chronic sinusitis seem to be associated with a reaction to yeast in the sinuses—something I proposed years ago. Nonetheless, as I already noted, this theory is controversial. Yeast are normal members of the body's "zoo." They live in balance with bacteria—some of which are helpful and healthy, and some of which are detrimental and unhealthy. The problems begin when this harmonious balance shifts and the yeast begin to overgrow.

Many things can prompt yeast to overgrow. One of the most common causes is frequent antibiotic use. Antibiotics kill off the good bacteria in the bowel along with the bad bacteria. When this happens, the yeast no longer have competition and begin to overgrow. The body is often able to rebalance itself after one or several courses of antibiotics, but after repeated or long-term courses—and especially if the body has an underlying immune dysfunction—the yeast can get the upper hand.

Other factors are also important. Studies have shown that animals who are sleep-deprived and/or have increased sugar intake develop bowel yeast overgrowth. Many physicians feel that eating sugar stimulates yeast overgrowth in people as well. Sugar is food for yeast. Yeasts ferment sugar in order to grow and multiply. Yeast overgrowth due to the overuse of sugar also seems to cause immune suppression, which facilitates bacterial infections, which then requires even more antibiotic use. Poor sleep also results in marked suppression of your immune function.

DIAGNOSING YEAST OVERGROWTH

There are no definitive tests for yeast overgrowth that will distinguish yeast overgrowth from normal yeast growth in the body. There is one test that may be useful, though. This is a urine tartaric acid test. Tartaric acid is a waste product of yeast growth. In fermenting wine, for example, it is critical to remove the tartaric acid. Otherwise, the wine could be toxic to people. William Shaw, Ph.D., head of the Great Plains Laboratory in Kansas City, Missouri, has found elevations in urine tartaric acid that decrease with antifungal treatment in both CFIDS/FMS patients and autistic children. Interestingly, both of these illnesses often improve with antifungals—specifically, itraconazole (Sporanox) or fluconazole (Diflucan) plus nystatin. Dr. Shaw likes to use the urine tartaric acid testing to decide when to treat yeast overgrowth and to follow up the effectiveness of treatment.

In my experience, however, using Dr. William Crook's yeast questionnaire (reproduced in Appendix C in this book) is still the most reliable way to tell if a person is at risk of yeast overgrowth. If the symptom score is over 140 points, I recommend treatment. In addition, anyone who has been on recurrent or long-term antibiotics (especially tetracycline for acne), or who intermittently has painful sores in different parts of the mouth that last for about ten days at a time and who has CFIDS/FMS, should be treated with antifungals. Bowel symptoms are some of the more overt symptoms that are caused by yeast. I feel that most people who have irritable bowel syndrome, or "spastic colon," have yeast overgrowth or parasites.

TREATING YEAST OVERGROWTH

A number of very effective methods can be used to take care of a yeast problem. Some involve dietary changes and supplements, others prescription medications. Combining both approaches may be more effective than any one method alone.

Natural Yeast Treatments

Primary among the methods for treating yeast overgrowth is avoiding sugar and other sweets. You can enjoy one or two pieces of fruit a day, but you should not consume such concentrated sugar sources as juices, corn syrup, jellies, pastry, candy, or honey. Stay far away from soft drinks, which have ten to twelve teaspoons of sugar in every twelve ounces. This amount of sugar has been shown to markedly suppress immune function for several hours.

Using stevia as a sweetener is a wonderful substitute for sugar. Stevia is safe and natural, and you can use all you want. (There are even cookbooks available for using stevia.) Another natural sweetener is made from the lohan fruit. Marketed under the brand name Sweet Balance, it is twelve times as sweet as sugar and appears to be safe. Although it contains some fructose (fruit sugar), you need only a small amount.

Be prepared to have withdrawal symptoms for about one week when you cut sugar out of your diet. Several excellent books have been written on the yeast controversy and offer additional dietary methods to try. One of the best is *The Yeast Connection and the Woman* by Dr. Crook, a physician who has done a spectacular job advancing the understanding of CFIDS/FMS.

Many people have found that acidophilus—that is, milk bacteria, a healthy type of bacteria for the bowel—helps restore balance in the bowel. Acidophilus is found in yogurt with live and active yogurt cultures. Indeed, eating one cup of yogurt a day can markedly diminish the frequency of recurrent vaginal yeast infections.[6] Acidophilus is also available in capsule form. Although many claims are made for one type of acidophilus being better than another, I am not sure this is so. I usually recommend taking a dose of 3 to 6 billion units a day (1 unit equals one bacterium) on an empty stomach. If you are on antibiotics (*not* antifungals), take the acidophilus at least three to six hours away from the antibiotic dose.

Caprylic acid is another natural remedy that can be helpful. The usual dose is 1,800 to 3,600 milligrams a day, with one-third of the dose being taken at each meal. Unfortunately, it often causes an acid stomach, with a "funky" tasting reflux. Oregano oil—make sure to get *enteric coated* oregano oil—may be more effective and better tolerated than caprylic acid, although both can cause stomach acid reflux. I recommend taking one to two capsules two to three times a day, with food. Fresh garlic, if you can handle it well, can also be very effective. Daily, crush one to three garlic cloves in olive oil, add salt, spread it on bread and eat it. It can be quite tasty—and lethal to whatever infections you have in your gut.

Olive leaf extract can be very helpful in treating yeast overgrowth. The recommended dose is two to four 500-milligram capsules three times a day, between meals. Pau d'arco is an herb that is helpful in suppressing yeast. You can take it in either tea or capsule form. Although I use pau d'arco infrequently for yeast overgrowth, many people report having found it helpful. Another popular natural treatment for yeast overgrowth is grapefruit seed extract, such as Citricidal. It tends to be well tolerated.

Medical Treatments for Yeast Overgrowth

Nystatin, an antifungal medication, has been helpful in the treatment of yeast overgrowth. Unfortunately, some fungi seem to be resistant to nystatin. In addition, nystatin is poorly absorbed, which means that it has little impact on the yeast outside of the bowel. Other antifungal medications, such as Diflucan and Sporanox, seem to be effective systemically (throughout the body) but they have two main drawbacks. First, they are expensive, costing more than $450 to $900 for a two-month course. Second, any effective antifungal can initially make the symptoms of yeast infection worse. Although it is uncommon, Diflucan and Sporanox can also cause liver inflammation. If you are taking Diflucan or Sporanox for more than six to twelve weeks, I would consider intermittently doing blood tests to check liver function—specifically, checking blood levels of alanine aminotransferase (ALT) and aspartate transaminase (AST), two compounds that are good indicators of injury to the liver. If you have preexisting active liver disease, you should be cautious about using Diflucan or Sporanox—or not use them at all. I strongly recommend taking 200 milligrams of lipoic acid a day whenever you take Sporanox or Diflucan. This is a natural supplement that helps to protect and heal the liver. For that matter, I also strongly recommend lipoic acid for anyone with *active* liver disease (for example, hepatitis), at doses up to 1,000 to 3,000 milligrams a day, as it may prevent and/or help treat cirrhosis.

Yeast Treatment Recommendations

If symptoms of yeast overgrowth are caused by an allergic or sensitivity reaction to the yeast body parts, symptoms may flare up when mass quantities of the yeast are suddenly killed off. This is called a yeast die-off reaction. If you get this reaction, start your treatment with acidophilus and a sugar-free diet for a few weeks, followed by oregano oil and/or olive leaf extract (1,500 to 2,000 milligrams three times a day, between meals) before beginning nystatin. Take nystatin in tablet or powder form. I generally recommend beginning with 500,000 international units a day for one to three days, and increasing the dosage by 500,000 international units every one to three days (slower if yeast die-off is a problem) until you are taking 1,000,000 international units two to four times a day. Take this dosage for five to eight months. (If you develop nausea, reduce the dosage.) One month after beginning the nystatin, I add 200 milligrams of Diflucan or Sporanox every morning for six weeks. If symptoms flare up, take just 100 milligrams each morning for the first three to fourteen days. If symptoms recur after you stop the Diflucan or Sporanox, I recommend continuing the medication for an additional six weeks at 200 milligrams a day.

Sporanox should be taken with food. If it is taken alone, its absorption is greatly reduced. When taking Diflucan or Sporanox, *do not* use quinidine (a heart medicine); cholesterol-lowering medications in the pravastatin (Mevacor) family, which also includes Baycol, Lescol Lipitor, Pravachol, and Zocor; or the bowel medicine cisapride (Propulsid). These combinations can be *deadly*. Also, antacid medications such as cimetidine (Tagamet), nizatidine (Axid), ranitidine (Zantac), and famotidine (Pepcid) prevent the proper absorption of Sporanox. At the high price of Sporanox per dose, you will want to absorb every last bit of the medication. If you need to be on an antacid medication, you should use Diflucan instead of Sporanox. Unfortunately, a less expensive antifungal, called terbinafine (Lamisil), at 250 milligrams a day, does not seem to work very well for candida yeast overgrowth, although it does work well for nail infections. I am currently trying patients on 500 milligrams of Lamisil a day to see if this dose works better.

Once the yeast has been effectively decreased and kept that way for six to twelve months, you can try adding *small* amounts of sugar back into your diet. If symptoms recur, however, stop the sugar again. Continuing to eat yogurt with live and active acidophilus cultures (unless you are lactose-intolerant) or continuing to take acidophilus capsules may also help.

Many books on yeast overgrowth, including Dr. Crook's, advise readers to avoid all yeast in the diet. This advice is based on the theory that an allergic reaction to yeast is the cause of the problem. The predominant yeast that seems to be involved in yeast overgrowth is *Candida albicans*, although I would not be surprised if researchers discovered that many other kinds of fungal infections are also involved. The yeast that is found in most foods (except beer and cheese) is not closely related to candida.

In my experience, trying to avoid all yeast in foods results in a nutritionally inadequate diet and little benefit. Although a few people do appear to have true allergies to the yeast in their food, they account for fewer than 10 percent of my patients with suspected yeast overgrowth. These people may benefit from the more strict diet recommended in Dr. Crook's book. Interestingly, once adrenal insufficiency and yeast overgrowth are treated, most people find that their allergies and sensitivities to yeast and other food products seem to improve or disappear.

Nutritional deficiencies such as low zinc or low selenium may also decrease resistance to yeast overgrowth.[7] A good multivitamin supplement should take care of these deficiencies. This is further evidence that all the factors involved in CFIDS are closely interrelated.

The best thing you can do to combat yeast overgrowth is to try to avoid it in the first place. When you get an infection, immediately begin treating it naturally. (See Treating Infections Without Antibiotics, page 65). Hopefully, you will be able to prevent it from turning into a bacterial infection that might require an antibiotic. Ask your doctor what measures you can take before resorting to antibiotics. Many good over-the-counter remedies are available. A knowledgeable compounding pharmacist can also be a wealth of information. Your local bookstore or health food store has books on natural infection-fighting measures as well.

If you find, however, that you must take an antibiotic, all is not lost. You can still lessen the severity of yeast overgrowth by avoiding sweets and by taking nystatin plus either taking acidophilus capsules (again, not within three to six hours of an antibiotic) or by eating one cup of yogurt with live and active acidophilus cultures daily. Don't use the yogurt (or milk) if you have sinusitis or pneumonia, because the milk protein causes mucus to thicken and makes it hard for the body to fight these infections.

What If the Yeast Comes Back?

It is normal for yeast symptoms to resolve after treatment. After six weeks on the Sporanox or Diflucan, most people feel a lot better. However, symptoms may recur soon after they stop taking the antifungal. If this happens, I would continue the Sporanox or Diflucan for another six weeks or for as long as is needed to keep the symptoms at bay. More frequently, people feel better after treatment and stay feeling fairly well for a period of six to twenty-four months. At that time, it is common to see a recurrence of symptoms, especially if they are eating too much sugar or are taking antibiotics.

The best marker that I have found for recurrent yeast overgrowth is a

Treating Infections Without Antibiotics

Many people do not realize how many things they can do before resorting to using an antibiotic to clear an infection. If you feel you are coming down with a respiratory infection such as a cold or the flu, I recommend that you try the following:

- Take natural thymic hormone. This is available as a product called ProBoost (it used to be Bio-Pro A), manufactured by Genicel, Inc., and is a very effective immune stimulant. Dissolve the contents of one packet under your tongue three times a day and let it absorb there (any that is swallowed is destroyed). A recent study in CFIDS patients with markedly elevated Epstein-Barr antibody levels showed a dramatic drop in the antibody levels after six weeks of treatment with thymic hormone. Many physicians are finding that thymic hormone has been very helpful for CFIDS/FMS patients with persistent viral, yeast, bowel, or other infections. I have found that using it for two or three days at the onset of an infection can shorten the length of the infection dramatically, and often stops it on the first day.
- Take 1,000 milligrams of olive leaf extract three times a day for three to seven days. Although probably not as effective as thymic hormone, olive leaf extract seems to be helpful against viral respiratory infections and, perhaps, yeast infections. It seems most helpful in fighting the common cold. In my experience, it has been very helpful for about half the people who try it—the cold is gone in twenty-four to thirty-six hours. If it causes nausea, cut the dose in half.
- Take 1,000 milligrams of echinacea a day. This is an herbal immune stimulant that can enhance your body's defenses. Use a standardized extract.
- Take 1,000 to 8,000 milligrams of vitamin C a day—enough to get diarrhea, then cut back to comfortable level.
- Suck on a zinc lozenge five to eight times a day. Make sure that the lozenges have at least 10 to 20 milligrams of zinc per lozenge. Less than this will not be effective. Zinc lozenges have been known to speed the time it takes to recover from a cold by about 40 percent. General Nutrition Centers sells a very good one.
- Drink plenty of water and hot caffeine-free tea (or hot water with lemon) and rest!
- Take Oscillococcinum, a homeopathic remedy available at most health food stores and some supermarkets, if you have flu-like symptoms such as chills, fever, achiness and/or malaise. It speeds healing and eases discomfort. It is best taken early in the infection—as soon as you have any symptoms.
- If you have a sinus infection, try nasal rinses. Dissolve ½ teaspoon of salt in a cup of lukewarm water. Inhale some of the solution about one inch up into your nose, one nostril at a

time. Do this either by using a baby nose bulb or an eyedropper while lying down, or by sniffing the solution out of the palm of your hand while standing by a sink. Then gently blow your nose, being careful not to hurt your ears. Repeat the same process with the other nostril. Continue to repeat with each nostril until the nose is clear. Rinse your nasal passages at least twice a day until the infection improves. Each rinsing will wash away about 90% of the infection and make it much easier for your body to heal.

- Take acetaminophen (in Tylenol and many other over-the-counter pain relievers) for muscle aches and use Cepacol or Chloraseptic mouthwash as a gargle for a sore throat. Gargling with salt water, mixed as described above for the nasal rinse, also helps a sore throat. If you use acetaminophen frequently, you should also take 500 milligrams of supplemental N-acetylcysteine (NAC) each day so you don't deplete your glutathione levels.
- Try using a humidifier or vaporizer in your bedroom. You can also make a steam room by running a hot shower in your bathroom and then breathing in the steam. Or try using a steam inhaler, such as the one available from Bernhard Industries (see Appendix J: Resources). This is also wonderful for chronic and acute sinusitis
- Take at least 500 milligrams of vitamin C a day for prevention.

If, despite these measures, nasal and lung mucus is yellow after seven to fourteen days, or if you are feeling worse after three to four days, you may have to consider taking a course of antibiotics. If you do, you should take nystatin while on the antibiotic. Erythromycin antibiotics such as azithromycin (Zithromax) and clarithromycin (Biaxin) are usually preferable to penicillin antibiotics. Interestingly, my patients have sometimes found that all their CFIDS symptoms (not just the cold) improve while they are taking an erythromycin or tetracycline antibiotic. If that happens, I recommend a twelve-week course of 500 milligrams of Biaxin or 100 milligrams of doxycycline twice a day. If you feel better on the antibiotic (take thymic hormone, echinacea, and the antifungal nystatin in conjunction with it), keep repeating six-week courses until the symptoms stay gone. I would also check for Lyme disease using a blood or urine test. And for most of my patients who repeatedly get respiratory infections that take forever to go away, I consider an empiric trial of prescription hydrocortisone (Cortef) at a dosage of $7\frac{1}{2}$ milligrams in the morning and 5 milligrams at noon for two to three months.

As a preventive for respiratory infections, the flu vaccine is a double-edged sword for people with CFIDS/FMS. In some CFIDS/FMS patients, it can cause mild flulike symptoms for a few days. In rare cases, it can cause a severe flare-up of symptoms. Still, unless you are one of the 10 percent of CFIDS/FMS patients who feel worse after the flu shot or other vaccinations, I would get a flu shot. For most people, the benefit can significantly outweigh the risk. Interestingly, a recent Scandinavian study showed that having frequent vaccinations against *Staphylococcus* bacteria significantly improved symptoms in fibromyalgia patients. The researchers felt that it helped by stimulating the immune system.

Taking at least 500 milligrams of vitamin C a day is also a very good idea. And dress warmly. A cold breeze blowing across your muscles or neck can make fibromyalgia symptoms flare up.

return of bowel symptoms, with gas, bloating, and/or diarrhea or constipation. If these symptoms persist for more than two weeks, especially if there is also even a mild worsening of the CFIDS/FMS symptoms, it is very reasonable to retreat yourself with six weeks of nystatin and perhaps Sporanox or Diflucan. In addition, I would also resume treatment if there is a recurrence of vaginal yeast or sinus infections. If a second round of treatment resolves the symptoms, you may opt to repeat this regimen as often as is needed, usually every six to twenty-four months. By using some of the natural remedies listed earlier in this chapter, however, you may be able to avoid repeated use of antifungals and the possible risk of becoming resistant to them.

Some people find that they need to stay on the antifungals for extended periods of time—years, in some cases—or the symptoms recur. If this is necessary, I add the natural remedies. I do, however, also use prescription medications when needed. The main risk of long-term use of the antifungals Sporanox and Diflucan is liver inflammation. As mentioned earlier, if these medications are used for extended periods, liver function should be monitored. Consider checking the ALT and AST liver tests (also called SGOT and SGPT test) every three to six months and anytime that a severe flulike feeling or worsening of symptoms occurs. In addition, it is very important to take 200 milligrams of lipoic acid a day as long as you are on the medication. Although I am not aware of any studies on using lipoic acid with antifungals, I have seen no worrisome liver tests in patients using this natural substance while taking these antifungals. As an alternative, instead of taking the antifungals every day, many people find they can get long-term suppression of the yeast by taking 200 milligrams of Sporanox or Diflucan twice a day, one day each week (for example, each Sunday).

Chronic Bladder Infections

Although we will be discussing some unusual infections, CFIDS/FMS patients also get more of the day-to-day variety of infections. These include urinary tract (bladder) infections (UTIs). The main symptoms of a UTI are dysuria (discomfort—for example, a burning sensation—when urinating), urgency (the feeling that you have to go very badly and right away when there is not much urine there), and frequent urination with low urine volume. This group of symptoms are also common in CFIDS/FMS patients in the absence of bladder infections and, when severe, is called interstitial cystitis (IC). However, I would not say that a person has interstitial cystitis unless this is the *major* symptom of their CFIDS/FMS, because almost everyone with this illness has some urinary urgency and frequency. The few people who have IC need to be careful, as many vitamin supplements can cause symptoms to flare up.

Because bladder symptoms can be seen in both UTIs and CFIDS/FMS, it is important to have a urine culture done before initiating treatment with antibiotics to make sure that it is infection, and not just muscle spasms in the bladder, that is causing these symptoms. If there is an infection, over 90 percent of the time it will be with *Escherichia coli* (*E. coli*). This bacteria is normally found in the intestines and, with the exception of a few rare, dangerous forms, is a healthy part of normal bowel bacteria. The problem occurs when the *E. coli* gets out of the bowel, where it belongs, and into the bladder. Most infectious organisms are washed out of the bladder when the urine comes out. *E. coli,* however, have little Velcro-like projections that stick to the bladder wall so that they cannot be washed out by urination.

Taking antibiotics will kill a bladder infection, but will also kill the healthy bacteria in the bowel. This sets you up for yeast overgrowth and other problems. Because of this, unless you have fever, back pain over the kidneys, or a toxic feeling, it is reasonable to try natural remedies for one to three days before going with the antibiotics. You can start these treatments while waiting for the results of the urine culture to come back.

There are two excellent natural remedies that can keep the *E. coli* from sticking to the bladder walls so they can be washed out. In addition, taking high doses of vitamin C (500 to 5,000 milligrams a day) can acidify the urine, making it inhospitable to the bacteria. Drinking a lot of water also helps to wash out the infection. The two natural remedies that keep the bacteria from sticking are cranberries and D-mannose. They can be very effective, but they work only for bladder infections caused by *E. coli* bacteria—approximately 90 percent of all bladder infections.

CRANBERRIES

Because approximately 20 percent of the female population suffers from UTIs, several studies have been done looking at this remedy. In an early study, forty-four female and sixteen male patients with acute bladder infections drank 16 ounces of cranberry juice a day for fifteen days. Of these patients, 53 percent had positive responses and another 20 percent showed modest improvement. Six weeks after stopping the juice, twenty-seven patients did have persistent or recurrent infections and eight of these had no symptoms. Seventeen patients had no symptoms and negative urine cultures.

In another study of elderly women (who are more likely than younger women to have bladder infections), 153 women either received 10 ounces of cranberry drink or placebo every day for six months.[8] The group that got the cranberry drink had 68 percent fewer bladder infections during that period. In this study, the juice was sweetened with saccharin instead of sugar. Other studies have also shown benefit using cranberry juice in bladder infections.

Cranberries help bladder infections because they contain compounds known as proanthocyanidins that prevent bacteria from sticking to the bladder wall. They may also decrease the risk of kidney stones, as well as possibly reducing urine odor.

Significant benefits can be achieved by using 6 to 16 ounces of cranberry juice a day. Because most cranberry juice products have a lot of sugar, which can promote yeast overgrowth and aggravate other symptoms in CFIDS/FMS, I think it is much better to use pure cranberry juice powder in capsule or tablet form. Choose a product that is standardized to contain 11 to 12 percent quinic acid. The therapeutic dose is one to two capsules a day. You can also use unsweetened cranberry juice and add stevia as a natural sweetener. In general, cranberry juice drinks and cranberry sauce are half as potent as the usual cranberry juice cocktails, fresh or frozen cranberries are four times as potent, pure cranberry juice is four times as potent, and cranberry capsules made from unsweetened cranberry juice powder are thirty-two times as potent.

D-Mannose

D-Mannose is even more effective for bladder infections than cranberry juice. Mannose is a natural sugar (not the kind that causes symptoms or yeast overgrowth) that is excreted promptly into the urine. Unfortunately for the *E. coli* bacteria, the fingers that stick to the bladder wall stick to the D-mannose even better. When you take a large amount of D-mannose, it spills into the urine, coating all the *E. coli*'s little "sticky fingers" so that the *E. coli* are literally washed away with the next urination. The nice thing about the natural approach, as opposed to antibiotics, is that cranberries and D-mannose do not kill healthy bacteria, thereby not disturbing the normal balance of bacteria in the bowel. In addition, D-mannose is absorbed in the upper gut before it gets to the friendly *E. coli* that are normally present in the colon. Because of this, it helps clear the bladder without causing any other problems. In addition, D-mannose even tastes good.

D-Mannose is quite safe, even for long-term use, although most people need it for only a few days. People who have frequent recurrent bladder infections may, however, choose to take it every day. The usual dose of D-mannose is ½ teaspoon every two to three waking hours to treat an acute bladder infection; and ¼ to ½ teaspoon three to four times a day to prevent severe chronic bladder infections. It is best taken dissolved in water. If you get bladder infections associated with sexual intercourse, you can take ½ teaspoon of D-mannose one hour before and then just after intercourse to prevent an infection.

The usual cost of D-mannose is approximately sixty dollars for 100 grams and thirty-five dollars for 50 grams. One-half teaspoon is approximately 2 grams. (For information on suppliers of this supplement, see Appendix J: Resources.) You should feel much better within twenty-four to forty-eight hours on D-mannose. If you don't, see a doctor for a urine culture (you may want to get the culture at the first sign of infection) and consider antibiotic treatment after two days if the culture is positive. Some evidence exists that the antibiotic nitrofurantoin (also sold under the brand names Furadantin, Macrobid, and Macrodantin) causes less yeast overgrowth than do other antibiotics.[9] Even with other antibiotics, most bladder infections are knocked out by one to three days of antibiotic use, instead of the old seven-day regimen.

Prostatitis

Although women tend to be the ones plagued with bladder infections, men don't get off unscathed. It is very common for men with CFIDS/FMS to have prostatitis, an inflammation or infection of the prostate that is usually seen in younger men between the ages of twenty and fifty. There are three main types of prostatitis:

1. *Bacterial prostatitis.* This is an acute or chronic infection in the gland that causes prostate swelling and discomfort, and in which an infection can be found by doing a culture.
2. *Nonbacterial prostatitis.* This is a condition that causes you to feel swelling of the prostate with no detectable infection. My suspicion is that it is not uncommon for nonbacterial prostatitis to be associated with yeast overgrowth or other infections that cannot be cultured.
3. *Prostadynia.* This is a general irritation of the prostate that causes a burning sensation with urination, urinary urgency, and frequency, without any infection or swelling of the prostate. This can come from a number of causes including, I suspect, chronic spasm or tightening of the muscles of the pelvic floor.

The symptoms of chronic prostatitis can come and go and be mild or severe. The symptoms include:

- Pain or tenderness in the area of the prostate. It is also common to have burning on the tip of the penis.
- Discomfort in the groin and, occasionally, lower back pain.
- Urinary urgency and frequency with pain on urination.
- Pain with ejaculation.
- In some cases, a slight discharge from the penis. If the discharge is cloudy and larger than one drop, or even a large drop, it is most likely bacterial prostatitis and I would then prescribe antibiotics. If a dis-

charge is present, I would also check to make sure that there is not also a sexually transmitted disease (such as chlamydia or gonorrhea) before beginning treatment.

Severe symptoms, with fever, chills and extreme fatigue, point to acute bacterial prostatitis, requiring treatment with antibiotics. The main medications used for bacterial prostatitis are tetracycline antibiotics (for example, doxycycline [Doryx, Monodox, Vibramycin, Vibra-Tabs]), ciprofloxacin (Cipro), or sulfa drugs (such as Bactrim or Septra DS). Unfortunately, since it is hard for antibiotics to be absorbed into the prostate, symptoms often recur, even after six weeks of treatment. I prefer to use doxycycline or Cipro because these may be effective against other hidden infections that can cause CFIDS/FMS.

Although there are a number of causes of prostatitis, excessive consumption of caffeine, alcohol, and spicy foods can also contribute to the symptoms. Sitting for long periods while traveling (for example, being a truck driver) can also cause irritation of the prostate. Although normal bacteria are the most common causes, some bacteria transmitted through sexual contact can also cause prostatitis. Some people feel that the main psychological component of prostatitis is shame.

Bowel Parasite Infections

A number of years ago, the news focused our attention on Milwaukee because of repeated outbreaks of an infection by a bowel parasite called *Cryptosporidium*. Scores of Milwaukeeans died from the outbreaks. A cartoon even made the rounds showing Mexican tourists being warned not to drink the water in Milwaukee! Although this infection usually resolves on its own within a week or two, it can persist in people with suppressed immune function. People with acquired immune deficiency syndrome (AIDS) are particularly susceptible.

Unfortunately, in many places throughout the United States, the water supply is contaminated, and parasites are no longer just a Third World problem. Doctors frequently see cases of infection by giardia, amoebae, and numerous other bowel parasites.[10] The symptoms of parasitic infections can mimic those of CFIDS and, in immune-suppressing situations like CFIDS, *all* parasites should be treated.[11]

DIAGNOSING BOWEL PARASITES

Most laboratories miss parasites when they do stool testing. I initially tested for bowel parasites by sending my patients' stool samples to a respected local lab. The tests kept coming back negative, so I eventually stopped testing. Finally, I started doing my own laboratory stool testing. Doing the testing properly was very time consuming, taking up to five hours per specimen. However, when my tests were processed properly, they frequently turned out positive. In my experience—and in that of other physicians as well—when you treat a patient for parasites, the person's fatigue and achiness often improve dramatically.[12]

If you would like your stool tested, make sure that the laboratory doing the test *specializes* in stool testing and that the sample is a purged specimen. A purged stool specimen is watery and loose. This is achieved by taking 1½ ounces of Fleet's Phospho-Soda, a laxative. The purpose of the stool purge is to get the best possible stool sample to check for bowel parasites and yeast. The laxative washes the organisms off the walls of the intestines so that they can be detected. The routine random tests performed in almost all standard laboratories are generally not adequate or reliable. In speaking with several lab technicians, I was told they had less than one hour of training in looking for parasites—which they found to be useless. In fact, a gastroenterologist friend once noted that during a certain bowel exam he had performed, he saw a large number of parasites swimming in the patient's bowel. He removed a big glob consisting of nothing but mucus and parasites and sent it off to the major local laboratory, just for confirmation of the infection and identification of the parasite. Even this sample came back negative for parasites! This is why I stress that stool testing must be done at a lab that specializes in parasitology. Because two excellent labs are available to mail specimens to, I no longer have to do the testing in my office. These labs are the Parasitology Center and the Great Smokies Diagnostic Laboratory. (For more information, see Appendix J: Resources.)

TREATING BOWEL PARASITES

The appropriate treatment for many bowel parasites depends on which organism is causing the problem. At this point, no consistently effective prescription medication is available for *Cryptosporidium* infections. The herb *Artemisia annua* (also known as Chinese wormwood), however, is an effective treatment. For most of my patients, I recommend using 1,000 milligrams three times a day for twenty days. Leo Galland, M.D., a parasite specialist, recommends an herbal formula containing *Artemisia* extract called Tricycline, produced by Allergy Research Group, for many parasitic infections. He recommends taking two tablets three times a day, after meals, for six to eight weeks. The cost of this preparation is about thirty dollars for fifty tablets. Some of these infections respond to treatment with 500 milligrams of paromomycin (Humatin) three times a day for ten days. An alternate treatment for *Cryptosporidium* is 250 milligrams of azithromycin (Zithromax) once a day for ten days, on an empty stomach, along with one tablet of sulfamethoxazole plus trimethoprim (Bactrim) twice a day for ten days and *Artemisia.*

For many types of parasites, I prescribe a ten-day course of 750 milligrams of metronidazole (Flagyl) three times a day—or, for *Clostridium difficile,* 250 milligrams of Flagyl four times a day *or* 500 milligrams three times a day. This is followed by 650 milligrams of iodoquinol (also sold under the brand name Yodoxin) three times a day for twenty days. Flagyl can cause nausea and vomiting—uncomfortable, but usually not worrisome. The extended-release (ER) form, 750 milligrams taken once or twice a day, is easier on the stomach, as are the name brand forms. You should not drink alcohol while taking this medication, as the combination will make you vomit. If you get numbness or tingling in your fingers (or it worsens if you usually have it), you should stop taking the Flagyl.

Lactoferrin is an iron-binding protein that helps fight parasitic infection, boost immune function, and benefit intestinal health. Taking one to three 350-milligram capsules at bedtime can be useful. Another natural supplement that can be helpful is colostrum (mother's milk). Take three capsules three times a day for eight to twelve weeks, on an empty stomach. Then stop or use the lowest dose needed to control symptoms. If nausea or indigestion occurs, lower the dose to a comfortable level for one to two weeks until it passes.

For the parasite *Entamoeba histolytica,* you can use tinidazole (Fasigyn), at a dosage of 2,000 milligrams once daily for three consecutive days, with food. This drug is not widely available, but it can be obtained (with a doctor's prescription) from Clark's Pharmacy (see Appendix J: Resources). Tinidazole can also be useful for for *Giardia lamblia* or *Dientamoeba fragilis.* Generally, three doses are taken at two-week intervals.

For blastocystis, taking 500 milligrams of Humatin three times a day or one tablet of Bactrim DS twice a day for ten days, *plus* 650 milligrams of Yodoxin three times a day for ten days, may be effective. You should not take folic acid supplements or a vitamin-B complex containing folic acid during these ten days. Yodoxin should be taken with food. For refractory blastocystis, you may need to take 100 milligrams of oral amphotericin B *plus* 500 milligrams of tinidazole *plus* one tablet of furazolidone (Furoxone) twice a day, with food, for five to seven days.

There are also a number of medications that may be useful if parasitic infection is suspected, but no parasites have been identified. One of these is albendazole (Albenza). The usual dosage is 400 milligrams a day for five days. Another drug that may be helpful (although somewhat controversial) is quinacrine, taken at a level of 100 milligrams a day for five days.

THE IMPORTANCE OF FILTERING YOUR WATER

As demonstrated in the Milwaukee example, drinking water can be a major source of parasitic infection. As the American water supply becomes more contaminated, parasitic bowel infections will likely become more common. These infections, as well as the overgrowth of yeast or toxic bacteria caused by the use of antibiotics, contribute to the problems of people with CFIDS/FMS.

Water filters can therefore be very helpful in the fight against parasitic infection, and can help to improve health in general. However, not all units are designed to filter out parasites. For a water filter to remove parasites, it must be rated by the National Sanitation Foundation (NSF) for cyst removal. A good example is the Multi-Pure filter (see Appendix J: Resources). Most filters on the market do not remove parasites and a wide range of contaminants. Solid carbon block filters and reverse-osmosis filters are the best types of units to use.

When shopping around for a water filter, request the NSF International Listing. The NSF is an independent, not-for-profit organization that tests and certifies drinking water treatment products. The unit you buy should meet both NSF Health Effects Standard 53 for cysts (giardia, cryptosporidium, entamoeba, toxoplasma), as well as their standards for the following contaminants: VOCs (pesticides, herbicides, and chemicals), endocrine disrupters (PCBs), trihalomethanes (cancer-causing disinfection byproducts), heavy metals (lead, mercury), MBTE (a gasoline additive), chloramines, and asbetos. Solid carbon block technology can reduce chlorine, taste and odor problems, particulate matter, and a wide range of contaminants. Solid carbon block filters do not remove healthful, naturally occuring minerals. They also require no electricity and add no salt or silver to the water. Any unit that does not meet all of these standards, particularly the health standard, is not adequate. Then contact the NSF (see Appendix J: Resources) to verify that any filter unit you are considering does indeed meet these standards.

In addition to verifying that a water filter meets the NSF standards, ask to see its Product Performance Data Sheet. Many states require that this sheet be given to all prospective customers of drinking water treatment devices. Also ask about the range of contaminants that the unit can reduce under NSF Health Effects Standard 53. Most units certified under Standard 53 list only turbidity and cyst reduction. The number of units that also reduce all of the contaminants listed above is very small. Make sure that the water filter you are considering can remove the specific contaminants that concern you without removing beneficial minerals. Beware of sales agents who tell you that NSF certification is not important.

Ask if the unit is licensed in such states as California, Colorado, and Wisconsin. These states have some of the toughest certification procedures in the United States. Finally, ask about the unit's service cycle, which is stated in gallons of water treated. Find out how often you will need to change the filter and what the replacement filters cost. If a filter unit can satisfy you on all these counts, it is probably a good product.

The Role of Other Infections in CFIDS/FMS

Many infections have been found in CFIDS. That people may have not just one, but several simultaneously, is significant. It suggests that although these infections may be a trigger, in most patients the immune system is suppressed, setting you up for unusual infections that persist. These infections may then drag you down, further suppressing your immune system.

Fortunately, most people improve (and often get very healthy) by simply treating the sleep, hormonal, nutritional, and yeast problems. Once these areas are treated, your body can usually eliminate any persistent infections by itself. Some people, though, have infections that need treatment with antivirals and/or antibiotics.

How can you tell if you need such treatments? First, I would try the other approaches discussed in this book. I would consider drug treatments if the following symptoms persist:

- Predominantly flulike symptoms, with debilitating fatigue and little or no pain or fever. People with these symptoms are more likely to have an underlying persistent viral infection, such as HHV-6, CMV, or EBV.
- A fever over 98.6°F—even 99°F—and/or lung congestion, sinusitis, skin pustules, or other chronic bacterial infections. People with these symptoms seem to be more likely to have bacterial, mycoplasmal, or chlamydial infections that respond to special antibiotics.

Let's look at these two situations and how to approach them.

Viral Infections

Human herpesvirus type 6 (HHV-6) is a virus that is related to the Epstein-Barr virus (EBV), cytomegalovirus (CMV), and also to the herpesviruses that cause cold sores and genital herpes. HHV-6 is transmitted like the common cold and many people have had it, as well as EBV and the cold sore virus, by the time they are twenty years old. The body usually gets rid of all of these viruses on its own. Because of this, if you did routine antibody testing, known as IgG testing, almost everybody would test positive for EBV and many will test positive for HHV-6 and CMV. The IgG test, however, does not tell you if you have an active infection unless another antibody test, the Ig*M* test, is also positive.

The IgM antibody is the one that increases in the first six weeks of an infection, so a positive IgM test suggests a new infection. This is followed by elevated Ig*G* antibodies, which stay elevated for the rest of your life and act as your body's surveillance system. Thus, all an elevated IgG means is that your body has seen this infection before and, if it sees it again, it's ready to knock it out quickly. This is how immunizations work. The immunization prompts the body to create the IgG antibodies, so that instead of taking one to two weeks to gear up to fight the infection, your body can eliminate that infection very quickly. Unfortunately, in CFIDS/FMS, you can have a chronic low-grade infection—even if your IgG antibody test is positive (elevated)—making the IgG antibody test for HHV-6, EBV, and CMV unreliable. In addition, IgM antibodies are not usually present in elevated levels in the low-grade infections with these viruses that may be seen in people with CFIDS and FMS.

What makes this important is that high doses of the drug valacyclovir (Valtrex) can eliminate EBV, but will not work if active HHV-6 or CMV infection is present. As I will discuss later, the only tests I would rely on to diagnose active HHV-6 are rapid cell cultures or polymerase chain reaction (PCR) testing. Because some insurance companies are more likely to pay for IgG than PCR testing, an argument can be made for checking IgG antibodies first. If the EBV IgG is positive and HHV-6 and CMV IgG are negative, one may choose to proceed with 1,000 milligrams of Valtrex four times a day for six months, without PCR testing. If the HHV-6 or CMV IgG antibodies are positive, then CMV and/or HHV-6 PCR tests should be done to be sure they are negative before proceeding with treatment.

HHV-6

Unfortunately there is no currently accepted standard treatment for HHV-6. Even though it is related to other herpesviruses, HHV-6 is resistant to acyclovir (Zovirax), Valtrex, famciclovir (Famvir), and the other antivirals that are commonly used for herpes infections. The only antiviral known to be effective against HHV-6 is ganciclovir (Cytovene). This drug has significant side effects, is very expensive, and has to be given intravenously—and possibly forever—to maintain the antiviral effect. Unfortunately, this is not a viable option in day-to-day life. Moreover, it has been only moderately successful when used. The main doctor who has been using ganciclovir to treat HHV-6 in the United States is Joe Brewer, MD, in Kansas City, Missouri. He also found that 140 of 207 CFIDS patients had positive HHV-6 cell cultures. Forty percent of CFIDS patients were positive on their first test and 70 percent were positive after three tests. This contrasts with sixty healthy patients he checked, in whom no HHV-6 tests were positive. Cultures are more likely to be positive during acute flare-ups of the infection, when the viral level in the blood rises.

As is often the case in CFIDS, there is conflicting data on infections in chronic fatigue syndrome. A study conducted at the National Center for Infectious Diseases of the U.S. Centers for Disease Control and Prevention examined twenty-six patients with chronic fatigue syndrome and fifty-two healthy patients.[13] In this study, several tests for HHV-6 and HHV-7 were done, including PCR testing. HHV-6 DNA was found in 11 percent of CFIDS patients and 28 percent of healthy patients, suggesting that the HHV-6 was actually less common in people with chronic fatigue syndrome than in healthy people. At this time, as the conflicting data shows, although HHV-6 may be one of many suspected infections in CFIDS, it is not yet clearly established as the cause of this illness.

When HHV-6 is present, it seems to infect the natural killer cells, important cells in your body's defense (immune) system that are critical in fighting infections. A number of studies have shown natural killer cells to be malfunctioning in CFIDS. HHV-6 infection does not necessarily decrease the *number* of the natural killer cells but does decrease their *function*. Natural killer cell function is described in what is called *lytic units*—which means the ability of cells to lyse, or break down, foreign invaders. An average person has a lytic unit level of 20 to 250, with over 80 percent of healthy people having over 40 units. Dr. Brewer finds that in people with CFIDS, the mean natural killer lytic unit level is 12 units. Dr. Brewer uses Specialty Labs in California for his natural killer lytic cell testing. He finds that the lytic level stays the same on repeat testing and seems to be a reliable test for natural killer cell function testing in CFIDS. Lytic unit levels do, however, decrease during flare-ups of symptoms. In Dr. Brewer's experience, this test is very specific for CFIDS and multiple sclerosis (MS). He has treated ten MS patients and five CFIDS patients with intravenous ganciclovir. He found that it helped to stabilize the MS patients. In the CFIDS patients, two to three were much improved, one still had a positive viral culture, and one had a poor response. Unfortunately, as noted above, maintaining patients on intravenous ganciclovir forever is not a viable option. Fortunately, a pill form of ganciclovir (Valganciclovir) is currently being developed. It should be noted that the HHV-6 virus is similar to CMV and that whatever is effective against one, tends to be effective for the other. This is a helpful bit of information as we follow new research looking for clues on how to eliminate HHV-6 infection.

EBV and CMV

The roles of EBV and CMV in CFIDS are not clear. It is not uncommon for antibody levels of these viruses to be elevated in people with chronic fatigue syndrome. However, it is not clear whether this simply reflects a previous or ongoing infection with these viruses. Research by a husband and wife team, Ronald Glaser and Janice Kiecolt-Glaser, at Ohio State University, suggests that EBV (the virus that causes mononucleosis) is still quite active and plays a role in many patients with these infections. In addition, work by A. Martin Lerner, MD, also suggests that EBV and CMV are active as well. He has found EBV and CMV to both be fairly common in patients with chronic fatigue syndrome, with and without pain. He found that about 20 percent had positive IgM and/or elevated early antigen (EA) tests to EBV with negative CMV. Of these, he reports that two-thirds improved with high doses of Valtrex. It takes about three to four months before patients *start* to improve, and after six months people can stop the Valtrex without the symptoms coming back. However, if there is no improvement in six months, consider it to be a negative result. They also found that, as noted above, IgM tests are almost always negative using the reagents used in most labs. They found that only Epstein-Barr IgM antibody testing using a reagent produced by the DiaSorin company (see Appendix J: Resources) has been useful in showing a significant number of positive tests. What was fairly common, though (and present in most patients) was either positive tests for EBV, CMV, or a combination of both, as noted above. When CMV or HHV-6 is present, the Valtrex is less likely to work because it is not effective against these viruses.

In another study done by Dr. Lerner, he found that patients who had elevated CMV IgG antibodies, but no significant evidence of associated Epstein-Barr virus (that is, negative IgM and EA antibody total less than 40), did improve with intravenous ganciclovir, at a dosage of 5 milligrams per kilogram of body weight, given intravenously every twelve hours for thirty days.[14] In this study, 72 percent (thirteen of the eighteen patients) improved markedly at the end of a month, without any significant side effects. As noted, an oral form of ganciclovir is currently in development as well. Thirty-six percent of the chronic fatigue patients Dr. Lerner checked (eighteen out of fifty) did turn out to have elevated CMV antibodies (albeit IgG—not a sign of recent or active infection) in the absence of IgM and EA antibodies to EBV (that is, no evidence of active Epstein-Barr virus). It should be noted, though, that 70 percent of healthy patients in the study also had positive IgGs for CMV, and it appears that the level of the IgG was not much higher overall in the chronic fatigue group than in the healthy controls. On the other hand, the higher the level of CMV antibodies in the chronic fatigue group, the more likely they were to improve with the intravenous ganciclovir.

What this means is that patients with chronic fatigue syndrome don't necessarily have different blood tests for antibodies to these viruses than healthy people. However, if you have a higher level rather than a lower level, you are more likely to improve with ganciclovir treatment. Previous research has not shown benefit from antiviral therapies in CFIDS.[15] Our experience using fairly high doses of Valtrex or Famvir (1,500 and 2,250 milligrams a day respectively) also showed no significant improvement on these regimens after six weeks, at which time we considered it to be ineffective. On the other hand, Dr. Lerner's research suggests that perhaps we gave these medications for too short a time and at too low a dose. When treating himself and a few other patients, he used Valtrex by mouth at a dosage of 1,000 milligrams four times a day for six months. Using the higher dosages and the extended period of time, as well as separating out groups that have Epstein-Barr virus (sensitive to the oral Valtrex) without CMV or HHV-6 (resistant to oral Valtrex but sensitive to intravenous ganciclovir), may make an important difference in making treatment effective. No major toxicity as a result of taking Valtrex was seen.

In addition, Dr. Lerner suspects that these viral infections affect the heart muscle, contributing to symptoms. I am not convinced that this is the case because changes in electrocardiogram (EKG) test results to evaluate heart function are common in people with CFIDS. This may occur because the autonomic (brain) dysfunction and hormonal changes seen in CFIDS can cause these same EKG changes without heart damage. Dr. Lerner reports that these changes went away with treatment. However, my experience in treating chronic fatigue syndrome has been that cardiac symptoms improve even without antivirals.

Although there is no currently accepted specific treatment for the CMV and HHV-6, there are still a number of things that may be very helpful in fighting these infections. Lithium tends to be antiviral and has been shown to decrease pain in FMS patients when added to treatment with amitriptyline (Elavil). Lithium is commonly used in manic-depressive illness. It is a natural mineral despite being sold by prescription. In high doses, it can cause some neurologic symptoms and suppression of the thyroid gland, but these can usually be treated by taking a small amount of essential fatty acids and thyroid hormone. Lithium may also worsen restless leg syndrome. Although we have no direct evidence that lithium is effective against HHV-6, it may well be effective, because it is known to work against a number of other viral infections. In my experience, 200 to 600 milligrams of lithium a day seems to be an effective dose for CFIDS/FMS patients. I check thyroid blood tests (a free T_4 and a total T_3, not TSH—see page 42) in my patients on lithium at three months, six months, and then yearly. The lithium level should also be checked at the same time to be sure that it is not above the upper limit of normal. The level can be below the normal range—this is fine as long as the treatment is effective. You may find that you can lower the lithium dose after you have been on it for several months. Heparin, a blood thinner, also has antiviral properties.

It is also worth considering a trial of high doses of Valtrex. It should be noted that doses of 1,000 milligrams three times a day are used for shingles in older adults and appear to be quite safe. On the other hand, higher dosing (8,000 milligrams a day) in AIDS patients did result in life-threatening problems in a few (under 2 percent of) individuals. This is common even with day-to-day drugs in AIDS patients, however; regular sulfa antibiotics have often resulted in severe toxicity in people with AIDS. Nonetheless, I would limit the dose to 1,000 milligrams four times a day. It is important to note that taking cimetidine (Tagamet) and/or probenecid (Benemid) raises the blood level of Valtrex. Tagamet has powerful immune-modifying properties and is very helpful for acute cases of Epstein-Barr infection (mononucleosis). Because of this, I add 300 milligrams of Tagamet four times a day (but *not* Benemid) to the Valtrex.

There are also natural remedies that may help with viral infections. Olive leaf extract is an herbal product that is known to have a wide spectrum of anti-infectious activity. Some doctors have found it to be effective in CFIDS, and in tests against HHV-6 and CMV virus, olive leaf extract did not just suppress the virus but killed it. I have not, however, seen studies testing its effect in human beings infected with HHV-6. Nonetheless, a number of physicians have found that using olive leaf extract in chronic fatigue syndrome is very effective. There is controversy over whether the form and source of the olive leaf is critical. I recommend that you use a standardized extract containing at least 6 percent oleuropein, which is one of the most active antiviral components in the olive leaf. The recommended dosage is three to four 500-milligram capsules three to four times a day, between meals. How long you need to take olive leaf for chronic fatigue syndrome is yet to be determined. Some people feel that it is important to use Mediterranean, not American, olive leaf extract. Other people argue that you should use a form that is organically grown, without pesticides. At this point, it is not clear whether this is simply marketing or important in day-to-day life. Nonetheless, I would be picky about the companies you buy the olive leaf extract from. (For recommended sources, see Appendix J: Resources.)

Thymic protein A, marketed under the brand name Pro-Boost (it used to be called BioPro), is a natural immune stimulant. Although not a hormone, thymic protein A mimics the natural hormone produced by the thymus, the gland that stimulates the immune system. I find it to be extraordinarily effective in fighting common infections of any kind that seem to pop up. For the more deep-seated infections of CFIDS, a higher dose (1 packet three times a day) will likely be needed. Once the infection seems to be in check and you are feeling better (that is, after six weeks), you can taper down to the lowest dose that maintains the effect.

Inositol hexaphosphate (IP_6; also known as phytic acid) is another natural immune stimulant. An extract of bran, it is less expensive, but likely less effective, than Pro-Boost, and is sometimes combined with vitamin C. The recommended dose of IP_6 is 5 to 8 grams (5,000 to 8,000 milligrams) a day. You should not take IP_6 within three hours of vitamin or mineral supplements.

A very concentrated mushroom extract marketed under the brand name MGN3 has been shown to stimulate natural killer cell immune function. In one study, it actually tripled natural killer cell function—an effect that could be very powerful, since HHV-6 can suppress natural killer cell function. Unfortunately, MGN3 is horribly expensive to use at the recommended dosage of two to four 250-milligram capsules four times a day for two weeks, followed by two capsules twice a day. Other mushroom extracts are cheaper, but may not be as effective.

High doses (15 to 50 grams) of vitamin C, administered intravenously, have been suggested to have antiviral effects in a number of other infections. They are often dramatically helpful for CFIDS when given in the intravenous nutritional therapy called Myers cocktails.

Lysine is an amino acid, one of the building blocks of protein, that inhibits oral and genital herpesviruses by depleting arginine, another amino acid that the virus needs to grow. It is not known whether it inhibits EBV, HHV-6, or CMV, but these viruses are all members of the herpes family. Lysine is safe and inexpensive. The recommended dosage is 1,000 milligrams three times a day.

I would take a combination of these natural remedies (as you can afford it—perhaps leaving the MGN3 for later if needed), for at least a six- to eight-week trial to see if they are effective. If you are feeling better at six weeks, you can then taper down the dose slowly as long as the benefit is maintained. When you are able, you can wean yourself off the treatments.

If symptoms recur, go back up to the dose that maintains the benefit or consider increasing the dose further.

In addition, your clotting system may be activated by several infections, making it difficult to eliminate them. Using the anti-clotting treatments that we will discuss later can also make it easier for your body to eradicate infections.

Mycoplasma and Chlamydia

Other infections have also been found to be very important in CFIDS. Mycoplasma and chlamydia are two types of microorganisms that can cause persistent infections and have similar characteristics. Dr. Garth Nicolson and his wife, Nancy L. Nicolson, who were both on-faculty in the Department of Microbiology and Immunology at Baylor University in Texas, are the leading proponents of treatment of these infections. Dr. Nicolson was also an endowed chair and department chairman at the M.D. Anderson Cancer Center of the University of Texas in Houston, and a professor of internal medicine at the University of Texas Medical School, also in Houston. Nancy Nicolson had chronic fatigue syndrome years ago. They were surprised that her test turned out to be positive for the organism *Mycoplasma incognitus* (also known as *Mycoplasma fermentans*). This type of mycoplasma was found to be resistant to the penicillin- and cephalosporin-family antibiotics, such as Keflex, that most doctors use, but was sensitive to long courses of doxycycline and Cipro. After an extended course of doxycycline treatment, she was much better. The Nicolsons then went on to develop their own tests for mycoplasma using PCR testing. In addition, when his stepdaughter came home after serving in operation Desert Storm, she came down with Gulf War illness (GWI). The Nicolsons tested hundreds of Gulf War veterans with GWI and found that 40 to 45 percent were positive for mycoplasma infections—almost all with *Mycoplasma fermentans*. This has been confirmed by other laboratories and a large Veterans Administration study. In contrast to this, fewer than 6 percent of soldiers who were not deployed to the Persian Gulf during the war tested positive for these infections.

Mycoplasma are a type of ancient bacteria that lack cell walls and are capable of invading a number of types of human cells. They can cause a wide variety of human diseases. These organisms can cause the types of symptoms seen in people with CFIDS and, according to Dr. Nicolson, tend to be immune-suppressing. Unfortunately, they cannot be readily cultured on a culture dish like regular bacteria can. In medicine, we have a bad habit of focusing on things that are easy to test for and making believe that things that are hard to test for do not exist. Because of this, bacterial infections such as pneumonia, bladder infections, and skin infections—in which one bacterium on a cell dish will rapidly turn into millions by the next day and be visible to the human eye—get all our attention. Unfortunately, mycoplasma and chlamydia, which cannot be easily cultured, tend to be ignored. It's like the old story about the person who was looking for a lost set of keys under the street lamp one night. His friends came by and asked him what was going on. He told them and they all looked for the keys under the light for about an hour. Finally, exasperated, they looked at the friend and said, "Where did you lose these keys?" The guy looked up and said, "Oh, about half a block down the street." They said, "Why are you looking for them here?" He said, "Because there is a light here and I can see!" This is kind of what it is like in medicine. If there is a test for something (such as cholesterol and bacterial cultures) that is easy to do, we focus our attention on that test and make believe that it finds the main problem. Unfortunately, in CFIDS and FMS, this is not the case.

Although mycoplasma and chlamydia are common in the environment, they usually are fairly noninvasive. It may simply be that once your immune system is weakened, these infections can get into cells where they don't belong. When that happens, even some of the common ones that are normally considered noninfectious can wreak havoc. When these infections reproduce slowly, they tend to be low-grade and chronic, as opposed to the acute and more prominent symptoms seen with bacterial and viral infections that multiply and divide rapidly.

Interestingly, the Nicolsons found that in patients with chronic fatigue syndrome or fibromyalgia, approximately 70 percent (144 out of 203 patients) had a positive PCR test for at least one—usually several—species of mycoplasma or chlamydia. When the Nicolsons tested 70 healthy patients, only 6 (less than 9 percent) were positive for any of the mycoplasma species. This is a highly significant difference. Only 2 of these 70 healthy people were positive for *Mycoplasma fermentans*. Similar results have been published by other doctors.

It is likely that there is a group of underlying problems and not a single one that triggers CFIDS/FMS. This applies to infections as well. This is why we see positive tests for both viral and mycoplasmal/chlamydial infections in so many people with this disease. For mycoplasma alone, when the Nicolsons checked for four different types of mycoplasma, over half of the ninety-three CFIDS patients that were positive had more than one type of infection. Over 20 percent of them had three out of the four mycoplasma infections test positive. The more infections they tested positive for, the worse their symptoms were and the longer they had had CFIDS/FMS.

The data suggest that many infections may trigger CFIDS/FMS or that CFIDS and FMS may cause immune suppression—which then sets you up to catch a whole bunch of different infections which your body has trouble clearing. This is why it is important to treat all the underlying processes simultaneously.

Diagnosing HHV-6, Mycoplasma, and Chlamydia

I had the honor of speaking with Konnie Knox, M.D., a major researcher on HHV-6 testing in CFIDS/FMS, who uses a technique called rapid cell culture. She actually infects different test tube cells with HHV-6, grows them, and then looks for signs of HHV-6 in the cell. In her experience, one out of three CFIDS/FMS patients is positive for active HHV-6 infection on the first blood test. When multiple testing is done (for example, three tests), 70 percent are positive. For the vast majority of people who are healthy, this test is negative. The other main illness where HHV-6 testing is often positive is multiple sclerosis.

HHV-6 and PCR testing by the Wisconsin Viral Institute or Dr. Nicolson's laboratory, International Molecular Diagnostics (see Appendix J: Resources), is the only HHV-6 test I recommend. The Nicolsons use very sensitive PCR testing that looks for DNA specific to mycoplasma, HHV-6, and other infections. Ordinarily, those DNA pieces are so microscopically small that to look for just one is much worse than looking for a needle in a haystack. With the PCR test, if that mycoplasma gene sequence is found, the technique multiplies it like a copying machine until millions of that sequence are present and can be picked up by testing. Because of this, PCR testing is exquisitely sensitive and can find the proverbial needle in a haystack. As noted above, IGG antibody testing is not reliable for proving the presence of mycoplasma and chlamydia infections in CFIDS. Another excellent lab is Immunosciences in California, run by Dr. Vjodani, another wonderful researcher in this field.

I can almost guarantee that if you do the mycoplasma or chlamydia tests at your local lab they will do the wrong tests and they will be useless for hidden CFIDS infections. I have never seen one come back with any useful information. What they usually do is check the antibodies—usually for the wrong mycoplasma infection—which simply shows that you, like virtually everybody else, have had a mycoplasma infection at some point in your life. It tells nothing about active infection and, again, is useless. Be sure to do the PCR testing and do it at one of the recommended labs.

Be aware that even with the best laboratories, it is not uncommon to have a false-negative report—where you have the infection but it does not show up on the test. Because of this, multiple tests may need to be done. There are good arguments for not doing the tests and simply going ahead and treating as if you have one of these infections. If you feel better after four months on the treatment, then you know you are hitting an infection and you can always intermittently stop the treatments to see how long you will need them. Also, there are many infections that are not tested for with these tests that would be effectively treated with the regimens that we are discussing. Many of these are likely to be infections that we don't even know exist. Because of this, if resources are limited, I sometimes simply treat the patient, based on clinical suspicion, without doing the tests.

Testing does have its benefits, however. If a test is positive, I am likely to treat more aggressively and it helps guide me on how long to give the treatment. For example, if after four months you are not better and the test is positive, I would be likely to go ahead and increase dosing or change to a different antibiotic. If the test was negative, I would be more likely to just stop treatment and suspect that the infection is less likely. This argues in favor of doing the tests. One simple thing to do is to go ahead and check with your insurance company to see if they cover these tests. This may make your decision much simpler.

Treating Mycoplasma and Chlamydia

Fortunately, both mycoplasma and chlamydia infections are usually sensitive to the right antibiotics. The antibiotics most likely to effect these organisms are the following:

- Doxycycline or minocycline (Dynacin, Minocin), usually at dosages of 100 milligrams three times a day. These two antibiotics are in the tetracycline family. They are very effective against a number of unusual organisms (for example, Lyme disease). They sometimes cause some stomach upset. If this occurs, take the medicine with food and a full glass of water or lower the dose. They should not be given to children under eight years old because they can cause permanent staining of the teeth. Do not use outdated or expired tetracycline prescriptions—they can kill you!

- Ciprofloxacin (Cipro), usually 750 milligrams twice a day. Although expensive, this is usually a well-tolerated antibiotic. It has a very wide range of effectiveness against a large number of organisms. When treating males, Cipro has the additional benefit of treating any hidden prostate infections, as does doxycycline. You should not take oral magnesium or any supplement containing magnesium within six hours of taking Cipro or you won't absorb the Cipro.
- Azithromycin (Zithromax), 600 milligrams a day, taken with food, *or* clarithromycin (Biaxin), 500 milligrams twice a day, taken on an empty stomach. These antibiotics are in the erythromycin family. Zithromax tends to be fairly well tolerated. Biaxin is more likely to cause a bit of nausea in some patients, but it is usually well tolerated. Both are quite expensive. They may work against infections missed by doxycycline and Cipro.

Although all of these antibiotics can be effective, it is not uncommon for infections that are sensitive to the erythromycin antibiotics (Zithromax or Biaxin) to be resistant to tetracycline antibiotics (doxycycline, minocycline) and Cipro, and vice-versa. Therefore, it is best to try either doxycycline or Cipro first. If they are not effective, then try the Zithromax or Biaxin. The antibiotic should be taken for at least six months. If there is no improvement in four months, switch to or add the other antibiotic or simply stop the treatment. It is helpful to check for low-grade fever. As mentioned earlier, I am more likely to use antibiotics for CFIDS patients who have temperatures over 98.6°F, even if it is only 98.8°F (I consider 98.8°F a fever because CFIDS/FMS patients usually have low body temperatures). If you do have low-grade, chronic temperature elevations, be sure that you monitor your temperature during treatment. If your temperature drops with the antibiotic, it suggests that you do have one of these nonviral infections and the antibiotic is helping. This would encourage me to continue the antibiotic trial—even if it takes up to eighteen months to see an improvement in your symptoms.

If you are clearly better, I would probably take the antibiotic for at least six to twelve months. It can then be stopped. If symptoms recur, keep repeating six- to eight-week cycles until the symptoms stay gone. It may take several years of treatment for the infection to be totally eradicated. To put this in perspective, this is how long children often take antibiotics for acne—which unfortunately, if not taken with antifungals, can lead to yeast overgrowth and possibly trigger CFIDS. You should therefore take two tablets of the antifungal nystatin twice a day, while on the antibiotics. It is a good idea to take an acidophilus supplement as well. Also, be aware that birth control pills may become ineffective while you take antibiotics, so be sure to use an alternative form of birth control. In addition, antidepressants, codeine, antacids, and mineral supplements (for example, magnesium) may block antibiotic absorption. Take these at least three hours away from the antibiotic (and don't take the antidepressant or codeine medications if they are not clearly helping).

It is very common to get what is called a Herxheimer (die-off) reaction that includes chills, fever, night sweats, and general worsening of CFIDS/FMS symptoms when the antibiotic first kills off the infection. These symptoms can be severe and last for weeks. Dr. Nicolson encourages patients not to abandon therapy prematurely. He notes that if you have been sick for years, it is unlikely you will recover in less than one year of treatment, so you should not be alarmed by symptoms that return or worsen temporarily.

The Role of the Blood Clotting System

Work done by David E. Berg, director of Hemex Laboratories in Phoenix, Arizona (see Appendix J: Resources), has shown that a number of infections can trigger the blood clotting system to become active, thus setting up a low-level, chronic clotting cascade. Some of the infections that can do this are HHV-6, mycoplasma, CMV, and chlamydia, which can trigger production of antibodies against clot-protective proteins on the inner surfaces of blood vessels, called antiphospholipid antibodies. One of these is called beta-2-glycoprotein 1. This then triggers the clotting cascade. Once the clotting system is triggered, a product called soluble fibrin monomer (SFM), which is like the polymers in plastic, is made. The theory is that they create long, thin sheets of a Teflon-like substance, similar to a scab that covers a cut, but microscopic in size, and that these sheets then coat the blood vessels. This makes it hard for nutrients and oxygen to get in and out of the blood vessels to the cells where they are needed.

WHY WOULD AN INFECTION TRIGGER THE CLOTTING SYSTEM?

Many infectious organisms do not survive well in the presence of oxygen. These are termed *anaerobic*. Mycoplasma (which can be anaerobic) and other organisms may trigger the clotting system to create a shell, which then acts like a suit of armor, protecting them from oxygen, your body's defense system, and antibiotics. This would explain why these infections may have evolved a way to trigger the clotting mechanism. The fibrin armor preventing antibiotics from getting to the infection could also explain why some people with these infections may not respond to antibiotics. Indeed, some physicians have found that the antibiotics work better once someone has been on a blood-thinning medication, which may dissolve the armor.

This is an interesting theory, but how do we know this is going on? Mr. Berg and others have done studies showing that blood tests to look for these clotting changes, called the immune system activation of coagulation (ISAC) panel, are abnormal in CFIDS/FMS patients, whereas they are normal in most other people. Results of two of these tests must be abnormal for the result to be considered positive. When this was done, fifty of fifty-four CFIDS/FMS patients had abnormal tests (that is, only 7.4 percent of the patients had normal blood tests). In healthy people, twenty-two out of twenty-three (96 percent) had normal blood tests. This means the test is both very sensitive and specific, picking up people with CFIDS and excluding healthy people. Almost everyone with CFIDS whom I have tested has turned out to have a positive ISAC panel, although I personally have not tested healthy people to see if this also occurs with them. Interestingly, this panel is also positive in many people with unexplained infertility (which can improve with the blood-thinner heparin) and may also be positive in people with multiple sclerosis, Parkinson's disease, autism, inflammatory bowel disease, and some other illnesses. This suggests that this test can be helpful in deciding whether to treat people with CFIDS/FMS with blood-thinners.

TREATING THE BLOOD CLOTTING SYSTEM

First of all, it is important to note that using heparin injections as a treatment for CFIDS/FMS is still controversial and experimental. I much prefer to use treatments that are as safe as possible. Although heparin is routinely used in the United States to treat blood clots, using it to treat CFIDS/FMS is very new. Most of the doctors that I have spoken with have only treated a few CFIDS/FMS patients with heparin and find that about half of these patients get better with treatment. The treatment protocol, developed by John Couvaras, M.D., includes the following:

1. Remove wheat, alcohol, and sugar from the diet, if possible.
2. Check the ISAC panel. If there are at least two abnormal results, then begin treatment.
3. Take an antifungal for fourteen days. (Dr. Couvaras uses 250 milligrams of Lamisil a day, but I find this to be poorly effective and would recommend using 200 milligrams of Sporanox or Diflucan instead.)
4. Get standard 4,000 to 8,000 units of heparin by injection subcutaneously (like an insulin shot) twice a day. A possibly safer low-molecular-weight heparin may also be used.
5. If the PA index part of the ISAC is positive, add an 81-milligram baby aspirin each day.
6. After being on heparin for one week, repeat the ISAC panel to adjust the dosages of heparin and aspirin. The goal is to move all the blood tests into the normal range but not past the normal range into therapeutic (blood-thinning) levels. If the values are still abnormal or you are still having symptoms, the heparin dosage should be increased, and if the PA index part of the ISAC is still high, you should increase the baby aspirin to twice a day.
7. If you feel better after one month of heparin therapy, you can switch to a low dose (2 to 3 milligrams a day) of warfarin (Coumadin), a blood-thinner in tablet form, and stop the heparin after four to five days of being on the Coumadin. Once you have been on Coumadin for two weeks, recheck the ISAC panel to make sure you are maintaining the blood tests in the normal range.
8. Take nutritional supplements as needed.

In my practice, because the ISAC panel runs over $320, I check a baseline ISAC panel but do not repeat the ISAC panels to adjust therapy. Instead, while a patient is on heparin, I check a partial thromboplastin time (PTT) test, which measures blood-thinning, and platelet count every three days for the first twelve days and then every two to four weeks. (An uncommon, but potentially very dangerous side effect of heparin is a severe drop in platelet count, which can cause life-threatening bleeding.) If the PTT is still within the normal range and the patient is not better, I increase the heparin to as much as 8,000 units twice a day (rarely, I will go up to 8,000 units, three times a day) and then also increase the aspirin to two a day. In comparison, hospital patients often require 1,000 units of heparin an hour (a total of 24,000 units a day) intravenously, while most CFIDS/FMS patients need only 4,000 to 5,000 units twice a day (8,000 to 10,000 units a day).

If the heparin is going to help, most patients feel better at about the ten- to fourteen-day point. At the end of four to twelve months, if the heparin helps, we switch to Coumadin (as noted above) and check an international normalized ratio (INR), aiming to keep it below 1.3 while adjusting the Coumadin to the optimum dose. It is very important to know that most medications can change the blood level of Coumadin and that anytime anything is added to, or deleted from, your regimen (including natural remedies) you need to recheck the INR four to seven days later to make sure that it is not getting too high. Heparin and Coumadin are powerful medicines and the main risk is bleeding. Although we are using very low doses that are usually very well tolerated, one can rarely see life-threatening bleeding occur. If you felt better on the heparin and then the symptoms come back on the Coumadin, you may need to go back on the heparin for several months to reestablish and maintain the benefit. Occasionally, people will need to be on heparin for an extended period. In this case, the PTT and platelet count should be checked every two to four weeks. All of this being said, most people tolerate these treatments quite well and many, many more people die from taking aspirin (for example, for arthritis) than from taking heparin each year. Still, heparin is riskier than the other treatments I recommend, and I tend to use it as a last resort.

In summary, there are a number of infections that can cause or occur because you have CFIDS/FMS. Once they occur, they can trigger the clotting cascade. This may keep the nutrients from getting to your body and create a "suit of armor" for the viral and mycoplasma infections. Using a blood thinner can break down these armor coatings that protect the infections from our treatment and allow nutrients to get where they need to go. Many tests can help. The one that I use to decide whether to use blood-thinners is the ISAC panel at Hemex Labs (see Appendix J: Resources). Testing for infections may be helpful, but can be expensive. If you can afford the tests and/or your insurance will pay for them, they are worth checking and will make it easier to adjust therapy over time. If you can't afford it, it is reasonable to treat empirically—that is, without testing—except for high-dose Valtrex therapy. If you have lung congestion and/or recurrent temperatures over 98.6°F, I would treat with the antibiotics. If you feel chronically flulike, I would consider the HHV-6 or (based on testing) the high-dose Valtrex regimen. It is also reasonable to treat with antibiotics and antivirals simultaneously—especially if you are taking anticoagulants.

Chronic Sinusitis—The Yeasty Beasties Revisited!

Years ago, we speculated that the chronic sinus congestion seen in CFIDS/FMS could be caused by yeast overgrowth. An interesting recent study reported in the *Mayo Clinic Proceedings* supports this thought.[16] In the study, researchers found that most people with chronic sinus infections had fungal growth in their sinuses. They felt that the inflammation was being caused by an immune response (the body's reaction) to the fungus. This research is interesting because more and more studies are showing that treating chronic sinusitis with antibiotics doesn't really do much and that shorter courses of treatment work just as well as the long courses. I find that conservative treatment is more effective than antibiotics for chronic sinusitis.

It's good that medicine is finally starting to catch up with reality. The report in the *Mayo Clinic Proceedings* noted that "fungus allergy was thought to be involved in less than 10 percent of cases . . . our studies indicate, in fact, fungus is likely the cause of nearly all of these problems and that it is not an allergic reaction but an immune reaction."[17] In this study, the researchers studied 210 patients with chronic sinusitis. Using new methods to collect and test sinus/nasal mucus, they found fungus in 96 percent of patients.

It's interesting to observe how medical research works. The researchers are now working with different drug companies to set up trials to test medications to control the fungus, but feel that it will be at least two years before any treatments will be available. In my experience, though, these problems often respond dramatically to either Sporanox or Diflucan—which, by no coincidence, are very powerful antifungal agents. It is not clear why the researchers did not simply try these medications.

It is important to distinguish between chronic sinusitis, which lasts for over three months, and acute sinusitis, which usually has been going on for a few days and less than a month. For these shorter attacks of sinusitis, bacteria are a more common cause and antibiotics (combined with natural remedies) can be helpful. Some researchers still continue to argue that fungus is not a cause of chronic sinusitis. They note that fungi are seen even in healthy noses, which is correct, but they neglect to discuss the immune changes that are also seen in these noses. Because so many people have responded dramatically to antifungals for the treatment of their chronic sinusitis, my suspicion is that the Mayo Clinic researchers are probably correct.

As you can see, your body's lowered defenses play a large role in CFIDS/FMS. The good news is that by treating the many underlying infections common in CFIDS/FMS and by treating any hormonal and nutritional deficiencies, you can bring your immune system back to a healthy state!

Important Points

- An important component of CFIDS is disordered immune function, which opens the door to repeated infections, repeated treatment with antibiotics, and yeast overgrowth.
- Treat yeast overgrowth by avoiding antibiotics and sweets. Many patients have found nystatin and other antifungal medications, such as Diflucan and Sporanox, to be helpful. Acidophilus (milk bacteria) and natural antifungals such as caprylic acid and garlic are also often useful.
- Bowel parasites are common in CFIDS patients, whose symptoms often respond dramatically to treatment. However, most laboratories do not adequately detect parasites through stool testing. To get an accurate test result, use a laboratory that specializes in stool testing (see Appendix J: Resources).

- Treat *Cryptosporidium* with the herbal antiparasitics *Artemisia annua* or Tricycline.
- Prevent parasitic infection by filtering your water with an effective filtration unit. I recommend the Multi-Pure filter.
- If you have body temperatures over 98.6°F and/or chronic lung congestion, try long-term treatment with Cipro or doxycycline. Take nystatin while on the antibiotic to prevent yeast overgrowth.
- If you have chronic flulike symptoms despite treatment for yeast and underactive adrenal glands, consider trying the antiviral, immune-stimulating protocol discussed in this chapter.

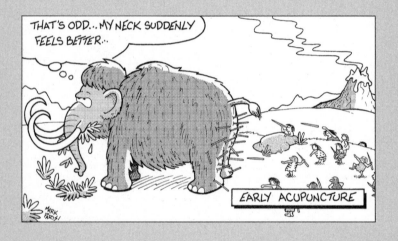

5

Fibromyalgia—
The Aching-All-Over Disease

FIBROMYALGIA, PREVIOUSLY KNOWN AS FIBROSITIS, is basically a sleep disorder characterized by many tender knots in the muscles. These tender knots, called tender and trigger points, are a major cause of the achiness that fibromyalgia and CFIDS patients feel. For most patients, fibromyalgia and CFIDS are the same illness.

Pain, unfortunately, is the major symptom of fibromyalgia and is often seen in chronic fatigue syndrome as well. Many people feel it's bad enough to not be able to work, get out of the house, or do much—but to have to sit at home and be in pain at the same time, adds insult to injury.

The good news is that the pain can usually be eliminated, or at least markedly improved. I have found that there are several key components underlying pain in CFIDS/FMS.

As noted above, the first and foremost component is disordered sleep. If you are not getting seven to nine hours of solid sleep, you will be in pain. Making certain that you get seven to nine hours of solid sleep without waking or hangover is a critical part of making your pain go away. Treating underlying infections (especially yeast infections), an underactive thyroid (regardless of whether the blood tests are normal or not), and magnesium deficiency are the other key players. In Chapter 6, I will discuss how to treat the sleep disorders seen in CFIDS/FMS so that you can get seven to nine hours of solid, uninterrupted sleep each night.

When we sleep, we usually have periods during which we stop moving and go into deep, very restful slumber. Unfortunately, the little muscle knots of fibromyalgia make it uncomfortable to lie in one position for an extended time, causing a return to light sleep. Because of this, people with fibromyalgia do not stay in the deep stages of sleep (stages 3 and 4) that recharge their batteries and during which the body produces growth hormone. In addition, the brain thinks it's daytime at night. Although a fibromyalgia patient may sleep for twelve hours every night, he or she may not have slept *effectively* for many years.

Fibromyalgia is a cousin to other muscle diseases, called myofascial pain syndromes. In 1990, the American College of Rheumatology put together a list of criteria for the classification of fibromyalgia. The diagnosis of fibromyalgia is made when the patient meets these criteria. To test yourself for fibromyalgia, see Criteria For Fibromyalgia on page 99. Most doctors don't know how to find and check the tender points (these are not necessarily the same as trigger points)—and the treatment works whether or not you have at least eleven of them anyway! That part of the exam will probably be eliminated when we have a good blood or urine test for FMS.

Perpetuating Factors

In their excellent 1,300-page review of muscle pain, *Myofascial Pain and Dysfunction: The Trigger Point Manual,* Drs. Janet Travell and David Simons review trigger points and their causes and patterns. The authors repeatedly note in their talks and writings that treating the underlying perpetuating factors—that is, the hormonal, nutritional, infectious, and other factors that cause the trigger points to persist—is extremely important. In their chapter on perpetuating factors in *The Trigger Point Manual,* they also address in depth the treatment of major structural problems, such as a short leg or short hemipelvis (an uneven pelvis).[1] It never ceases to amaze me how quickly a case of fibromyalgia can resolve once these underlying problems are treated. The duration of the disease does not seem to affect how responsive it is to treatment.

Fibromyalgia becomes self-perpetuating as soon as sleep is disrupted. Even if the underlying trigger, such as a trauma that occurred years before, has resolved, the sleep deprivation of the illness can cause suppression of the hypothalamus. Thyroid and adrenal suppression may also be present,

Criteria for Fibromyalgia

According to the American College of Rheumatology, a person can be classified as having fibromyalgia if he or she has:

- *A history of widespread pain.* The patient must be experiencing pain or achiness, steady or intermittent, for at least three months. At times, the pain must have been present:
  - on both the right and left sides of the body.
  - both above and below the waist.
  - midbody—for example, in the neck, midchest, or midback (or headache).
- *Pain on pressing at least eleven of the eighteen spots on the body that are known as tender points.* (See Figure 5.1, below.)

The presence of another clinical disorder, such as arthritis, does not rule out a diagnosis of fibromyalgia.

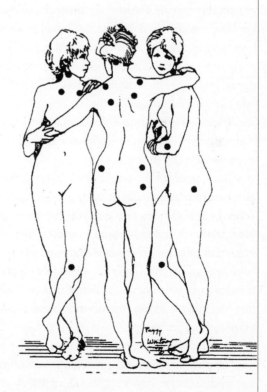

Figure 5.1.
Tender point locations on the body.

Criteria and illustration adapted from F. Wolfe, et al., "The American College of Rheumatology 1990 Criteria for the Classification of Fibromyalgia: Report of the Multicenter Criteria Committee," Arthritis and Rheumatology 33 (1990): 160–172. Used with permission.

despite the usual blood tests coming back normal.[3] The alteration of sleep then causes fairly marked changes in immune system functioning.[4]

I have found that my fibromyalgia patients tend to recover when *all* of the major underlying perpetuating factors are treated. It is important to understand that fibromyalgia is *both* a common endpoint for many of the problems we have discussed thus far *and* a cause for these problems. Infections, nutritional deficiencies, and hormonal deficiencies can all, individually and in concert, trigger and perpetuate fibromyalgia. Fibromyalgia can also cause the hormonal and immune dysfunctions and, perhaps by leading to malabsorption, the nutritional deficiencies.

TREATMENTS FOR FIBROMYALGIA

A number of treatments currently exist for fibromyalgia that are both necessary and helpful. Among the most important are treatments that increase deep sleep.[5] *Getting seven to nine hours of deep sleep a night without waking or hangover is critical!* Although most fibromyalgia patients look at me like I'm insane when I tell them this is possible, they happily come back feeling better—and *sleeping seven to nine hours a night without waking or hangover* using our protocol. Chapter 6, on sleep treatments, will tell you how! Although this book describes how to get rid of fibromyalgia, I've listed some other approaches for pain relief below.

Treat your nutritional deficiencies or the illness will persist. Taking a high-potency B-complex supplement with minerals, especially magnesium, is critically important.

Some people find gentle physical measures to be very helpful. A form of neuromuscular reeducation called Trager, developed by Dr. Milton Trager, has been *very* beneficial for my more severe fibromyalgia patients. Many patients, though, do not need these measures. If your fibromyalgia persists despite the treatments discussed in this book, however, you should consider calling the Trager Institute (see Appendix J: Resources) to locate the closest practitioner. The best kinds of Trager practitioners are instructors and tutors. These practitioners have reached a very high level of expertise in the technique.

Rolfing is another technique that can be very effective for FMS pain. Also known as structural reintegration, Rolfing is deep-tissue manipulation and massage. Powerful, it is designed to relieve and rebalance muscular and emotional tension. If done right, it can be comfortable. If done incorrectly, it hurts. A lot of people who say they do Rolfing were not fully trained in the technique. If someone does something that hurts, tell him or her to stop. The one exception to this is a technique called ischemic compression, in which the practitioner pushes on a spot with thirty pounds of pressure for forty-five seconds. It hurts like hell, then feels better. You can also do this on your own (more comfortably using a device called a Thera Cane). To locate a Rolfing practitioner in your area, contact the Rolf Institute (see Appendix J: Resources). Many patients have also found a technique called myofascial release to be very effective. If you decide to see a physical therapist, make sure that you pick someone who is both knowledgeable and gentle. If they know the "stretch and spray" technique of Dr. Travell, it's a good sign! I have seen too many patients made worse by physical therapists who were too rough. With fibromyalgia, gentleness is often much more powerful than roughness.

Acupuncture is another type of treatment that can be very helpful. Because it approaches health and illness from a very different perspective than traditional medicine does, it can often be very effective for illnesses that resist traditional measures. Many practitioners combine acupuncture with herbal and homeopathic remedies to make their treatments even more effective.

Chiropractic also can be very helpful in releasing the muscles. Unfortunately, however, if you don't treat the perpetuating factors that caused the muscles to shorten in the first place, they'll go right back to being shortened a few days after the treatment. That's why so many excellent chiropractors add nutritional, hormonal, antifungal, and other natural treatments to their practices. A special form of chiropractic, called Atlas chiropractic, focuses on the "Atlas" vertebrae in your neck. This may be especially helpful if you have overactive knee reflexes or your symptoms get worse when you turn your head upward to look at the ceiling for twenty seconds (if you have these symptoms, also be sure to read the discussion of cervical stenosis and Chiari malformations in Chapter 10). Yoga and many other forms of body and energy work have been very helpful for our patients. Try several and see which feels best to you.

Some people with fibromyalgia find that taking supplemental coenzyme Q_{10}, a nutritient used as an energy source by the muscles, can be helpful. I recommend taking 100 to 200 milligrams a day. Take it with some oil (for example, 400 units of vitamin E or essential fatty acids) to improve absorption. Coenzyme Q_{10} is somewhat expensive but can often be obtained at a discount (see Appendix J: Resources).

Some people use aspirin or ibuprofen (in Motrin, Nuprin, and other products) for the achiness of fibromyalgia. If it helps, it is worth using. Most often, however, aspirin products are minimally effective and can worsen food sensitivities or ulcers. Most patients find that a bedtime dose of zolpidem (Ambien), cyclobenzaprine (Flexeril), carisoprodol (Soma), clonazepam (Klonopin), amitriptyline (Elavil), or trazodone (Desyrel) is effective for pain without aspirin. Klonopin is useful if pain is severe, but it is potentially addictive. Many natural remedies, such as valerian, lemon balm, kava kava, 5-HTP, passionflower, and low doses of melatonin, can decrease the need for sleep medications (more about these in Chapter 6). If daytime pain relief is needed, many medications, including metaxalone (Skelaxin) and celecoxib (Celebrex)—which are not sedating—or baclofen (Lioresal), gabapentin (Neurontin), and tramadol (Ultram)—which are sometimes sedating—can be very helpful. (How to treat pain is discussed at length in Chapter 7.)

Treating structural problems is also critical in fibromyalgia. If the top of one hip is just one-quarter to one-half inch lower than the other, the entire gait can be thrown off and the muscles put into spasm. If a straight line is drawn from just above the top of the right hipbone to just above the left hipbone, that line should be parallel to the ground *when both feet are together.* If the hip tops are not parallel to the ground, the shoulders also are often uneven. For example, if the left hip is higher than the right hip, the left shoulder is often lower than the right shoulder. This is the body's attempt to maintain balance, but it puts a significant strain on the other muscles. Using a small insert (for example, a heel lift or orthotic) in the shoe of the short leg to make the hips the same height can make a world of difference. First, however, you should see a chiropractor who does a lot of hands-on work, as opposed to one who mainly uses machines. A series of good chiropractic treatments can often balance the hips and resolve the leg-length difference.

If you find that one hip is lower than the other when you sit, try using a butt-lift, a support that goes under the low side to make the hips even. Often, a chiropractor or a physiatrist (physical therapy physician) can be of benefit. As noted above, Rolfing can also help correct structural problems.

Many patients find that bodywork also releases suppressed feelings and memories from the muscles. Experience, feel, and embrace these. Your awareness, experience, *and release* of these feelings is an important part of the healing process.

As you can see, the underlying causes of the disease processes, and indeed the disease processes themselves, are often the same in fibromyalgia and chronic fatigue syndrome. By treating these underlying nutritional, hormonal, and infectious problems, as well as the underlying sleep disorder, most people can eliminate their pain!

Important Points

- Fibromyalgia is a sleep disorder characterized by multiple tender areas in the muscles. Treat it with medications that increase deep sleep, such as Ambien, Desyrel, Klonopin, and/or Elavil or Flexeril. Natural remedies, such as passionflower, kava kava, 5-hydroxy-L-tryptophan (5HTP), or a combination of valerian root and lemon balm, may also help, as can supplemental melatonin (a hormone).[6]
- Treat nutritional deficiencies with a daily multivitamin that is high in the B vitamins and magnesium with malic acid.
- Consider massage or body work, such as chiropractic, Trager, Rolfing, or myofascial release.
- Acupuncture and yoga are sometimes helpful.
- Coenzyme Q_{10} has helped some patients.
- For extra pain relief, try Ultram, Lioresal, Neurontin, or other treatments recommended in Chapter 7, on relieving pain.
- Treat structural problems. Orthotics, chiropractic treatment, or Rolfing can be very helpful.

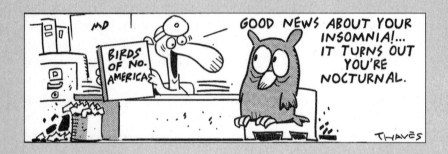

6

A Good Night's Sleep—
The Foundation of Getting Well

THE MOST EFFECTIVE WAY TO ELIMINATE PAIN IN CFIDS/FMS is to get seven to nine hours of solid, deep sleep each night on a regular basis. Disordered sleep is, in my opinion, the underlying process that drives CFIDS/FMS. Usually, when I lecture, I ask, "How many of you who have CFIDS/FMS get at least seven to nine hours of solid sleep a night without medications?" Generally, out of about 300 to 400 people in the audience, only one or two people, if any, raise their hands. My suspicion about those people who do raise their hands is that they have another illness going on and not chronic fatigue syndrome and fibromyalgia.

As we saw in Chapter 3, hypothalamic dysfunction (a major player in CFIDS/FMS) affects sleep, as well as blood pressure, hormonal systems, and temperature regulation. In animals with hypothalamic dysfunction, sleep is either disordered or, in very severe cases, simply no longer occurs. In animal studies done by Carol Everson, Ph.D. at the University of Tennessee, sleep deprivation resulted in immune suppression, resulting in multiple infections (including yeast overgrowth in the gut).[1] Many other abnormalities also occurred based on the sleep disorder. These same processes seem to occur in people with CFIDS/FMS.[2]

Disordered sleep was first demonstrated by Dr. Harvey Moldofsky, a Canadian researcher, who noted that the quality of deep sleep in fibromyalgia was poor. This was described as alpha wave intrusion into delta wave sleep. To put this into English, sleep has its own architecture and is not a single state. REM sleep, a light-sleep period during which we have our dreams, is the best known part of the sleep architecture. There are also other stages of sleep, designated simply by number. Stages 1 and 2 sleep are fairly light stages, while stages 3 and 4 (or delta wave) sleep are the deeper stages of sleep. My experience, and that of many other clinicians, suggests that what are inadequate in fibromyalgia and chronic fatigue syndrome are stages 3 and 4 sleep. This is supported by Dr. Robert Bennett's research at the University of Oregon Health Services Center. Dr. Bennett is one of the world's foremost researchers in fibromyalgia. He found that growth hormone deficiency occured in fibromyalgia and that treating this deficiency resulted in improvement of symptoms after four to five months. However, he felt uncomfortable recommending routine growth hormone treatment for fibromyalgia because of its cost (approximately $15,000 per year). What is interesting, though, is that growth hormone is released during stages 3 and 4 sleep.[3] Therefore, the loss of these deep stages of sleep may be what accounts for the growth hormone deficiency that has been observed. My own suspicion is that not only does hypothalamic dysfunction cause disordered sleep, but, by some yet-unknown mechanism, the poor sleep then causes further hypothalamic suppression. It is because of this that breaking the cycle of poor sleep and maintaining quality sleep for at least six to nine months is critical to breaking the cycle of fibromyalgia.

Growth hormone is responsible for many of the repair processes that go on in our muscles and in the rest of our body. It may be that it is the loss of this repair function, which normally occurs during deep sleep, that contributes to the pain of fibromyalgia. Several studies have shown that if you wake up people whenever they go into deep sleep, or even shake them lightly, so that they go from deep sleep into light sleep, they will develop classic fibromyalgia-like pain within one to two weeks and often within one night.[4]

It is absolutely critical that people with CFIDS/FMS get seven to nine hours of solid sleep each night, without waking or hangover. Sound sleep is the goal and, hard as this may be to believe, it is very attainable using the suggestions I will give you in this chapter.

The Basics: Good Sleep Hygiene

Although poor sleep hygiene is not a major problem for most people with this disease, it is the major cause of poor sleep for most Americans, and it is important to address this first. The following are some important things to consider:

- Consume no alcohol before bedtime.
- Do not consume any caffeine after 4:00 P.M.
- Do not use your bed for problem solving or doing work. If you are in the habit of using your bed for doing work, it is best to change your work area to another area of the house. *If it helps you to fall asleep,* you can watch *relaxing* television (perhaps on a timer that turns the television off if you fall asleep while watching) or read a *relaxing* book in bed until you can no longer stay awake.
- Take a hot bath before bed.
- Keep your room cool.
- If your mind races because your brain thinks it is daytime when it is really nighttime, continually focus your thoughts on things that feel good and do not require much "thinking energy." If you find that you cannot help but to continue to problem-solve, get out of bed and write down all your problems on a piece of paper until you can think of no more—then set them aside and go back to bed. Do this as often as you need to. It may be helpful to schedule thirty minutes of "worry time" early in the afternoon or evening when you can update a checklist of your concerns.

   Personally, I list my problems and projects on the left side of a page, and what I eventually plan to do about them (if anything) in the middle of the page. I consider these two columns to be what I leave in the hands of God or the universe. As CFIDS/FMS patients, we seem to think that we're responsible for making everything happen, like making our body heal or making sure the sun rises in the morning! Every so often, I move a problem from the "universe's" columns over to a third ("my") column on the right side. The items in the third column are the one or two things that I want to work on now. I am constantly amazed at how the things that I leave in the "universe's" hands progress (on their own) as quickly as the things that I've put in "my" column.

I also have a separate list for day-to-day errands. I put a star by those items that *must* get done soon. I do other items, if and when I *feel* like it. It is helpful to remember that neither you nor anyone else will ever get everything done! Just do those things that feel good to do on any given day (even if it's nothing). It will usually *feel* good to do the things that *really* have to get done. When I was doing general hospital internal medicine, I never heard a dying patient bemoan not having worked enough, or not having completed all the errands on his or her checklist!

- If your partner snores, get a good pair of earplugs and use them. The wax plugs that mold to the shape of the ear are often the best ones. It may also be useful to have either a sound generator that makes nature sounds or, better yet, a tape that induces stage 4 sleep (more about this later). Spouses of people with sleep apnea and/or snoring often also have severely disturbed sleep. You may need to sleep in a separate bedroom (after tucking in or being tucked in by your partner) until you find a way to sleep soundly through the snoring.

- If you frequently wake up to urinate during the night, do not drink a lot of fluids near bedtime. Most patients with CFIDS/FMS have frequent waking during the night. Like most people, their bladders are full at night. Because of a full bladder, they think they are waking up because they have to urinate. This is not the case. They are waking up because of their CFIDS/FMS.

  If you were to wake up your spouse when you woke up and asked, "Honey, is your bladder full?" He or she would moan, "Uh-huh," and roll over and go back to sleep. Unfortunately, most people have learned to get up and go to the bathroom when they wake up at night. The bladder is kind of like a baby—if *you* teach the baby to wake up to play in the middle of the night (that is, if you go to the bathroom frequently), pretty soon *it* will wake you up to play at night. There is a simple way to remedy this problem. If and when you wake up during the night and you notice your bladder is full, just talk to it (in your mind, so your spouse doesn't think you're nuts) and tell it, "Nighttime is for sleeping. We will go to the bathroom in the morning when it is time to wake up." Then roll over and go back to sleep. If you still have to urinate five minutes later, then you can go to the bathroom.

Most of you will find that your bladder will happily go back to sleep, and when you wake up in the morning, you won't even have to urinate as badly as you did when you woke up in the middle of the night.

Because of the bladder muscle spasticity that is common in fibro-myalgia, you may be afraid that you will wet yourself if you don't get up to urinate. The *large* majority of people with CFIDS/FMS will not experience incontinence. If this concerns you, the first couple of nights you may want to use an incontinence protection product such as a Depend undergarment just so you don't worry about wetting yourself. After a few nights, you will be comfortable sleeping without protection. Although this sounds like a very low-tech approach to treating sleep, you will be amazed at how beneficial it is. Try it and see!

- Put the bedroom clock out of arm's reach and facing away from you so you can't see it. Looking at the clock frequently aggravates sleep problems and is frustrating.

- Decrease the amount of time you spend in bed. Although you might think that you would increase your deep sleep time by spending extra time in bed, this is *not* what happens. When people routinely stay in bed longer than they need to, they may get their usual deep sleep in the beginning of the night and then have long awakenings and very shallow sleep during the middle of the night. Then they may sleep soundly again when it is time to wake up. When such people consistently decrease the amount of time spent in bed to the length actually needed for sleep, they gradually squeeze out the long middle-of-the-night awakenings. Two of the medications discussed later in this chapter (Ambien and Sonata) are especially helpful for this.

- Have a light snack before bedtime. Hunger causes insomnia in all animals, and humans are no exception. Adding foods high in the amino acid tryptophan, such as milk and turkey, also contributes to sleep. (A discussion of the natural tryptophan supplement 5-HTP can be found on page 113).

- Get out of bed at the same time each morning, even after a poor night's sleep. Regular rising supports a healthy circadian (day/night) rhythm and can be helpful. You can nap up to one and a half hours a day, but try not to nap much after 2:00 P.M. if possible. Set an alarm clock for one to one and a half hours of nap time and splash cold water on your face when you wake up.

If you follow the suggestions above, you can be sure that poor sleep hygiene is not your problem. This is important because your doctor may want to blame your problem with insomnia on poor sleep hygiene. It is important to let him or her know that your problem is not poor sleep hygiene, it is hypothalamic sleep center suppression.

Sleep Medications and Remedies

Although I much prefer natural remedies to prescription medications, the hypothalamic sleep disorder in CFIDS/FMS is often too severe to be dealt with by natural remedies alone. However, natural remedies can be very helpful and usually decrease the amount of medication you need. In addition, once you come off sleep medications (usually after nine to eighteen months, although they can be used indefinitely, if needed) you may find that all you require are the natural remedies. Whatever treatments you use, though, it is important that they not only increase the duration of sleep but also maintain or improve the deep stages (stages 3 and 4) of sleep. Unfortunately, most sleeping pills in common use (for example, Dalmane, Halcion, and Valium) actually worsen the quality of sleep by increasing the amount of light stage (especially stage 2) sleep and decreasing the deep stages of sleep even further. You want to be certain that the treatments and medications you use leave you feeling better the next day, not worse.

There are several approaches to using sleep treatments in CFIDS/FMS. Some doctors prefer to use a single medication or treatment and push it up to its maximum level. If that works, great; if not, they stop it and switch to another medication. Other doctors prefer to use low doses of many different treatments together until the patient is getting good, solid sleep regularly. I strongly prefer the latter approach, for two main reasons. First, my experience is that people with fibromyalgia can be very medication-sensitive if high doses of medications are used. Most of a medication's benefits occur at low doses and most of the side effects at high doses. Second, each medication is cleared out of the body on its own schedule, regardless of whether it is taken with other medications. If you take a low dose of a sleep medication, so that it is out of your body when it is time to wake up eight hours later, the blood level may not be high enough to keep you asleep at night. If you increase the dose to the level at which it does keep you asleep all night, it may not be cleared out of your body until 2:00 P.M. the next day, leaving you feeling very hung over. If, however, you combine low doses of four or five different sleep aids, each of them will be cleared out of your body by morning. Meanwhile, the effective blood levels that you have during the middle of the night from each treatment are additive and will keep you asleep. Because of this, most people find that it takes anywhere from three to seven different treatments combined to get seven to nine hours of solid sleep each night without waking or hangover. (You'll notice that I keep repeating this phrase!)

GETTING STARTED

My treatment checklist, elements of which are reproduced later in this chapter, lists a number of natural and prescription sleep aids. Depending on your preference, you may want to start with the natural aids, see how those work, and then use the prescription ones as needed (or available). My preference is to start with at least one of the sleep medications (Ambien and/or Desyrel) combined with some of the natural remedies. However you choose to do it, on the first night, simply begin with one of the remedies at a low dose.

For most of the treatments recommended, by the next morning you will know the effects (both beneficial effects and side effects) that the medication is going to have. It may, however, take four to six weeks to see the full effect of 5-HTP and St. John's wort. In rare cases, some of these treatments have the opposite of their normal effect, activating you instead of putting you to sleep. If this happens, don't use that treatment.

Once you have tried a low dose of a single treatment, increase the dosage each night until you either get seven to nine hours of solid sleep without waking or hangover or until you get side effects (for example, next-day sedation), or until you are at the maximum dose on the checklist. It is worth noting the lowest dose that gives you the most benefit. In other words, you may find that 50 milligrams of Desyrel is just as effective as 150 milligrams, in which case there is no need to take the higher dose. Once you have tried one treatment, you can go ahead and add in a second one in the way I just discussed, and then a third one, and so on. You may choose, when you add them in, to initially drop the other treatments, using each of them by itself so you can see what each one does by itself. Or you may choose to add one treatment to the next. Basically, you are trying the treatments on to see what "fits," in the same way you would try on shoes to see which ones *feel* the best. Once you have found the combination of treatments that feels the best, you can simply stay on that combination. If you need to (to get seven to nine hours of solid sleep a night) you can take *all* the medications on the checklist together at the maximum dose noted on the list.

It is not uncommon to see your sleep worsen again during periods of increased stress—whether physical or emotional—and the flaring of your illness. During these times, increase the treatments as needed to maintain seven to eight hours of solid sleep without waking or hangover. I find that patients do not have a problem with continually having to escalate the dose, so don't worry about increasing the treatments during periods of stress or flaring of your illness. The best way to need less medication in the long run is to use *as much as it takes* to get seven to eight hours of solid sleep each night without waking or hangover for six months. When you are sleeping well and feeling better for six months, you can then decrease the treatments as long as you continue to get seven to eight hours of solid sleep each night without waking or hangover. Most people find that they can taper off all sleep medications after about eighteen months. Other people need to take some of the sleep treatments for years. This is okay.

For all of the medications listed below, any side effects that you may notice will occur the same day that you take the medication. I have not seen any "fly now, pay later" side effects from prolonged use. I will note that for Ambien, and possibly for Sonata, the computerized information sheet from the drugstore may note a recommendation from the U.S. Food and Drug Administration (FDA) that the medication be used for only seven days. This is not because problems have been seen with long-term use, but because it is FDA policy for any sleep medication. (Most of the other treatments discussed below are not considered by the FDA to be sleep medications.) The FDA wants people to learn proper sleep hygiene instead of taking medication for their insomnia. This is very reasonable—except for people with CFIDS/FMS, in which the sleep problem is hypothalamic suppression, not poor sleep hygiene.

Natural Sleep Remedies

Most of the natural sleep remedies discussed here are not sedating, yet they help you fall asleep and stay in deep sleep. Some are available in combination formulas as well. Consider the following natural sleep aids:

- Magnesium and calcium. Taking at least 75 to 150 milligrams at night is a good idea because it can help your sleep. Taking 600 milligrams of calcium at bedtime also may improve the quality of your sleep.

- Valerian and lemon balm. A double-blind research study showed that taking a combination of 180 to 360 milligrams of valerian and 80 to 160 milligrams of lemon balm (also known as melissa) a night improved deep stage sleep.[5] It did this without being sedating. For about 10 percent of people, valerian is energizing and may keep them up. If this happens to you, you can use valerian during the day instead of at night. It is nontoxic and would be hard to overdose on. Valerian does have a calming effect, though, and can be used during the day for anxiety as well.

- Passionflower. Taking 100 to 200 milligrams at night can also help sleep. It is also helpful for anxiety during the day.

- Delta wave sleep-inducing compact disks or cassettes. To fall asleep, you can play deep sleep-inducing tapes or CDs. If you wake up during the night, you can push your sound system's replay button. Better yet, get a CD or tape player that can replay continuously throughout the night.

- 5-Hydroxy L-tryptophan (5-HTP). Take 100 to 400 milligrams at night. When used for six weeks, a 300- to 400- milligram dose has been shown to decrease FMS pain and often helps people to lose weight. 5-HTP is what your body uses to make serotonin, a neurotransmitter that helps improve the quality of sleep. The one caution I would note is that if you are taking a number of treatments that increase serotonin (these include antidepressants like Prozac, St. John's wort, Ultram, Desyrel, and the like), taking high doses of 5-HTP can result in a serotonergic reaction, a life-threatening reaction caused by a too-high level of serotonin. This is very, very rare, however. I have never seen such a reaction myself, nor have I talked to anyone who treats CFIDS/FMS who noted that they have ever seen one. A serotonergic reaction feels like "the panic attack from hell." Because panic attacks are common in CFIDS/FMS, this is almost always what it will turn out to be. If a reaction does happen, you should be checked out in a hospital emergency room to be safe. If you are taking any of the serotonin-raising treatments, it is reasonable to limit the 5-HTP to 200 milligrams at night.

- Kava kava. This is a South Pacific herbal remedy. I recommend using a 30-percent extract, and taking anywhere from 200 to 750 milligrams at night. With prolonged use, a rash will uncommonly occur. The rash will sometimes resolve by taking a 50-milligram vitamin-B complex. I would stop or decrease the dose or frequency of kava kava use if the rash continues, despite the use of the B-complex.

- Melatonin. This is a hormone made by the pineal gland. Although it is natural and available over the counter, this does not mean that it is without risk. My concern with any hormone is that although it might be quite safe when used within the body's normal range, I worry about toxicity when people take more than the body would normally make. For most people, all it takes to restore melatonin to normal levels is ³⁄₁₀ milligram. The usual dose you find in stores, however, is 3 milligrams, which is ten times the level I recommend. Except for a small subset of people, who likely have trouble absorbing it properly, the ³⁄₁₀ milligram is every bit as effective for sleep as higher doses. Moreover, high levels of melatonin may raise the level of another hormone, prolactin, which is often high in people with CFIDS/FMS, aggravating the risk of depression or infertility. Although I don't know of any danger yet from using melatonin in higher doses—and it may even have immune stimulating and antioxidant effects that could conceivably be beneficial—I would use a dose higher than ³⁄₁₀ milligram only if it *clearly* helps you feel better than the lower dose.

- St. John's wort. Although it is used as an antidepressant, I suspect this herb also helps sleep. Take 600 to 900 milligrams at night and another 600 to 900 milligrams during the day. As noted above, St. John's wort can raise serotonin levels, so I would limit the dose to 900 to 1,200 milligrams a day if you are also taking Prozac or a similar antidepressant. Give it six weeks to help.

- Breathe Right adhesive nasal strips. These are very helpful in treating the nasal congestion that often accompanies chronic fatigue syndrome because of yeast overgrowth. There is a school of thought that suspects that much of the fatigue in chronic fatigue syndrome also comes from the nasal congestion, so it is very reasonable to leave the nasal strip on for about two days to see whether opening up your nasal passages helps your overall energy level. If so, you might consider wearing a strip during the day to boost energy as well as during the evening to help you sleep. Breathe Right strips are available in two sizes—large ones for those with larger noses and smaller ones for smaller noses. If nasal congestion persists after you are treated for yeast overgrowth, I would consider using methylsulfonylmethane (MSM) nasal spray for ten days along with the nasal strips. MSM is a sulfur compound. In nasal spray form, it can be helpful with nasal congestion, allergies, and snoring.

- Wild lettuce pills. These also can aid sleep.
- Dr. Teitelbaum's Sleep Formula, a combination of valerian, lemon balm, passionflower, kava kava, 5-HTP, and low-dose melatonin (see Appendix J: Resources for more information).

PRESCRIPTION MEDICATIONS

Although I prescribe medications in different orders for different people, depending on their symptoms, the most common order I use is that below. If something is mentioned as especially good for a certain condition, you may want to try that medication first. Do not drive or operate hazardous equipment if you are sedated from the medications. As with almost everything, do not get pregnant during treatment. Although in my experience it is quite uncommon, even for CFIDS/FMS patients, it is possible to get unusual reactions from combining these medications. If a medication causes recurring nightmares, change the dose or medication.

- Zolpidem (Ambien). I like Ambien because it is short-acting (that is, less likely to leave you hung over) and less likely to cause side effects than many other medications. Because it is short-acting, it may not keep you asleep all the way through the night, but will likely give you four to six hours of good, solid sleep as a foundation. The normal dosage is one-half to one 10-milligram tablet, taken at bedtime. If you wake up in the middle of the night you can take an extra one-half to one tablet (leave it by your bedside with a glass of water) and any sedation is usually worn off by the time you are ready to wake up in the morning. One-half tablet is usually enough for the middle of the night. If you find that taking an additional dose in the middle of the night leaves you hung over, use Sonata (see below) instead.

  Do not take more than 15 milligrams of Ambien at one time. I usually don't see improved sleep with the higher doses, and I have seen a case of sleepwalking that occurred when a patient took 20 milligrams as a single dose. Studies have not shown a wearing-off effect with Ambien or Sonata in most people, nor have they found addiction with long-term use.[6] What does occur, though, is rebound insomnia when you stop using this medication—that is, the need to use something else to assist your sleep for a week. Because of this need for sleep assistance, if you have taken Ambien for more than four months, when you stop it, use one of the other medications or natural sleep remedies discussed in this chapter for a week or so to assist sleep during the adjustment period. In my experience, Ambien can be helpful for restless leg syndrome as well.

- Zaleplon (Sonata), 10-milligram tablets. Sonata is a comparatively new sleep medication. It helps people to fall asleep and the sedating effect generally wears off within four hours, making next-day hangover uncommon. It is best used in the middle of the night (for example, at 4:00 A.M.) if you wake up and need something to help you fall back to sleep, or if you have trouble *falling* asleep but not staying asleep. Sonata is not like any other medication—that is, it is the first drug in its class, and therefore of a unique type. It affects receptors for the neurotransmitter gamma-aminobutyric acid (GABA). This makes it seem very promising for people with CFIDS/FMS. In research studies on patients who were awakened four hours after taking the medication, they showed no evidence of impairment of waking function. The most common side effects are headache, dizziness, or sedation, but these were found to occur as frequently in patients taking this drug as in people taking a placebo (dummy pill). There is no evidence of withdrawal symptoms, even if the medication is stopped abruptly. The recommended dose is one to two 10-milligram capsules. Most FMS patients require 20 milligrams (two capsules). It is recommended that Sonata not be taken with, or immediately after, a high-fat or heavy meal, as this decreases its effectiveness. If you are taking Tagamet, you may need to take a lower dose of Sonata because it is cleared out of the body more slowly while on Tagamet (although this can also be a good thing). Overall, though, most FMS patients I have treated with Sonata have *not* found it to be helpful. I think Ambien is better.

- Trazodone (Desyrel). Desyrel is marketed as an antidepressant, but its main use in CFIDS/FMS is to treat disordered sleep. It has the added benefit of being helpful for anxiety and can be used during the day for this as well. Desyrel comes in 50-milligram tablets, and the usual recommendation is to take one-half to six tablets at bedtime (most patients need no more than two tablets). If you take more than two tablets, you can get Desyrel in 150- to 300-milligram tablets as well. Your *total* daily dose should not exceed 450 milligrams. If you are on other antidepressants, limit the dosage to 150 milligrams a day to avoid the risk of excessive serotonin levels (see page 113). The main side effects of Desyrel are next-day sedation (if this happens, either lower the dose or take it earlier in the evening) or priapism in males. Priapism is a condition characterized by a painful erection that does not go away. I would note, however, that I have never seen this, despite prescribing Desyrel for hundreds of patients. Most men find that while it causes an improvement in the strength of their erections, it does so at a comfortable level, as opposed to an erection that will not go away after a normal amount of time. If you develop an erection that does not go away after an hour (despite a cold bath), stop taking the medication and go to a hospital emergency room. If the erections are not lasting extraordinarily long but seem to be even the least bit uncomfortably long, you should stop the Desyrel and switch to the other medications.

- Clonazepam (Klonopin). Although in the Valium family, and therefore potentially addictive, Klonopin can be *very* helpful for people with FMS. When used at doses of less than 3 milligrams at night, I have not seen any problem with addiction. Most people do not need to go above this dose. Klonopin can be especially helpful in the presence of severe pain, as well as for patients with restless leg syndrome. Start with half of a 0.5-milligram tablet and work your way up slowly as needed. The main side effect is next-day sedation, which is fairly common. If this occurs, take a lower dose or take it several hours before bedtime. Most people find that they can slowly increase the dose over time as the next-day sedation wears off. Because it is potentially addictive, do not suddenly stop taking Klonopin if you have been on it for over six weeks. Instead, taper off by decreasing the dosage by 0.25 to 0.5 milligrams a day every week or so. It is excellent for restless leg syndrome.

- Doxylamine (Unisom for Sleep). This is an antihistamine that is available over the counter. The standard dose is 25 milligrams at nighttime. It is worth trying, especially if you tend to have a stuffy nose that interferes with your sleep. However, if you have trouble with severe dry eyes and mouth, this may not be a good medication for you because it can aggravate these symptoms. Some people find that the effect wears off with continued use and that it works best when used intermittently (for example, two days on, then two days off the medication).

- Carisprodol (Soma). This is predominantly a muscle relaxant and I would use this earlier in treatment if there is severe pain. The usual dose is one-half to one 350-milligram tablet at bedtime. Soma is potentially addictive, although I have never seen this in patients who are only using one to two tablets at bedtime (as opposed to people taking it four times a day for pain). The main side effect is sedation.

- Cyclobenzaprine (Flexeril). This is a muscle relaxant. It can be a very helpful medication for many people, especially if the pain is severe. The usual dose is one-half to one 10-milligram tablet at bedtime, but some people need to take two tablets at bedtime. Because Flexeril is related to Elavil, it poses some risk for people with abnormal heart rhythms. Rarely, it leads to weight gain, though much less often than Elavil does. This medication also can also cause dry mouth and eyes.

- Mirtazapine (Remeron). This medication is unrelated to any of the other medications discussed above. One doctor has noted that it seems to be especially helpful in patients who seem to "hibernate" during the day. Generally, Remeron is well tolerated and can be very helpful. The usual dosage is one to three 15-milligram tablets, taken at bedtime.

- Amitriptyline (Elavil). Technically an antidepressant, Elavil was one of the first medications to be studied for fibromyalgia and was found to be effective. It is also the only medication that many doctors have heard of for treating fibromyalgia. Although Elavil can be very helpful, it has significant side effects and has therefore been moved down to the bottom of my list. These side effects include weight gain, dry mouth, sedation, and aggravation of restless leg syndrome, neurally mediated hypotension, and abnormal heart rhythms. It is, however, especially good for nerve pain, vulvadynia (pain in the vulvar area), and, perhaps, interstitial cystitis, characterized by severe urinary frequency and burning without infection. You can take one-half to five 10-milligram tablets at bedtime. If you take more than two tablets, it should be tapered off and not stopped suddenly. I would not use more than 80 milligrams at bedtime (unless you have to) because of the side effects it can cause.

- Alprazolam (Xanax). This is a short-acting cousin of Valium that gives a good three to five hours of sleep with less hangover in the morning.

I was pleasantly surprised to find that it improves sleep quality, because it is a cousin to Valium, which usually seems to worsen this in most people. It is very good for anxiety as well, and tends to be very well tolerated. It can be addictive, however. The usual dosage is one-half to four 0.5-milligram tablets at bedtime or during the night.

- Levodopa plus carbidopa (Sinemet 10/100). This is an anti-Parkinson's medication and I use it (one each evening) only in patients with restless leg syndrome. It can be very helpful, but I use Klonopin and Ambien for this problem first. Using other anti-Parkinson's medications (for example, pergolide) may be safer than Sinemet in the long term.

In addition to the prescription medications above, the serotonin-raising antidepressants known as SSRIs can help improve sleep, in addition to having many other benefits for CFIDS/FMS, even if there is *no* depression present. These medications include fluoxetine (Prozac), paroxetine (Paxil), and sertraline (Zoloft). Experience suggests that by lowering elevated levels of the pain transmitter called substance P, they can decrease pain. In addition, many people find that SSRIs assist with weight loss. Because it is common for patients with CFIDS/FMS to gain thirty to fifty pounds at the beginning of the disease—because of metabolic changes, not because of overeating—anything that helps in weight loss is appreciated. SSRIs also improve neurally mediated hypotension (NMH), which is often seen in this disease.[7] They take six weeks to start working. Most patients find that these antidepressants energize them and do best taking the medication in the morning. Some patients find the medication sedating and these patients should take it at night. Occasionally, the increased energy interferes with sleep.

If needed, you can add 300 to 900 milligrams of gabapentin (Neurontin) (see page 138) at bedtime. If all else fails, in rare cases I prescribe 10 milligrams of a medication called olanzapine (Zyprexa, an antischizophrenia medication) at bedtime. For many people, this can improve sleep dramatically after two weeks. Unfortunately, Zyprexa can cause significant weight gain and a flattening of emotions that some patients find to be uncomfortable. I tend to save this medication as a last resort.

By using a combination of the treatment discussed above, almost all people with CFIDS/FMS can get seven to nine hours of solid sleep a night without waking or hangover. It can take a lot of trial and error to find out exactly what is best for you, but it is worth being persistent. Once you are feeling well for six to nine months, or you find you need less medication to get seven to nine hours of solid sleep without waking or hangover, you can go ahead and decrease the medication. If I have a patient who has been feeling better and then finds that his or her pain is coming back, one of the first things I ask is, "How is your sleep?" The usual answer is, "Not good." Many people, because of fear of addiction and having to use constantly escalating doses of sleeping pills, are afraid to take enough medication to get adequate sleep. They are so grateful to get five hours a night that they settle for that. That's a bad idea! I recommend taking whatever it takes to get seven to nine hours of solid sleep without waking or hangover, even if this means taking six of these medications at one time—or even all of the above medications.

If you had high blood pressure, your doctor would not put you on blood pressure medication and then, two weeks later—when your pressure was normal—tell you that you had to stop them quickly so you don't get addicted. The doctor would also increase them if your blood pressure went up. With hypothalamic dysfunction, it is equally inappropriate to stop taking medications prematurely. If you have high blood pressure, your doctor would not hesitate to let you stay on your medications (in fact, you'd be required to do so) for years, if needed. The same approach should also be used for sleep medications for CFIDS/FMS patients. Fortunately, most people are able to discontinue most of the medications after about twelve to eighteen months of getting solid sleep. Keep in mind that if you use adequate medication to get seven to nine hours of solid sleep a night for six to nine months, you will actually need less sleep medication in the long run!

After you're better, you may occasionally find that your sleep worsens for a while during physical and/or emotional stresses. If this occurs, increase or resume your sleep medications for as long as you need and then taper them back down or stop them when the problem is resolved. If difficulty sleeping persists, look for the cause. If the cause is not obvious, it is often recurrent yeast. Please be sure to do what you can to achieve the goal of adequate good-quality sleep. You'll be very happy you did!

Sleep Apnea

Sleep apnea is a condition in which you repeatedly stop breathing during the night. There are two main types of apnea. One type is obstructive. In this condition, the pipe that carries air into the lungs gets blocked intermittently. The other type is central, which means that the trigger in the brain that signals breathing intermittently stops working. Obstructive sleep apnea (OSA) is the condition that we are most concerned with in CFIDS/FMS.

In OSA, the pharynx (throat) repeatedly collapses during sleep. The person with OSA fights to breathe against a blocked airway, resulting in decreased oxygen levels in the blood. Eventually, the sense of suffocation wakes the person, the throat muscles contract, the airway opens, and air rushes in under high pressure. When the airway is opened, the rushing air allows the patient to once again drift back into sleep, but creates a loud gasping sound. People with OSA are generally not aware that this is happening, although their partners often have severely disrupted sleep from the snoring and gasping. This cycle repeats itself many times throughout the night, and this constant waking from deep sleep, as well as the loss of oxygen in the blood, can cause next-day sleepiness, brain fog, poor concentration, and mood changes. Another side effect of OSA is high blood pressure. I generally recommend that any CFIDS/FMS patient who has high blood pressure (most of them have low blood pressure) and is overweight consider testing for sleep apnea.

There is a lot of controversy about how common OSA is. As is the case for other illnesses (including CFIDS/FMS!) there is not even an agreement about how to define it. Generally, if the throat closes off for at least ten seconds, with no air flow, it is considered to be an apneic episode. This lack of breathing for ten seconds is enough to cause the oxygen level to drop in the blood and to cause one to go from deep sleep into light sleep. Many sleep specialists define sleep apnea as having five or more episodes of decreased breathing per hour in association with daytime sleepiness. Although some specialists estimate that OSA is present in only 3 percent of the adult population, a recent study of all patients in five general medicine doctors' offices suggested that approximately 17 percent of adults had *clinically significant* sleep apnea (defined as having at least *fifteen* episodes an hour of non-breathing during sleep). This study shows that when a doctor looks for it, sleep apnea is very common.[8]

Although sleep apnea is diagnosed by a positive overnight sleep study, fewer than 8 of the 10,000 patients at these practices had been referred for a sleep study in the previous year, though it would be expected that as many as 1,700 of them had sleep apnea. This is because doctors simply have not been trained to look for OSA. In fact, as noted in an editorial in a recent issue of the *Annals of Internal Medicine,* "The real problem is the lack of education at all levels about all sleep disorders.[9] Physicians have been shown to receive, on average, a total of only 2.1 hours of formal education in sleep medicine during their medical school training. Sleep history is typically skipped in the general history." When physicians did receive training about sleep apnea, the number of patients they sent for sleep apnea testing increased dramatically.

CAUSES OF SLEEP APNEA

The main reason for OSA is being overweight. If more fat deposits develop in the rest of your body, they also occur in the tissue surrounding the throat. When you get into certain positions, the placement of your head can actually cause compression of the pipe that carries air into the lungs. As noted above, because of the (often large) weight gain caused by the metabolic disturbances in CFIDS/FMS, OSA can occur and complicate treatment of these illnesses. The primary symptoms associated with sleep apnea are snoring and daytime sleepiness. Having a neck circumference of seventeen inches or more also predisposes one to OSA. Because we inherit certain physical characteristics of the throat, there also appears to be a genetic predisposition to sleep apnea.

There are other problems that occur besides the daytime sleepiness in sleep apnea. As noted above, high blood pressure is common. A number of studies have also shown that patients with severe sleep apnea are at a two- to seven-fold increased risk of having an automobile accident. There is also a possible risk of heart and lung damage as a result of untreated OSA. Although some doctors do not consider OSA to be significant until there are fifteen or more apneic episodes per hour of sleep, evidence suggests that even five or more episodes per hour are associated with increased risk of auto accidents and high blood pressure.

DIAGNOSING SLEEP APNEA

Symptoms that suggest sleep apnea are snoring, being overweight, hypertension, daytime sleepiness, periods where breathing stops at night, and frequent auto accidents. If you have several of these symptoms, you should have an overnight sleep study done. During this test, several aspects of sleep are measured. An electroencephalogram (EEG) measures the brain wave patterns that tell the depth of sleep and gives a printout of how much time is spent in the various stages of sleep. It can also tell how long it takes to fall asleep, how many times you wake during the night, and how many actual hours of sleep you get. Respiratory monitors can measure air flow and tell if the blood oxygen level is dropping, which demonstrates the apnea. The test should also be able to check for leg movements to look for restless leg syndrome (more about this later in this chapter) and to monitor for snoring as well.

These tests can be very expensive, costing approximately two thousand dollars. Because of the cost, insurance companies are sometimes hesitant to pay for it. It is a good idea to have the sleep laboratory get preauthorization from your insurance company before the test is done. Because of the high cost, it is common to have what is called a *split-night study*. When this is done, the technician spends the first half of the night looking for evidence of clinically important sleep apnea. If they find it, they put a mask on you that gently keeps up the pressure in your throat, which in turn keeps your airway from collapsing. This is like gently blowing into a balloon to keep the opening open. They will do a continuous positive airway pressure (C-pap) titration to determine the optimum mask pressure needed to keep your airway open. Because of the study's cost, it is certainly reasonable to do a split-night study all in one night, rather than coming back for a second night to do the C-pap titration, which would double the cost.

For sleep testing, the lab will often recommend that you be off of all sleep medications for several nights before doing the test. If you have not yet started sleep medications, this is reasonable. However, I recommend that patients who have been on sleep medications stay on them during the test. I suggest this for several reasons. First, because most CFIDS/FMS patients need the sleep medications, I need to know whether they are developing sleep apnea from the medication, even though I think this is uncommon, because most of my patients (even with sleep apnea) feel better on the sleep medications. The second reason is that, during testing, it is often difficult to fall asleep in a strange environment, being hooked up with wires, and hearing the noise of the technician. It is not uncommon to have inadequate sleep studies where the person is simply not able to sleep for a significant amount of time during the night. This results in a very expensive and useless study where, at best, the doctor recognizes that this study was not effective, and at worst (because the person did not sleep much and therefore had no periods when he or she stopped breathing), the lab incorrectly concludes that sleep apnea is not present.

Some sleep testing machines can be used at home. These machines are often more effective (even though they monitor fewer variables) because you are more likely to be able to have a normal night's sleep in the familiarity of your own home. One of my patients used a video camera one night to look for sleep apnea, snoring, and restless leg syndrome—an interesting approach.

TREATING SLEEP APNEA

There are several treatments for sleep apnea and they fall into three main treatment categories: behavioral, pharmacologic, and mechanical. Let us consider each in turn.

Behavioral Treatments

As noted above, being overweight is the main cause of OSA. Because of this, weight loss is one of the most effective ways to treat it. When you are treated for your CFIDS/FMS, it often becomes easier to lose weight. In fact, it is not uncommon to lose twenty to thirty pounds. Markedly cutting back on your carbohydrate intake and increasing your protein intake can help as well. I often prescribe medications that help to treat CFIDS/FMS and that also assist with weight loss, among them phentermine (also sold as Fastin and under other brand names), dextroamphetamine (Adderall, Dexedrine), thyroid hormone, and certain antidepressants.

Avoid sleeping in positions that cause you to snore and have sleep apnea, especially lying on your back. Sleep apnea can often be decreased by taking a tennis ball, putting it into a cloth pocket and then sewing it into the mid-back of your pajama shirt. Then, when you lie on your back, the tennis ball makes it uncomfortable, forcing you to roll onto your side or stomach without waking you. Finally, avoid bedtime alcohol and other substances that can aggravate sleep apnea.

Pharmacologic Treatments

A number of drugs have been used for OSA, but with limited success. A few patients have also been helped by supplemental oxygen. This is especially helpful if you live at high altitude.

Drugs that contribute to weight loss (including the ones noted above), as well as antidepressants that help weight loss, such as Prozac, can also be useful. It is important, though, to not take these drugs later in the day if they interrupt sleep.

Mechanical Treatments

There are several mechanical devices that change the shape of the upper airway and help to prevent the throat from collapsing. *Orthodontic devices* can help to keep the lower jaw and tongue forward. These are most likely to be helpful for mild cases of sleep apnea and for people who who cannot tolerate the C-pap machine. A nasal C-pap is a mask that is kept over your face while you sleep. It keeps constant pressure in your airway and, as noted above, helps to keep the airway inflated and open while sleeping. Unfortunately, many (if not most) people are not willing to continue with the C-pap treatment because of the noise of the machine, the discomfort of wearing the mask, and the cost. Most patients find that if they can tolerate the C-pap for three to six months, the treatment becomes second nature and comfortable.

Another possibility is surgery to reshape the throat so it stays open during sleep. Removing the tonsils, nasal surgery, and surgically trimming back the soft palate and the uvula (the tiny thing that hangs down in the back of your throat) are the most common treatments performed. Although these surgeries can be very helpful for snoring, they are less likely to help the sleep apnea. A new technique, in which high-frequency radio waves are used to heat and scar areas in the soft palate and tongue and thus shrink them, shows promise. Unfortunately, this technique is too new to evaluate its effectiveness.

It is controversial whether using more aggressive treatments for sleep apnea are worthwhile for people who have fewer than fifteen episodes of apnea per hour. The more conservative approaches (for example, weight loss and avoiding sleeping on your back) are a more reasonable way for those with mild apnea to begin treatment.

Narcolepsy

Narcolepsy is a sleep disorder characterized by excessive sleepiness during the day and a condition called cataplexy. Cataplexy is a sudden temporary loss in muscle strength. It is often triggered by strong emotions, such as anger or happiness, and can last for seconds or minutes. In severe cases, the person may collapse to the floor. More commonly, the head may sag and the mouth may droop, with only a momentary feeling of weakness. During cataplexy episodes, the person is fully conscious and can see and hear but may not be able to speak. Some people with narcolepsy also have sleep paralysis, an inability to move any muscles when initially falling asleep or waking. This can be frightening but it is not dangerous. About 70 percent of patients with narcolepsy have only daytime sleepiness, with no cataplexy. Narcolepsy is believed to affect 1 out of 1,000 people. A recent study done in New Zealand suggested that narcolepsy is fairly common in CFIDS/FMS, although I am not certain if I agree with that finding.

DIAGNOSING NARCOLEPSY

A diagnosis of narcolepsy can be made with multiple sleep latency testing (MSLT) done in combination with sleep apnea testing. A person with narcolepsy often falls asleep repeatedly in less than five minutes if put in a quiet environment. If REM (dream) sleep occurs in two or more of four or five naps, a diagnosis of narcolepsy is confirmed.

TREATING NARCOLEPSY

Stimulants (specifically Dexedrine, also commonly used in patients with hyperactivity) can be very helpful for many people with CFIDS. The amount of Dexedrine (methylphenidate) needed to maintain adequate alertness varies from person to person. Once the proper dose is found, it does not need to (and should not) be raised. The maximum dose is 10 to 30 milligrams of Dexedrine taken three times a day, up to 60 milligrams a day. Most CFIDS patients find 5 to 7.5 milligrams in the morning and 0 to

5 milligrams at noon to be optimal. I become more concerned about addiction if a patient needs over 30 milligrams a day, and I rarely prescribe these higher doses.

A newer drug, modafinil (Provigil), has also been found to have a beneficial stimulant effect in chronic fatigue syndrome and in narcolepsy as well. The usual dosage is 200 to 600 milligrams a day. Provigil is not considered to be an amphetamine, like Dexedrine, and there are fewer legal restrictions concerning its use. It is also unlikely to cause addiction (which I see in rare cases with high-dose Dexedrine). Some patients find that their cataplexy and narcolepsy also improve with 20 to 60 milligrams of Prozac a day.

Restless Leg Syndrome and Periodic Leg Movement Disorder

People with restless leg syndrome (RLS) have the sensation that they need to continually move their legs while sleeping. Occasionally, RLS also occurs during the day. Limb movements tend to be repetitive and most frequently involve the legs. A person will often extend his or her big toe while flexing the ankle, the knee and sometimes even the hip. This can occur with the arms as well and sometimes even with the whole body.

Another pattern consists of a disagreeable leg sensation and sense of restlessness that is brought on by rest and often relieved by movement. It is not uncommon for your bed partner to be very aware that your legs are kicking much of the night or are constantly moving. You may or may not be aware of your own movements. It has been estimated that as many as one-third or more of fibromyalgia patients have RLS. Although the cause of RLS is not clear, experts suspect it comes from a deficiency of the neurotransmitter called dopamine. RLS can also be aggravated by iron deficiency (having blood ferritin levels less than 50, even though over 9 is considered normal), nerve injuries, vitamin B_{12} and folic acid deficiency, hypothyroidism, and other problems. In some people, RLS may be associated with hypoglycemia. Some medications (especially Elavil and perhaps lithium) can aggravate RLS.

Diagnosing RLS

If you tend to scatter your sheets and blankets, and especially if you tend to kick your bed partner or if you note that your legs tend to feel jumpy and uncomfortable at rest at night, you probably have RLS. You can also have a sleep study done to look for leg muscle contractions. If contractions occur every twenty to forty seconds and last for about one-half to five seconds each, you have RLS. The sleep study will determine if these leg movements are associated with waking from deep sleep into light sleep to a degree that would be expected to cause daytime fatigue. Leg movements are not considered significant unless one has associated daytime sleepiness—for example, CFIDS/FMS.

Treating RLS

There are both natural and prescription approaches to treating RLS. Following are summaries of those that have been found to be most successful.

Natural Treatments

Natural remedies for RLS focus on diet and nutritional supplementation. Avoiding caffeine is important.[10] Because RLS may be associated with hypoglycemia, eating a sugar-free, high-protein diet with a protein snack at night may decrease episodes of cramping and RLS at night.[11]

An estimated 25 percent of RLS patients have low serum iron levels.[12] As noted above, if your serum ferritin score is under 50, I would take an iron supplement. I recommend the prescription iron supplement Chromagen FA because it also contains folic acid and combines iron and vitamin C, which helps the iron to be absorbed. Take iron supplements on an empty stomach. Vitamin E can also be very helpful, although it takes six to ten weeks of treatment to help.[13] Take 400 international units a day. If you have RLS in which pain, numbness, and lightning stabs of pain are relieved by movement or local massage, taking 5 milligrams of folic acid three times a day (available by prescription) is helpful. However, folic acid does not help cases of RLS where there is no discomfort.[14]

Finally, a few case reports have suggested that taking the amino acid L-tryptophan can be effective. Because it is hard to get this without a prescription, I recommend using the related compound 5-HTP (see page 113).

Prescription Treatments

Ambien and Klonopin are the first two medications I use to treat sleep in patients whom I suspect have RLS. These medicines usually do a superb job in suppressing RLS. I tell patients to adjust the dose to not only get adequate sleep, but to also keep the bedcovers in place and to avoid kicking their partners.

If these medications do not fully control RLS, I would add Sinemet 10/100 or 25/100, to be taken one hour before bedtime. This is a anti-Parkinson's medication that raises dopamine levels. Pergolide (Permax), another anti-Parkinson's drug that increases dopamine's effectiveness, can be started as well (and may be safer), at a dosage of 0.05 milligrams before sleep and increasing to 0.6 to 0.8 milligrams as needed. Opioids such as codeine or propoxyphene (Darvon) can also be effective.

Important Points

- Getting seven to nine hours of solid, deep sleep a night without waking or hangover is critical to getting well.
- Ambien, Desyrel, and Klonopin are the three best prescription sleep medications. Most regular sleeping pills make you worse by keeping you in light sleep.
- Valerian, lemon balm, kava, passionflower, 5-HTP, melatonin, and other natural remedies can help sleep.
- Treat sleep disorders such as sleep apnea, narcolepsy, and/or restless leg syndrome, if they are present.

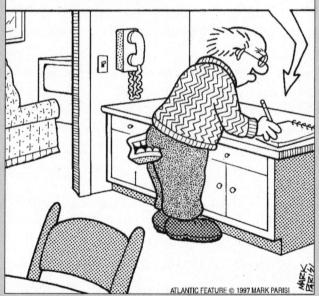

CHAPTER 7

Pain, Pain, Go Away—
Natural and Prescription Pain Relief

As noted earlier, treating sleep loss, under-
lying infections, nutritional deficiencies, low thyroid function, and low
estrogen levels can get rid of most, if not all, fibromyalgia pain. Unfortunately, though, we sometimes cannot get to the underlying cause of the
pain. This may be because of a viral infection we cannot fully treat yet or
because we simply don't know what the trigger was. In such cases—and
even in routine cases—it is important to have tools early in treatment that
can be used to decrease or eliminate your pain.

The source of fibromyalgia pain varies from person to person. In most
cases, it is caused by chronic muscle shortening that causes the muscles to
be chronically achy. In such cases, muscle relaxants can be very helpful.
Other pain is caused or aggravated by elevations in spinal fluid levels of
substance P, the chemical messenger that transmits the sensation of pain.
Changes in cell structures called N-methyl-D-aspartate (NMDA) receptors in the brain, which play an important part in sensing pain, can also be
involved in FMS and may give us another avenue to fight the pain. Nerve
pain is also sometimes seen. Elavil, Neurontin, and lidocaine are especially
helpful for treating nerve pain.

For most people, the pain is a mix of the above, and many treatments
described in this chapter will help several kinds of pain. Antidepressants
such as paroxetine (Paxil), fluoxetine (Prozac), and sertraline (Zoloft) can

sometimes be very effective in treating fibromyalgia pain. It is very reasonable to start using these medications when first beginning treatment because it takes six weeks to see their full effect. Many people need to start with low doses of antidepressants (for example, 10 milligrams of Prozac a day) and sometimes need to work up to fairly high doses (such as 60 milligrams of Paxil or Prozac) to see the optimum effect. It should be noted that most of the CFIDS/FMS patients I treat with Prozac are *not* depressed. Although drug interactions are possible, I have not found this to be a major problem. Be careful with these medications, though. Long-term use of acetaminophen (in Tylenol and many other over-the-counter medications) and/or nonsteroidal anti-inflammatory drugs such as aspirin, ibuprofen (Advil, Motrin, and others), or naproxen (Aleve) can cause liver and kidney damage. I would especially avoid acetaminophen because it depletes the body's glutathione—an amino-acid compound that is a critical antioxidant for people with CFIDS/FMS.

Many physical therapy measures can be very helpful in treating fibromyalgia pain. The best of these therapies include trigger-point injections with lidocaine, acupuncture, Dr. Janet Travell's stretch and spray technique, chiropractic treatments, many massage modalities, and prolotherapy. Prolotherapy consists of injecting weak ligaments with a substance that causes inflammation, which causes scarring in the ligament, actually strengthening it and often reducing pain. Prolotherapy is especially effective for people with loose ligaments who can hyperextend their joints and have "loose," elastic skin.

Let us look at a number of treatments that have been found to be very helpful for treating fibromyalgia pain.

Natural Pain Treatments

There is quite a selection of natural treatments available to help with pain. Some are taken internally, others applied externally. Most can be used in conjunction with conventional medical treatments.

Homeopathic Remedies

Rhus toxicodendron (Rhus tox) is a homeopathic treatment that helps a small percent of fibromyalgia patients with their pain. Because it is homeopathic, it has almost no side effects and is inexpensive, so it may be a good place to begin. Follow the directions on the bottle. The tablets are probably the easiest form to use. Be sure to let them dissolve under your tongue—don't chew them. You can take a tablet every fifteen minutes for the first two hours and then four to six times a day. If it does not help within a week, it is likely not going to.

HERBAL TREATMENTS

Ginger is an herb that can be very helpful for pain.[1] It also helps with the nausea and dizziness often experienced by people with CFIDS/FMS. You can take 1,000 milligrams of dried ginger extract one to four times a day or make ginger tea. To make the tea, boil 10 grams (⅓ ounce) of chopped fresh ginger (about a quarter-inch slice) and add stevia to sweeten it, as desired. Some people find it works better if they allow the ginger slices to dry out before using them (you can keep a bag of ginger slices in your refrigerator). Once you finish drinking the tea, eat the ginger that remains. I like to use packets of ginger tea crystals. If you like the sharp taste of ginger, you can eat candied ginger that is mostly ginger with a little bit of sugar. I wouldn't worry very much about the small amount of sugar in these products relative to the amount of ginger—as long as ginger is the first listed ingredient in the product.

Another herbal remedy for pain is capsaicin cream. Capsaicin is a compound that comes from hot peppers. It works by depleting substance P, the messenger that the body uses to transmit pain signals, in the skin. When the cream works, the area of the skin that the cream is on can no longer send a pain signal. Capsaicin cream can be very helpful for arthritis and for some people with fibromyalgia pain. It sometimes causes stinging when first used and must be used regularly (at least three or four times a day) to be effective. It may take several days to a week or two to see the effect. If you only use it once in a while, it may make the pain worse, instead of better.

Phytodolor is an herbal product made by PhytoPharmica that is available in many health food stores. Taking 30 drops three times a day can be helpful but it takes one to two weeks to work.

Dietary Supplements

The supplement 5-hydroxy-L-tryptophan (5-HTP), a form of the amino acid tryptophan, raises serotonin levels and can be very helpful for pain. In two studies in which fibromyalgia patients were given 100 milligrams of 5-HTP three times a day, their symptoms markedly improved, so it is well worth trying. It can also help you to lose weight. Give it six to ten weeks to work.

Glucosamine sulfate is a form of another natural compound that can help with pain. It tends to be more helpful for arthritis pain than for fibromyalgia pain, but it is worth trying. Be sure to get glucosamine *sulfate* rather than just glucosamine, because the sulfur can also be helpful. Take 500 milligrams three times a day for six weeks—it takes six weeks to find out if it is going to help. When the maximum benefit is seen, lower the dose to whatever maintains the benefit.

Methylsulfonylmethane (MSM) is another form of sulfur that is very helpful for wound healing and allergies. It may also help arthritis pain and, in high doses, has been reported to be very helpful for some people with fibromyalgia. Unfortunately, it can take as much as 12 to 15 grams a day (12,000 to 15,000 milligrams, or twenty-four to thirty capsules) to see the benefit. I usually use 6 grams a day in the beginning. If MSM helps within three to four weeks, then you can reduce the dose to the lowest dose that maintains the benefit. Taking it with vitamin C probably helps the absorption of the MSM.

Essential fatty acids (EFAs), which are the building blocks of fats and oils, have an anti-inflammatory effect and can be beneficial for pain. If you have dry eyes, dry mouth, dry hair, and/or dry skin, these symptoms may suggest an essential fatty acid deficiency. Taking essential fatty acids in the form of expeller-pressed oils can be very helpful. Good sources of essential fatty acids include fish oils, flaxseed oil, and primrose oil. These oils are available through several companies that specialize in chronic fatigue products. For flaxseed oil, the Barlean's company makes an excellent brand. Follow the dosage directions on the bottle. Some people find cod liver oil useful as well. Take ½ tablespoon (5,000 milligrams) a day. You should not use this oil if you are pregnant or about to get pregnant, however, because it may have too much vitamin A.

BODYWORK

There are many forms of bodywork that can be very helpful. Two of my favorites are Trager and Rolfing—if Rolfing is done by a *certified* Rolfer with a lot of experience (some people with minimal training claim that they do Rolfing and can work too aggressively). Myofascial release is also a very effective technique for fibromyalgia pain, as are chiropractic treatments and acupuncture. Some physical therapists are much too aggressive and can aggravate symptoms. If any bodywork therapist hurts you, let him or her know so that he or she can ease back and work more gently. Remember, "No pain, no gain" is stupid!

There is one exception to this rule, however—a technique for pain relief that is temporarily painful but can be helpful. This is *ischemic compression,* in which twenty to forty pounds of pressure is put on each of the tender spots for about forty-five to sixty seconds. The pain and tenderness can be quite significant, but is less after the pressure is released than it was before the pretreatment. If a therapist is doing ischemic compression, you may choose to grin and bear it, but you should only do so if you find that you feel better after the session than you did before the session. You can do ischemic compression of your own tender points by using a device called a Thera Cane (see Appendix J: Resources). Dr. Travell's stretch and spray technique, which is also done by some physical therapists, is pain-free and more effective.

BRACELETS AND MAGNETS

Although very low-tech, copper bracelets have withstood the test of time simply because they often are helpful. Several patients who tried a number of pain medications without success have reported feeling better when they wore copper bracelets. If a copper bracelet has a shiny coating, use nail polish remover to remove the coating in areas where the bracelet comes into contact with your skin.

Magnets have been very helpful for a large number of my patients with pain. I generally recommend starting with spot magnets for localized areas that hurt a lot, as well as magnet shoe insoles and the universal chair pad. If the spot magnets help in two months, then consider purchasing a mattress pad. The mattress pads are more expensive and, for some patients, too strong to start with. Many people, though, have been pleased that they started with a mattress pad because it offered substantial relief. There are a number of different companies that sell magnets (see Appendix J: Resources).

Prescription Medications

In Chapter 6, I discussed using clonazepam (Klonopin), carisoprodol (Soma), and cyclobenzaprine (Flexeril) for sleep. These medications can also be very helpful for pain. There are many other medications that can be very effective for pain relief. They can be used together and as needed, and include:

CELEBREX

Celecoxib (Celebrex) is a drug designed to combat inflammation, swelling, stiffness, and joint pain. The usual recommendation is to take 100 to 200 milligrams once to twice a day. You should know within two weeks, and probably within a few days, what the effect will be.

Do not use it if you are allergic to sulfa or aspirin products—for example, you get hives or a rash after taking these drugs. It is okay to use Celebrex if you get an upset stomach from aspirin, but no other symptoms. If you are allergic to sulfa drugs, you can use a cousin to Celebrex called refecoxib (Vioxx), one-half to one 25-milligram tablet a day. Do not use over 200 milligrams a day of Celebrex or 12.5 milligrams of Vioxx if you are on Sporanox or Diflucan.

ARIZONA PAIN FORMULA CREAM

Arizona Pain Formula Cream is a cream that contains several different pain medications. It is available by prescription from Ron's Pharmacy (see Appendix J: Resources) or from other compounding pharmacies. By rubbing a pea-sized amount into the skin over painful areas three times a day, you can often eliminate your worst pain spots. Sometimes using the cream for a week to ten days in one spot will make that spot of pain go away—then you can march through other pain spots, eliminating them as you go. You can use the cream on up to three or four silver-dollar-sized areas at a time, three times a day. The cost is approximately sixty-six dollars for a 30-gram tube, which lasts quite a while. If you have nerve pain, have the pharmacist add 10-percent gabapentin (Neurontin) and 8-percent lidocaine to the cream, and rub it on on the source of the pain and along the line or full area of pain.

ULTRAM

Tramadol (Ultram) is a cousin of the narcotic family that is minimally addicting. The recommended regimen is one to two 50-milligram tablets up to four times a day as needed for pain. This medication rarely causes seizures or elevated serotonin levels when combined with antidepressants. The most common side effects are nausea, vomiting, and sedation. These effects generally wear off with continued use, and can often be avoided altogether by starting with a low dose and *slowly* working up.

SKELAXIN

Metaxalone (Skelaxin) is a muscle relaxant. The good thing about it is that it tends to be nonsedating. Take one to two 400-milligram tablets four times a day as needed for pain. You will usually know within one week what the effect of Skelaxin will be.

ZANAFLEX

Tizanidine (Zanaflex) is a muscle relaxant that helps to relieve pain, spasms, muscle cramps, and tightness. The usual dose is one to two 4-milligram tablets three times a day for pain. It can be sedating, so some people choose to take it at nighttime. The main problem with Zanaflex is that it can sometimes cause nightmares. If it does cause nightmares, stop taking it because the problem usually does not go away with continued use.

BACLOFEN

Baclofen (Lioresal) is a muscle relaxant that can be *very* helpful for fibromyalgia pain. Take one-half to one 20-milligram tablet one to three times a day. For some people, it is very sedating, causing a "pleasantly drunk" feeling. Other people find that it makes them more awake. The benefit of baclofen should be seen within a day, and is often seen within thirty minutes.

NSAIDs

Nonsteroidal anti-inflammatory drugs (NSAIDs) are a family of medications that includes aspirin and its relatives, such as ibuprofen (in Motrin, Nuprin, and other products) and naproxen (in Aleve and Naprosyn). Some are available over the counter, others by prescription. These medications work in only a small subset of fibromyalgia patients. However, many people do get benefit from NSAIDs for arthritic and some muscle pains.

When taken regularly, NSAIDs create a risk of developing stomach bleeding that can become life-threatening. NSAIDs are responsible for approximately 10,000 to 20,000 deaths a year in the United States. The two medications in this class that I have found to be the most helpful for fibromyalgia—with the least stomach upset—are oxaprozin (Daypro) and diclofenac sodium (Voltaren). With Daypro, the recommended dosage is two 600-milligram caplets each morning; with Voltaren, you take 50 milligrams two to three times a day. The effects of these medications should be seen within two weeks.

ELAVIL

Technically an antidepressant, amitriptyline is especially good for nerve pain, pelvic pains, vulvadynia (pain in the vulvar area), interstitial cystitis (see page 68), and proctalgia fugax (episodic rectal pain due to muscle spasm). The main side effects are weight gain, sedation, restless leg syndrome, heart palpitations, and dry mouth. Elavil can also worsen neurally mediated hypertension (NMH), a type of low blood pressure syndrome experienced by some people with CFIDS/FMS.

Neurontin

Though it is primarily used in the management of seizure disorders, gabapentin (Neurontin) can be very helpful for both diabetic and shingles nerve pain, reflex sympathetic dystrophy (a chronic, potentially disabling pain disorder of a hand or foot, in which the sympathetic nervous system mistakenly sends pain messages), vulvadynia, and the more common tingling and muscle pains seen in fibromyalgia. It is best to start with a low dose, such as 100 milligrams, and slowly work your way up to 300 to 800 milligrams four times a day, up to a maximum of 6,000 milligrams a day. Neurontin comes in 100-, 300-, and 400-milligram capsules, and in 600- and 800-milligram tablets. Some people find that taking 300 to 900 milligrams a day does a superb job in helping pain. For other people, 2,400 milligrams a day is the threshold dose, although it can be taken at doses of 5,000 to 6,000 milligrams a day. Such high doses are rarely needed, however.

In rare cases, I have seen some neurological side effects, such as impaired speech, that might be a result of taking Neurontin. The most common side effects are sedation, dizziness and headache. The sedation tends to go away over a period of time. Neurontin is expensive, but can be a godsend for patients with neurological pain.

LIDOCAINE

Intravenous treatment with the anesthetic lidocaine, especially when given with intravenous nutritional therapies such as Myers cocktails, can be a blessing for both easing muscle and spastic colon pain and helping to raise energy levels in people with CFIDS/FMS. (More information about Myers cocktails can be found in Appendix G.) Many people who have severe, intractable pain have found intravenous lidocaine to be wonderful. It may first be given in a test dose of 40 to 50 milligrams infused over a thirty-minute period. The Myers cocktail can be given at the same time, in a different IV bag but through the same needle. If the lidocaine is well tolerated, you can take up to 100 milligrams the first day, as long as your blood pressure remains stable and there are no severe side effects. The treatment can be sedating—a wonderful sleepy feeling is common, and I often let patients take a nap on the table afterwards—and you should not drive if you feel sedated after a lidocaine infusion. It is generally a good idea to have someone drive you home after a lidocaine treatment.

If the first treatment is well tolerated, you can take a maximum of 100 to 120 milligrams an hour to a dose of 300 to 400 milligrams at a sitting, if needed. The effect seems to increase over the first four times that it is given. I usually infuse at least a dose of 200 milligrams during a single two-hour session before deciding that it is not effective for a particular patient.

Intravenous lidocaine can be taken as often as needed. Many people find that they need to take a treatment every one to three weeks. Too high doses of lidocaine (usually much higher doses than those mentioned here) can be associated with abnormal heart rhythms or seizures, so it is sometimes administered with a patient hooked up to a heart monitor. However, most doctors I know who infuse lidocaine do not use a heart monitor while giving it, and neither do I. One dose administered in my office costs approximately $72 for the initial infusion of a Myers cocktail or lidocaine, and ninety-two dollars if given together. In comparison, when given while on a heart monitor by Johns Hopkins pain specialists, the cost is approximately $700 per treatment. Some people feel that giving lidocaine without a monitor is controversial, but in my experience it has been quite safe. In one study done using intravenous lidocaine for fibromyalgia treatment, researchers gave subjects 240 milligrams over a period of thirty minutes (over four times the speed I recommend—I don't recommend giving it that fast) without significant problems.

Lidocaine can also be used externally in pluronic-lecithin-organogel (PLO gel). This gel is mostly helpful for people with nerve pain such as reflex sympathetic dystrophy or neuropathies. Simply rub it on painful areas as needed. The lidocaine gel must must be an 8- to 15-percent concentration in PLO gel. One source for this product is Ron's Pharmacy (see Appendix J: Resources).

NORFLEX

Orphenadrine (sold under the brand name Norflex, among others) is another muscle relaxant. It is also used to control tremors in people with Parkinson's disease. The recommended dose is one tablet twice a day.

DEXTROMETHORPHAN

Dextromethorphan (DM) is another medication that works via the NMDA receptors (see page 131). It is especially helpful when taken with narcotics because it makes narcotics work better and helps to prevent them from losing their effectiveness. I strongly recommend that anyone taking narcotics take DM with it. I also recommend DM for people who are taking Ultram. The recommended dose is 25 milligrams one to three times a day. DM is available over the counter in many cough and cold medicines, but it is usually mixed with decongestants and/or other cough medications. It can be obtained in pure form by mail from Cape Apothecary (see

Appendix J: Resources). Although, theoretically, high doses of DM can decrease short-term memory, I have not seen this problem. If memory loss does occur, simply lower the dose.

LITHIUM

Although lithium is usually used to treat manic episodes and manic depression, research and my experience have found that it can have quite a dramatic effect on eliminating refractory pain in CFIDS/FMS, especially when combined with antidepressants. Although I am not sure why it happens, lithium has many actions, including an antiviral effect. The recommended dose is 300 milligrams two to three times a day.

The main side effect of lithium is tremor (if the dose gets too high) or sedation. If tremor is a problem, taking 2 teaspoons of expeller-expressed safflower oil daily or lowering the dose of lithium may help. Use safflower oil from a health food store and take it uncooked, as in salad dressing. Lithium can also cause a drop in thyroid function. Your T_4 thyroid hormone level should, therefore, be checked every six to twelve months, as should your lithium blood level.

KETAMINE

Ketamine is an anesthetic agent that also works on the NMDA receptors (see page 131). Although I have not used it very often (mostly because most people's pain will go away without it), it is something that can be quite helpful and has been shown to be effective in reducing fibromyalgia pain.

There are two ways to administer ketamine:

1. Intravenously, at a rate of 0.3 milligram per kilogram (2.2 pounds) of body weight, given over ten minutes by a physician familiar with its use. This usually gives relief for up to one week.
2. Topically, in the form of an 8-percent PLO gel. A total of one-half to one inch of the cream is put on one or several painful areas and rubbed in. You then wait thirty minutes and then increase the dose up to a maximum of four inches of the cream as needed. It can be used up to three times a day if it relieves pain.

The main problem with ketamine is that, being an anesthetic, it can cause people to have disassociative (very spaced out) feelings. This is a normal side effect and not dangerous—it has even been reported to be enjoyable—but some people find it unpleasant. If this occurs, lay down and sleep the feelings off. Lower the dose if the side effects are uncomfortable. Ketamine can also have an effect on short-term memory.

CALCITONIN

Calcitonin (Calcimar, Miacalcin) is a hormone most often used in the treatment of bone diseases. Although I have not needed to prescribe it, it has been reported to be helpful for fibromyalgia pain. It also tends to improve bone strength and is a treatment (albeit quite expensive) that is used for osteoporosis as well.

NARCOTICS

Norco is a medication that combines hydrocodone, a codeine-family narcotic, with acetaminophen, the active ingredient in Tylenol. It is often used for severe cancer pain. The recommended dose is one-half to one 10-milligram tablet, one to three times a day.

Like any other narcotic, Norco can be quite addictive. Because it contains acetaminophen, you should generally not take more than four tablets a day, as it is possible to develop liver toxicity and/or glutathione deficiency from the acetaminophen at higher doses. The benefit of Norco over most other similar codeine-and-acetaminophen products in common use (for example, Vicodin or Percocet), is that it has *less* acetaminophen in it. If you need to use products containing acetaminophen, also take 500 to 1,000 milligrams of the supplement N-acetylcysteine (NAC) a day and 1,000 milligrams of vitamin C a day to raise your glutathione levels. Also consider taking a denatured whey protein supplement such as Imuplus—it is effective but expensive.

There is a small subset of patients with fibromyalgia who require narcotics for their pain. Interestingly, these people often find that their mental clarity is *improved* when on narcotics, unlike most people, who feel drunk and sleepy on them. Norco should be used with dextromethorphan (DM) to prevent it from losing its effectiveness. I usually start with a set dose that controls the pain, usually a *maximum* of four tablets a day, and the patient must agree that the dose will *not* be increased over time. People who require narcotics for pain relief may need to take them long-term. Patients who are on narcotics for chronic pain, however, are less likely to become addicted than people who use them to get high.

Methadone is a synthetic narcotic that is also very helpful. It is probably better for chronic pain than other narcotics. Unfortunately, the government paperwork and regulations surrounding it make it too difficult for most doctors to use. It may be available from chronic-pain management centers. Most doctors are hesitant to talk about the use of narcotics for treatment of fibromyalgia pain because they don't want to attract government regulators or people who are seeking drugs. Being a bit of a troublemaker, I asked a group of pain specialists at a recent lecture I gave to raise their hands if they used narcotics for fibromyalgia treatment. At first, no hands went up. After I put my hand up, most of the doctors also slowly put their hands up, too. I do list narcotics last, though, because they can be quite addictive and I prefer to use the other medications first.

Miscellaneous Pains

Using the treatments described above will eliminate most, if not all, of the pain for most people with fibromyalgia. If needed, all of these medications (except if two are listed together in the same section, such as Voltaren and Daypro) can be tried sequentially or in combination to eliminate pain. There are also effective strategies to help with some of the "miscellaneous" painful problems that often affect people with CFIDS/FMS, including mouth sores, irritable bowel syndrome, and arthritis pain. *You can be pain-free!*

MOUTH SORES

Sores in the mouth usually come from several different sources. If they are usually in the same place and on the lips (that is, cold sores), they are generally caused by the herpes virus. I recommend taking 500 milligrams of famciclovir (Famvir) three times a day at the first sign of an outbreak, beginning at the start of the first tingling sensation (the indicator that an outbreak will be coming in a few days), before the sore emerges. This will usually nip the attack in the bud. If attacks are very frequent, taking 250 milligrams twice a day on an ongoing basis will usually prevent most of them. The above also applies to genital herpes.

Taking 1,000 milligrams of the amino acid supplement L-lysine three times a day is also helpful for suppressing cold sores. This works by decreasing the level of arginine, another amino acid, which the cold sore virus feeds on. The one concern is that arginine is needed to make growth hormone, which is already deficient in many people with CFIDS/FMS (see Chapter 3), so it might be worth limiting the L-lysine to 1,000 milligrams a day to suppress the herpes, and then using Famvir at first sign of a sore to knock it out. This applies to both mouth and genital herpes infections.

If you have sores *in* your mouth, these are usually aphthous ulcers, often known as canker sores. In people with CFIDS/FMS, most of these come from yeast infections. For these, get prescription Mycelex Troches (oral lozenges). The first day of the attack, suck on a lozenge five to six times a day for ten to fifteen minutes. Then leave the piece(s) sitting right up against the sore(s) for thirty minutes or so, or until you are tired of them being there. This can usually make the pain go away within twenty-four hours instead of the usual ten days. If you begin treatment in the first two days of the attack and the pain does not markedly improve within two days of treatment, then the problem is not fungal. In that case, using either a cotton swab dipped in tetracycline or a prescription cream called Kenalog in Orabase applied to the sores can often help. Treating vitamin B_{12}, folic acid, and/or iron deficiencies, and occasionally food allergies, can also be helpful.

IRRITABLE BOWEL SYNDROME

Also known as spastic colon, this is a condition in which irregular contractions of the intestines results in constipation and/or diarrhea, often alternating, as well as gas, pain, cramping, and bloating. This usually resolves when bowel infections are treated. For example, treating yeast infections is very important. This can be done with nystatin and either itraconazole (Sporanox) or fluconazole (Diflucan).

Natural remedies for yeast infections include the following:

- Caprylic acid. Take 1,800 to 3,600 milligrams a day.
- Acidophilus. Take 4 to 6 billion units a day.
- Oregano oil. Take two capsules three times a day for three to four months and then twice a day as needed. Take this on an empty stomach.

- Olive leaf extract. Take one to three 500-milligram capsules three to four times a day, between meals.
- Garlic.
- Grapefruit seed extract (Citricidal).

These can be taken singly or in combination with each other. Treating any parasites or other infections that are present in the colon is also important. If spastic colon pain persists despite treatment, or while you are waiting for the treatment to work, peppermint oil capsules can be very helpful. Take one to two enteric-coated capsules containing 0.2 cc of peppermint oil each three times a day, between meals—not with food. Simethicone (found in Mylicon and other over-the-counter products), which is available at most grocery stores and pharmacies, can help gas pains as well. Chew a 40- to 80- milligram tablet three times a day as needed for gas.

Another herbal remedy that can be helpful is Iberogast. This is a digestive-system herbal produced by PhytoPharmica (see Appendix J: Resources). Take 20 drops three times a day in warm water with meals. Iberogast is very helpful for indigestion but takes four to eight weeks to work. In addition, betaine HCl (which are hydrochloric acid capsules) can be very helpful if you have poor digestion caused by inadequate stomach acid. This often manifests itself as gas or bloating after meals, especially meals with meat in them. Try taking two to six capsules with each meal, along with pancreatic enzymes, for a week to ten days to see if this helps digestion. If you get a worsening acid stomach, cut the dose back. Do not take betaine HCl if you have a history of ulcers or severe stomach acid problems, and do not take it within three hours of a dose of nicotinamide adenine dinucleotide hydrogen (NADH). Many people who think they have acid stomach actually have very little stomach acid but instead have bile reflux.

If you have a history of having had parasites, you might be reinfecting yourself. A good water filter system, such as Multi-Pure, can be very helpful. (See Appendix J: Resources.) Most other filters, except for reverse osmosis filters, are not very effective.

ARTHRITIS PAIN

Arthritis pain can affect anyone, including people with CFIDS/FMS. For relief of arthritis pain, try the following combination of natural remedies:

- Glucosamine sulfate. Take 500 milligrams three times a day.
- Methylsulfonylmethane (MSM). Start by taking 6 to 12 grams (6,000 to 12,000 milligrams) a day, then drop down to 2 to 6 grams (2,000 to 6,000 milligrams) a day as needed to maintain the effect.
- Vitamin E. Take 400 international units a day.
- Ginger. Take 1 to 4 grams a day.

These treatments can be very helpful for arthritis, but it takes about six weeks to see the effect.

Important Points

- Most CFIDS/FMS pain can be eliminated.
- Getting eight hours of solid sleep a night, and treating low thyroid function, nutritional deficiencies, and underlying infections (especially yeast) often eliminate the root causes of the pain.
- Celebrex and Skelaxin are two of many potentially helpful medications for daytime use.
- Klonopin and baclofen are also good, although sedating, pain medications for CFIDS/FMS.
- Try natural and prescription treatments individually and/or in combination, as needed.

8

Jump-Starting Your Body's Energy Furnaces

IN PREVIOUS CHAPTERS, WE HAVE LOOKED AT THE role of lifestyle factors, hormonal disturbances, sleep disruptions and disorders, infections, and other likely contributors to CFIDS/FMS. Mounting evidence suggests that there may be other important factors in this syndrome as well. One of the most interesting is the possibility of trouble in the body's production of energy at the cellular level.

Each cell in the body contains structures called *mitochondria*. The mitochondria are the tiny furnaces in each cell that produce energy by burning calories. In this chapter, I will look at evidence that suggests mitochondrial problems in CFIDS/FMS and an integrating theory that explains why this occurs. I will also examine how the mitochondria work, discuss treatments that can help the mitochondrial furnaces work properly, and explain how you can use this information to feel better.

The Consequences of Mitochondrial Dysfunction

Besides the fact that fatigue in itself suggests low energy production, a large number of clinical findings common in CFIDS/FMS can be explained by mitochondrial furnace malfunction. For example, if the mitochondrial furnaces are working poorly, this would affect the brain, and could account for that common CFIDS/FMS symptom known as brain fog. In addition, mitochondrial dysfunction can cause decreases in levels of neurotransmitters in the brain, specifically low dopamine and acetylcholine, and possibly low serotonin. Particularly severe changes in the hypothalamus have been seen in mitochondrial dysfunction syndromes. This could account for the hypothalamic suppression characteristic of CFIDS/FMS.[1]

In the liver, you would see a decreased ability to eliminate toxins and medications. This could contribute to sensitivities to both medications and environmental factors. In the muscles, mitochondrial dysfunction would lead to low energy production and accumulation of excessive amounts of lactic acid during exercise. Lactic acid is the compound that causes your muscles to ache after exercise, so this can cause achiness and may cause postexertional fatigue.

The kidneys also could be affected. Specifically, there might be a defect in the filtration and detoxification process. CFIDS/FMS researcher Dr. R. Paul St. Amand, postulates that fibromyalgia is caused by a genetic defect in phosphate excretion by the kidneys. It is conceivable that poor kidney function resulting from mitochondrial dysfunction may also be involved.

Mitochondrial dysfunction would also cause digestion to suffer. This could be related to the bowel problems that plague so many people with chronic fatigue and fibromyalgia. Finally, in the immune system, you would expect to see poor white blood cell function and therefore a decreased ability to fight infection. Thus, mitochondrial dysfunction might well be the root cause of—or at least a contributing factor to—the hypothalamic, immune, neurotransmitter, nutritional, detoxification, sleep and other disorders seen in CFIDS/FMS. (For a visual representation of the interrelationships between all these factors, see Figure 8.1, The CFIDS/FMS Cycle.)

Improving Mitochondrial Function

If mitochondrial dysfunction is an underlying or contributing cause to CFIDS/FMS, the next question is whether anything can be done to make those cellular energy furnaces work better. Fortunately, there are a number of natural treatments available to do just that. Let us now look at some of the treatments that can improve mitochondrial energy production.

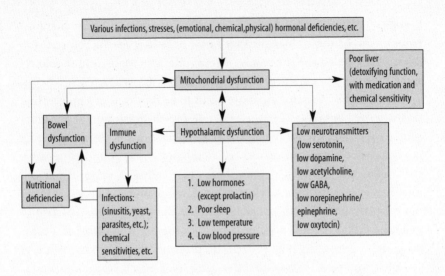

FIGURE 8.1 *The CFIDS/FMS Cycle*

ASPARTATES AND MALIC ACID

Aspartates and malic acid are compounds that are needed to "rescue" part of the Krebs cycle when levels of the nutrient thiamine pyrophosphate (TPP) are low. (More about TPP later in this chapter.) The Krebs cycle is series of chemical reactions that take place in the body's cells and allow glucose to be used for the production of energy. It is also sometimes referred to as tricarboxylic acid (TCA) cycle.

As dietary supplements, aspartates and malic acid have at least three excellent qualities: They are very effective; they are safe and nontoxic, even for those with chemical sensitivities; and they are cheap! Although the other supplements I will discuss in this chapter are also safe and usually have no side effects, they can be expensive.

Aspartates are compounds based on the amino acid aspartic acid. Many studies show aspartates to be helpful for various fatigue syndromes. Over 3,000 patients have been studied, with many in placebo-controlled trials.[2] To achieve the desired effect, the potassium and magnesium needed to be *chemically attached* to the aspartate. Studies using each component separately or in various combinations did not show the desired effect.[3]

When the proper type of aspartate was used, about 70 to 85 percent of patients improved, compared with to 25 percent of patients given a placebo.[4]

Results often begin in ten days. The usual dose is 1 gram (1,000 milligrams) twice a day (or 500 milligrams four times day) after meals. You can stop taking the supplement after twelve weeks. If fatigue recurs, you should resume the aspartate for six- to eight-week periods as needed.

As noted above, a true aspartate needs to be subjected to a process that creates a solid bond between the aspartate and the potassium and magnesium. This makes sense, because aspartate plays a role in transporting potassium and magnesium across cell membranes—the boundary between the insides and outsides of cells. There is evidence to suggest that cell membranes may malfunction in CFIDS. If magnesium and potassium are not properly bound to aspartate, it is more difficult for the aspartate to carry them into the cell, and, perhaps, into the mitochondria.[5] If a company says a product is fully reacted, it's probably the real thing. If it says "aspartate complex," it may not be as effective. General Nutrition Centers has a product containing 250 milligrams each of magnesium aspartate and potassium aspartate—that is, a total of 500 milligrams of aspartates in the *same* tablet—that has the proper ratios to suggest it is chemically reacted.

The combination of magnesium and malic acid is also critical. Malic acid is a compound that occurs naturally in foods, in fruits in general and in especially high levels in apples. (Remember the old saying: An apple a day keeps the doctor away.) When levels of malic acid and the other compounds discussed in this article are low, the body often has to shift to a very inefficient (anaerobic) means of generating energy. This contributes to the abnormal buildup of lactic acid (noted above) that occurs after exertion in CFIDS/FMS.[6] This causes muscle pain, achiness, and fatigue.

Malic acid is critical both during healthy (aerobic) and inefficient (anaerobic) muscle metabolism. Interestingly, malic acid can be converted to aspartate as well. My favorite *tablet* forms of magnesium with malic acid is Fibrocare, made by a company called To Your Health (see Appendix J: Resources). Each tablet contains 75 milligrams of magnesium glycinate, which is better tolerated than most magnesium preparations; 25 milligrams of vitamin B_6, which increases magnesium cell membrane transfer and utilization; 300 milligrams of malic acid; 25 milligrams of vitamin B_1 (thiamine); 50 milligrams of vitamin C; and 2½ milligrams of manganese. I recommend taking two tablets two to three times a day for eight months, and then decreasing to two tablets a day. Take less if diarrhea is a problem. An even better recommended source of magnesium and malic acid is the From Fatigued To Fantastic powder formula (see Appendix J: Resources).

THIAMINE PYROPHOSPHATE (TPP)

Thiamine pyrophosphate is the activated form of vitamin B_1 (thiamine). It is essential for many steps in the process of energy production. For example, it is needed to get carbohydrates to burn efficiently. It is also needed to clear out excess lactic acid, which makes muscles ache. I suspect that TPP is another key player in mitochondrial dysfunction. Dr. Jean Eisenger and his associates in Toulon, France, have done brilliant research in this area. He has found significant impairment of thiamine (vitamin B_1) function in FMS. Thiamine must be converted to its activated form (TPP) to do its job.

A compound called adenosine triphosphate (ATP) is the "currency" used by the mitochondria in the cells of living things to generate energy. Anything that depletes ATP (for example, infections, toxic exposures to the liver, chronic muscle shortening from any cause, and, possibly, brain ATP loss) may prevent the formation of TPP, which in turn further diminishes ATP production. This can effectively shut down the functioning of those mitochondria, resulting in a Catch-22—energy is like the body's money and, as the old saying goes, It takes money (energy) to make money (energy)!

The good news is that Dr. Eisenger has found that several treatments can help. First, receiving 50 milligrams of TPP by intramuscular injection three times a week for six weeks decreased pain in over 76 percent of FMS patients he studied.[7] This is not yet readily available in the United States, but it can be imported for personal use from Lab ISI in Italy, which sells it under the trade name CoCarboxylase (see Appendix J: Resources). I would use the 100-milligram vials (about two dollars each wholesale) three times a week. These shots do cause a sore bottom.

Taking 25 to 100 milligrams of vitamin B_6 (pyridoxine) and 300 to 450 milligrams of magnesium is helpful. Vitamin B_6 is critical to thiamine function. However, if magnesium is not added, thiamine can aggravate magnesium deficiency.[8]

Phosphocreatine (and, I suspect, creatine) also helps if you need a quick burst of energy. I will discuss creatine below. Finally, using the other treatments suggested in this chapter to promote ATP production will likely result in the body making its own TPP.

L-Carnitine and Acetyl-L-Carnitine

Low levels of the carnitine compound acylcarnitine in the blood or muscles of people with CFIDS/FMS have been found by two different research centers.[9] Carnitine plays many roles in the body. It has the critical function of preventing the mitochondria from being shut down when the system backs up. It does this by keeping a substance called acetyl coenzyme A from building up and shutting down the TCA cycle and the electron transport system, the cell's effective energy burning systems. (More about the electron transport system later in this chapter.) Also, without sufficient carnitine, the body cannot burn fat (and, in fact, makes excess fat), resulting in large weight gains.

L-Carnitine is a naturally occurring form of carnitine that is only found in animal flesh. Beef is high in carnitine. Carnitine can also be synthesized in the body. This process requires adequate amounts of the amino acid lysine, which is low in rice-based vegetarian diets (which also have no carnitine).[10] I suspect that the real reason many CFIDS patients who take lysine to prevent herpes outbreaks see their symptoms improve may be that this increases the body's carnitine production.

In my experience, and that of other clinicians, taking supplemental L-carnitine has *not* been very helpful, and D-L-carnitine can actually worsen symptoms.[11] Taking 500 to 1,000 milligrams of *acetyl*-L-carnitine milligrams three times a day, however, can be very helpful. It has no side effects except for its cost, usually $1.50 or more for 1,000 milligrams. Adding 500 to 1,000 milligrams of L-lysine, which is cheaper, can decrease the amount of acetyl-L-carnitine you need to take by helping your body to make its own carnitine. The body also requires vitamin C (I recommend 200 milligrams a day) and B-complex vitamins to make carnitine.[12] I suspect that most people can lower their dose of acetyl-L-carnitine after eight to twelve weeks—for example, to 500 milligrams a day—or even stop it. Any brand is fine as long as it is *pure* acetyl-L-carnitine.

NADH

Nicotinamide adenine dinucleotide plus high-energy hydrogen (NADH), also known as coenzyme 1, is necessary to carry the energy made by burning carbohydrates, proteins, and fats from the TCA cycle to the electron transport system in the mitochondria, so that it can be converted into ATP energy "dollars." NADH's ability to be turned into energy depends proper functioning of various enzymes and other compounds.

In people with CFIDS/FMS, the body has difficulty producing NADH. Because NADH has many other functions, a lack of it is disastrous for the body. One major function of NADH is in stimulating the production of the important neurotransmitters dopamine, norepinephrine, and serotonin. These neurotransmitters appear to be low in people with CFIDS/FMS; low NADH may contribute to these deficiencies. Serotonin is important for sleep and emotional balance. Norepinephrine is responsible for alertness, concentration, and mental activity. Dopamine is also responsible for a sense of well-being and for energizing the body. It stimulates strength, coordination, cognition (mental functioning), mood, sex drive, and the secretion of growth hormone, which is also low in people with CFIDS/FMS. In addition, serotonin needs NADH and ATP to get into the cells where it does its job. NADH stimulates the enzyme tyrosine hydroxylase (TH), which is the key enzyme for the production of dopamine. Taking supplemental NADH can stimulate the production of dopamine and norepinephrine by up to 40 percent.

In addition to the functions mentioned above, dopamine lowers levels of prolactin, a hormone that is often elevated in people with CFIDS/FMS. It also lowers appetite.[13] Work being done by Dr. Dan Malone of the University of Wisconsin, using medications that raise dopamine and/or serotonin, suggests that dopamine plays a very important role in CFIDS/FMS and, like serotonin, appears to be low in people with this disorder.[14]

Indeed, NADH has been found to improve depression in a study of 205 depressed patients, with 93 percent of the patients showing a beneficial clinical effect.[15] Because of NADH's effect on dopamine levels, it is also very helpful in treating Parkinson's disease and may help restless leg syndrome.[16]

The Georgetown University Medical School did a placebo-controlled study of NADH treatment of CFIDS under the direction of Dr. Joseph A. Bellanti, who is the director of Georgetown's International Center for Interdisciplinary Studies of Immunology, and Dr. Harry Preuss. Dr. Bellanti proposed that NADH works by replenishing depleted cellular stores of ATP, thus improving the fatigue and cognitive dysfunction. In their study, patients were given 10 milligrams of NADH a day for one month. In that time, thirty-one of the CFIDS patients showed at least 10 percent improvement. Outside the study, they continued the NADH for a second month, and found that 80 percent of CFIDS/FMS patients felt somewhat improved after two months. (Because of this, you should not try NADH unless you are willing to give it at least a two-month trial.) Increasing the dose to 20 milligrams each morning sometimes increased the effect. Dr. Preuss feels that NADH is a safe natural compound. Georgetown researchers are also studying NADH in the treatment of Alzheimer's disease and hope to begin studies on the drug's use for treating depression and obesity. NADH certainly seems to be a promising new treatment for CFIDS/FMS.

Unfortunately, NADH is very sensitive to stomach acid. I use only NADH that is made by the company that produced it for the Georgetown study—the Menuco Corporation. Their brand name for NADH is Enada. I recommend a dosage of 10 milligrams daily. It is critical that NADH be taken first thing in the morning on an empty stomach, one-half hour before taking any food or supplements, except for thyroid hormone. The reason for this is that anything that is in the stomach could stimulate the production of stomach acid, which makes it harder for NADH to survive and also binds the NADH in the stomach, preventing its absorption. Since NADH costs about $1.80 for a 10-milligram daily dose, it is important that it be taken under optimum conditions. If it doesn't help after two months, you can stop taking it or try increasing the dosage to 20 milligrams a day for six weeks.

Sometimes, after two to three months, the dose can be reduced to 5 milligrams a day, and after four to five months, it may be possible to stop taking it altogether, especially if NADH is taken as part of the complete program described below. Hopefully, this will jump-start the mitochondrial furnaces so that they can function on their own without any further aid. Overall, about 25 percent of my CFIDS/FMS patients have found that NADH helps enough for them to want to stay on it.

CREATINE

Although I have spoken about ATP being the body's main energy source, the body does not store much ATP—it makes it as it needs it. During the initial stages of exercise, the body's main energy source—the main thing it uses to create ATP—is a compound known as phosphocreatine. This maintains ATP levels while the body gears up to burn food to make ATP, a process called glycolysis.[17]

Creatine is also important for brain function.[18] As noted earlier in this chapter, the muscles of people with CFIDS/FMS make more lactic acid during exercise than do those of healthy people. Creatine acts as a buffer to reduce lactic acid buildup and allow sluggish mitochondria to kick in.[19] Otherwise, *low* creatine will prevent you from getting up to peak exercise—even if this means simply walking across the room—or will result in aggravated next-day muscle pain. Its main effect is to supply the initial burst of energy for an activity. This may increase endurance and enhance your ability to exercise without fatigue or achiness.[20]

Creatine is a naturally occurring protein that, like carnitine, is found in animal muscle (for example, in meat, fish, and poultry). Because of this, supplemental creatine is even more helpful for vegetarians.[21] Cooking tends to destroy creatine. The body can also make creatine from the amino acids arginine, glycine, and methionine.

Supplemental creatine may be taken with a small amount of sweets to enhance its absorption. It should be taken on an empty stomach with a lot of water and a bit of honey.[22] It can be taken in the form of creatine monohydrate, at a dosage of 5 grams (5,000 milligrams) four times a day for five days (the so-called loading dose), and then 2 grams (2,000 milligrams) a day (the maintenance dose). Alternatively, you can begin with and stay on 3 grams (3,000 milligrams) a day. The loading dose is more effective, however.[23] Another form of supplemental creatine, phosphocreatine, is available overseas, but this form may not get across cell membranes as well as creatine.

COENZYME Q_{10}, IRON, SULFUR, AND COPPER: THE ELECTRON TRANSPORT SYSTEM

Coenzyme Q_{10}, iron, sulfur, and copper are critical for the electron transport system (ETS) to do its job of harvesting over 75 percent of the ATP energy from food. Since most cellular functions are dependent on an adequate supply of ATP, the health of the entire body is therefore dependent on an adequate supply of coenzyme Q_{10}, iron, sulfur, and copper.

A great deal has been written on coenzyme Q_{10} and CFIDS/FMS. I will simply note that studies have demonstrated it can do the following:

- Enhance immune function.[24]
- Assist weight loss when dieting.[25]
- Improve exercise tolerance in sedentary people.[26]

In addition, coenzyme Q_{10} may decrease allergies.[27] I recommend taking 100 to 200 milligrams of coenzyme Q_{10} a day. Take it with some kind of oil (butter, olive oil, salad dressing, vitamin E, or an oil supplement). This may significantly enhance its absorption.

Iron, sulfur, and copper are also critical to ETS function. Iron deficiency is easy to test for and treat. Ferritin levels should be kept over 40 and iron percent saturation over 22 percent. Adequate amounts of copper (1 to 3 milligrams a day) are present in the multivitamins I recommend, as are the B vitamins. Sulfur is harder to come by. A good form of supplemental sulfur is methylsulfonylmethane (MSM). Early experience suggests taking MSM may be very helpful for some people with chemical sensitivities, allergies, muscle and joint pain, and poor wound healing. I recommend taking four to six 500-milligram tablets twice a day, with meals, for six to eight weeks, then as needed.

Treating Mitochondrial Dysfunction Summarized

To sum up, following is my recipe for treating mitochondrial dysfunction and jump-starting your body's energy production. The supplements are listed in order of priority, in case cost is an issue (some of them can be expensive).

1. Take a good multivitamin daily.
2. Take two magnesium/malic acid two tablets three times a day (less if it causes diarrhea) for eight months, then cut back to two tablets a day.
3. Take 100 to 200 milligrams of coenzyme Q_{10} daily.
4. Take 2,000 to 3,000 milligrams of magnesium-potassium aspartate a day for three months, then stop. Be sure to take a brand that is *fully reacted,* such as the General Nutrition Centers brand.
5. Get vitamin B_{12} shots, especially if your B_{12} level is under 540 picograms per milliliter (pg/mL) of blood. I recommend getting 3,000 micrograms intramuscularly one to three times a week for ten to twenty shots. If injections are not available, take 1,000 to 5,000 micrograms a day in tablet form.
6. Get injections of thiamine pyrophosphate (TPP, available as CoCarboxylase). I recommend getting 100 milligrams intramuscularly three

times a week for four to six weeks. This is not yet available in the United States, but individuals (perhaps with their doctors' help) can import it for personal use from Lab ISI in Italy (see Appendix J: Resources).

7. Take 500 to 1,000 milligrams of acetyl-L-carnitine three times a day for three months. Then take 500 to 1,000 milligrams a day as needed or discontinue it. Add 1,000 milligrams of L-lysine three times a day for three months to help the body make its own carnitine. Then you can reduce the lysine to 1,000 milligrams a day.

8. Take two 5-milligram tablets of nicotinamide adenine dinucleotide plus high-energy hydrogen (NADH) each morning for six to twelve weeks. It *must* be the Enada brand. It also *must* be taken first thing in the morning on an empty stomach—at least one-half hour before any food, medications, or supplements.

9. Take 5 grams (5,000 milligrams) of powdered creatine monohydrate four times a day for five days, then cut back to 2 grams (2,000 milligrams) a day. Mix it with water, and, if you tolerate it well, add 1 teaspoon of honey or sugar to the glass to help absorption. Get one that is assayed as 99+ percent pure.

10. Get injections of adenosine monophosphate (AMP). I recommend 100 milligrams given intramuscularly three times a week. Alternatively, you can take 50 milligrams of My-B-Tabs (AMP) from LeGere Pharmaceuticals dissolved under the tongue three times a day. Give AMP six to twelve weeks to have an effect. It is most likely to help if you have a lot of flu- or mono-like symptoms. The tablets help only infrequently, however.

11. Take four to six 500-milligram tablets of methylsulfonylmethane (MSM) twice a day for six to eight weeks, then as needed—for example, one to three tablets two times a day.

12. If your ferritin test is under 40 or your percent saturation is under 22 percent, take an iron supplement. I prefer the prescription product Chromagen-FA, although there are many other good forms. Take the iron on an empty stomach. Do not take it within six hours of taking any hormones.

Although the treatments listed above work best if used together, you can probably get a good effect, even if the TPP, NADH, AMP, and MSM are left out. Except for the multivitamin and magnesium/malic acid, which should be taken forever, the above supplements can all be stopped after eight to twelve weeks. They can also be used safely, though, for long periods of time if needed, though you probably will not need the full dose.

Important Points

- The mitochondria are the energy furnaces in your cells that burn food for energy. Many studies and findings suggest that these furnaces are functioning inefficiently in CFIDS/FMS.
- Due to mitochondrial dysfunction, a person with CFIDS/FMS can lose over 75 percent of the energy in carbohydrates because they are shunted into the inefficient burning system. As a result, the body cannot burn fat and makes more fat. The furnace is turned down and the body becomes unable to make the "tools" the furnace needs to work well—a vicious cycle that occurs throughout the body, affecting the brain (fatigue, brain fog), liver (chemical and other sensitivities), bowel (malabsorption of nutrients) and muscles (pain and postexertional fatigue).
- A number of substances that are available in supplement form appear to be low, and, especially when used together for eight to twelve weeks, may get one's energy furnaces up and running. These include thiamine pyrophosphate (TPP), aspartates and malic acid, acetyl-L-carnitine, nicotinamide adenine dinucleotide plus high-energy hydrogen (NADH), sulfur, coenzyme Q_{10}, iron, copper, adenosine triphosphate (ATP), the B-complex vitamins (including B_{12}), and magnesium.

CHAPTER 9

More Natural Remedies

HAVING SURVIVED THE HIGHLY TECHNICAL INFOR-
mation in the last chapter, I think you'll be happy to join me in exploring
more down-to-earth natural remedies. These treatments are (often dramatically) helpful for CFIDS/FMS.

It pleases me that there has been a wonderful increase in the use of
herbal remedies. This renaissance has been especially true in Europe and
Asia, where the explosion of interest in herbal remedies has been associated
with a major increase in scientific research. In Europe, the German government's Federal Health Agency has created the Commission E, an independent group that evaluates the safety and effectiveness of various herbal
therapies. They have published a series of over 400 monographs that help
physicians to make informed decisions on how to use these tools. As a result, Germany and Japan each use over three times as many herbal remedies as are used in the entire United States. Hopefully, the United States
will eventually catch up with both Europe and Japan. While the German
government actually promotes education and awareness for its physicians,
the U.S. Food and Drug Administration (FDA) has prohibited manufacturers from making any therapeutic claims for herbal remedies or directly
supplying the scientific data or information on the herb's proper use with
the products. This chapter will supply this information for you.

Because the quality control of herbals is quite variable, a movement is underway to standardize herbal preparations by making sure that they have a specific amount of the active agent. So if the label says *standardized,* you have a better chance of the herbal being effective. If it has the complex wording I use in discussing that herbal product—for example, *24 percent glycosides*—better yet! Except for looking to see if these complex words are on the label of the herbal remedy, feel free to ignore the few complex names in this chapter.

Ginger—Great in CFIDS/FMS

Ginger can have wonderful health benefits for people with CFIDS/FMS. Although ginger is native to Asia, Jamaica is now its major producer, exporting over 2 million pounds a year. Sometimes, fresh ginger (high in the compound gingerol) and dried ginger (high in shogaol) have different effects. I will note the uses where this distinction is important. The benefits of ginger include the following:

- Relief of muscle and/or joint pain. Many components of ginger are, like aspirin and ibuprofen, potent inhibitors of inflammatory substances such as prostaglandins). Ginger is also thought to inhibit substance P, a pain mediator that is known to be elevated in FMS. For substance P inhibition, dried ginger seems to be most effective. In a study of ten patients with muscle pains and forty-six patients with arthritis (both rheumatoid and regular "wear and tear" osteoarthritis), 100 percent of muscle pain patients and 75 percent of arthritis patients noted relief. The recommended dose was 1,000 milligrams of powdered ginger a day. Many patients took 3,000 to 4,000 milligrams a day and noted quicker and better relief using the higher dose.[1] Try using the fresh ginger, as discussed below, and then try using a slice of dried ginger and see which works better for you.
- Decreased nausea and vomiting. Taking 500 to 1,000 milligrams of ginger is effective for this. Ginger also decreases bowel spasm while improving gastric motility (moving food out of the stomach to the bowels). These are often major problems in CFIDS/FMS, resulting in bloating after eating. Ginger can also inhibit diarrhea. In several studies, fresh (for example, roasted), but not dried, ginger was found to inhibit stomach ulcers caused by aspirin and ibuprofen.

- Increased thermogenesis (warming of the body). Fresh ginger works much better for this.
- Relief of migraine headaches.
- Dysequilibrium (for example, motion sickness). Although likely not as effective for vestibular (inner ear) dizziness, in which you feel like you are spinning in a circle, ginger inhibits the nausea associated with dizziness. For motion sickness, it works best when you take 1,000 milligrams four hours before travel.
- Increased blood pressure. This can be helpful for people with CFIDS/ FMS, who often have low blood pressure. Only dried ginger works for this purpose.

In addition to these benefits, ginger can decrease the risk of heart disease by platelet inhibition (like aspirin and vitamin E do) and by lowering cholesterol. It is a strong antioxidant and can inhibit certain bowel infections (*Salmonella* and Vibrio) and, in 5-percent and 25-percent aqueous extracts, can be effective against vaginal *Trichomonas* infections.

Side effects of ginger are minimal. Very high doses (for example, 6,000 milligrams of *dried* ginger) on an empty stomach can cause stomach problems. It is rare that such a high single dose is needed. The optimal dosing is not yet clear. Most research studies have used 1,000 milligrams of dry powdered ginger root. This is the form I used when I specifying doses above. This is equivalent to about 10 grams (one-third ounce, or about a quarter-inch slice) of fresh ginger root. Higher doses can be more effective initially for pain—for example, 500 to 1,000 milligrams of dry powder three to four times a day—with the dose lowered to the lowest effective dose in four to six weeks.

Although they have not been used in studies, minced ginger in a liquid base for cooking (similar to jarred minced garlic) and ginger tea granules, supplying 5,000 milligrams of ginger per cup of tea, are available. If you use fresh ginger in cooking or to make tea, do not peel it until just before use or some of the volatile (active) oils will evaporate.

Gingko Biloba—For Memory and Circulation

Ginkgo biloba extract has been shown to have multiple benefits for memory and depression. These include:

- Improving the decreased libido and erections and the delayed orgasm sometimes seen with antidepressant use. Dosages of 60 to 80 milligrams of ginkgo three times a day for six weeks are required for this.
- Decreasing the breast tenderness and mood shifts of premenstrual syndrome (PMS).[2]
- Helping to settle down dysequilibrium and vertigo.[3]
- Improving memory. This effect has been shown in healthy young volunteers and in older adults in many placebo-controlled studies.[4] Many CFIDS/FMS patients also find that ginkgo helps their memory. In twelve healthy males, electroencephalogram (EEG) testing showed that taking 120 to 240 milligrams of ginkgo biloba extract improved alpha brain wave activity in a way that supported improved cognitive function.
- Improving circulation. In general, ginkgo improves circulation in the brain and legs. More than forty controlled studies have shown this. By improving circulation, ginkgo may also decrease tinnitus (ringing in the ears) and headaches, as well as Raynaud's syndrome, in which spasms in the arteries of the fingers in response to cold cause pain and extreme coldness. This is sometimes seen in people with CFIDS/FMS. Ginkgo may also lower cholesterol and help angina.
- Helping asthma and bronchitis. In China, ginkgo is made into a tea for this purpose.
- Helping depression. Doses of 80 milligrams, taken three times a day, may be effective for this.

The ginkgo you buy should be a 50:1 extract standardized to contain 24-percent glycosides (it will say this on the label). For most purposes, 40 milligrams three times a day is the standard dose. Treating depression, however, requires 80 milligrams three times a day. It takes six weeks to see the effect of treatment. Serious side effects are quite uncommon, as are drug interactions. In fact, the side effects seen with ginkgo in studies were often *less* than the side effects seen with placebo.

Kava Kava—For Sleep and Anxiety

Kava kava (or, simply, kava) a member of the peppercorn family, has been one of the South Pacific's most revered herbs and intoxicants. Used in most tribal Oceania cultures for hundreds of years, it was central to many social celebrations and often used as a remedy for a number of physical ailments, as well as being a part of daily life. In many South Pacific cultures, kava has also been used medicinally. Uses include soothing the nerves, counteracting fatigue, inducing relaxation, aiding in weight loss and treating cystitis, urinary tract congestion and rheumatism. Hawaiian *kahunas* (medicine men) used it extensively for ailments such as "general debility (especially in children), weary muscles (a great restorer of strength), chills and head colds, difficulty in passing urine and sharp blinding headaches." Overall, kava was "found to reduce fatigue, allay anxiety and to produce a generally pleasant, cheerful and sociable attitude. . . [sometimes] bordering on intoxication."[5]

Kava was traditionally prepared as a drink from the ground-up herb. When used ceremonially, kava was usually taken on an empty stomach in the evening. Since the root needed to be softened, it was usually prechewed (traditionally, by virgins) or grated first.

In the United States, it is usually taken in capsule form. A single dose containing 150 to 210 milligrams of kava pyrones is the usual dose to induce sleep. Most capsules contain 30 percent kava pyrones, so a 250-milligram capsule has 75 milligrams. Thus, to get 150 to 210 milligrams of the pyrones, you would take 500 to 750 milligrams of the extract at night for sleep. At this dose many people find that it relieves insomnia and induces a deep, restful sleep with clear, epic-length dreams. Upon waking, they feel rested.[6]

When used for anxiety, the usual dose is one 100-milligram capsule three times a day. The effect begins in about one week and increases over the next eight weeks. Interestingly, while several placebo-controlled studies have shown kava to be as effective for anxiety as prescription medications like amitriptyline (Elavil) and diazepam (Valium), unlike the sedating prescription medications, it was not found to cause any significant side effects. Surprisingly, it actually improved mental functioning and clarity! Research also shows kava to be an excellent muscle relaxant. It seems to work by a mechanism similar to that of lidocaine (Novocain), which has been shown to be very beneficial for CFIDS/FMS.[7]

Although most people do not get any side effects when using kava alone for short periods, there are several cautions. Kava may strongly potentiate (increase) the effect of other sedative medications. This can be a good thing, however, if you are not too sedated. Although a study combining a blood alcohol level of 0.05 percent with kava did not show problems in humans, mice who took both together showed ten times the increase in sleep time. If you do combine kava with other sedating medications, you should do so only if it is not too sedating, and you should begin slowly, with very low doses. The German Commission E monograph on kava suggests it *not* be used in pregnancy or nonsituational depression (that is, depression for no apparent reason).[8]

A second concern with kava is that taking prolonged high doses may cause a dry, scaly rash that begins on the face and moves downward. Visual sensitivity to bright light may also occur. Taking the B vitamins may decrease this, as can staying in the dose range discussed above. If a rash occurs, stop taking the kava or lower the dose.[9]

Tyrosine—For Occasional Energy Boosts

Tyrosine is an amino acid (one of the building blocks of protein) that is used to make the neurotransmitter norepinephrine. This brain chemical is thought to be low in people with CFIDS/FMS. Tyrosine can be considered for *occasional* use, at a dose of 4,000 milligrams, to enhance performance. In one placebo-controlled study, twenty male marines took 35 milligrams of tyrosine per pound of body weight twice a day during a night of sleep deprivation. Tyrosine acted as a stimulant without significant side effects. The effect lasted for three hours.[10]

Lemon Balm—For Sleep

For people with CFIDS/FMS, the main use of lemon balm (also known as melissa) is to improve sleep. One study demonstrated that when combined with valerian (see below), in a dose of 90 to 180 milligrams of lemon balm plus 180 to 360 milligrams of valerian, taken at night, lemon balm improves deep sleep.

Used topically, lemon balm can have an antiviral effect against cold sores if used early in the outbreak. Loma-hephan cream, applied two to four times a day for five to ten days, was the product used in the study.[11] This corroborated previous studies showing antiviral effects of lemon balm.

Valerian—For Sleep and Anxiety

Valerian is another very useful herbal remedy for CFIDS/FMS. It has been used for at least 1,800 years. The Greeks named it *phu-,* which derives from the same word as the word *pew* that we use in response to something stinky. The name was well earned, as valerian has—to put it kindly—quite a distinctive odor (it is very stinky)! Cats seem to love it, though, and will go after it like catnip. Fortunately, there are valerian products with a coating that eliminates the smell.

Valerian is a mild sleep aid that has the interesting effect of calming you if you are anxious but acting as a stimulant if you are fatigued. Although not strong enough by itself to normalize sleep in the early stages of treating CFIDS/FMS, it decreases the amount of sleep medication needed. When symptoms have been resolved for six months and sleep medications are weaned off, some patients like to continue using it to ensure good sleep.

In a study using valerian for anxiety, at a dosage of 100 milligrams three times a day for three weeks, it was found to be more effective than placebo. Because valerian decreases fatigue, it is a helpful calming agent in CFIDS/FMS. Valerian also eases bowel spasms and may decrease menstrual cramps, fluid retention, and seizures.

The main problems with using valerian for sleep occur if you use an inappropriate dose (taking less than 180 milligrams is unlikely to be effective and taking over 450 milligrams is unlikely to add much benefit). Also, because it can be a stimulant for people who are fatigued, about 5 to 10 percent of CFIDS/FMS patients find they can't use it for sleep because it makes them hyper at night and keeps them up. Although considered safe for short-term use, even at high doses (and no significant toxicity has come to my attention with long-term use), I would likely limit the dose to 600 milligrams a day unless a higher dose shows clear benefit. Although it is used as a flavoring in the production of such processed foods as soft drinks and baked goods, I would *avoid* using valerian supplements during pregnancy. Valerian interacts well with other sleep medications and can also be taken with 300 micrograms of melatonin at night.

Peppermint Oil—For Bowel Spasm

Peppermint, native to Europe, has been a popular American remedy for treating colon spasm for at least 200 years. Patients with CFIDS/FMS often have symptoms of irritable bowel syndrome (IBS), or spastic colon, which include abdominal pain, alternating diarrhea and constipation, gas, and bloating. Although treating the yeast and/or parasite infections can often resolve these symptoms, peppermint oil can also be helpful. This was demonstrated in a successful placebo-controlled study using peppermint oil for IBS.[12] If nausea is present, it can be taken with ginger (see page 160).

Peppermint oil may also suppress intestinal candida and may dissolve gallstones. It is important to be aware that even though it eases spasms in the colon, peppermint oil can cause indigestion in the stomach. Because of this, I only use *enteric coated* peppermint oil—that is, capsules that are specially made not to dissolve until after they are past the stomach. They should be taken between meals, not with food. Use one to two capsules containing 0.2 cc each three times a day as needed.

Menthol, one of peppermint oil's principal constituents, can also be used topically for pain relief. It acts as a counterirritant, stimulating the nerves that perceive cold, while suppressing those for pain. Use it in a cream or ointment with 1.25 to 16 percent menthol applied to the affected area up to three to four times a day in the affected area. Be aware that it can cause a rash, especially if a heating pad is used over it.

Glutathione—For Detoxification and Immunity

Glutathione is a critical antioxidant. It is a protein compound made up of three amino acids. Although some glutathione comes from the diet, most is made by the body. Its production requires energy molecules that may be low in people with CFIDS/FMS. The body requires adenosine triphosphate (ATP) and nicotinamide adenine dinucleotide phosphate hydride (NADPH, which in turn requires the active form of vitamin B_1 called thiamine pyrophosphate [TPP] to make glutathione). Because these compounds may be low in people with CFIDS/FMS, glutathione activity may be low.

Glutathione is needed to protect the cells' mitochondrial energy furnaces from damaging themselves. This function is critical. The mitochondria make a steady stream of damaging free radicals as an unavoidable byproduct of using oxygen to make energy. Glutathione acts here, like vitamins C and E, as a very potent antioxidant. This activity is so important that the mitochondria are the first areas to be damaged if glutathione deficiency occurs. A body of evidence is also building that suggests that the cumulative effect of these free radicals are major causes of degenerative diseases and the aging process.

Similarly, glutathione helps the liver detoxify compounds made by the body—what the liver was made to do—and the thousands of new chemicals and medications that modern society exposes us to. Dealing with all these new chemicals is not something the human liver was expecting to do. Detoxifying cigarette smoke, chemicals, alcohol, or the medications one takes (especially acetaminophen [Tylenol]) can markedly deplete the body's glutathione. This can result in later chemical and medication sensitivity, in addition to damaging the mitochondrial energy furnaces.

A third major function of glutathione is in aiding proper immune function. Strenuous aerobic exercise can deplete muscle antioxidants. Many chronic infections also can cause depletion of glutathione (and thus mitochondrial damage). Many CFIDS/FMS patients have found that taking glutathione, especially by intravenous injection, has been very beneficial. In fact, it has often been ranked as one of the single most effective supplements. Taking 1,000 milligrams of vitamin C plus 400 international units of natural vitamin E each day may augment its effectiveness. While the average diet supplies about 150 milligrams of glutathione a day, the majority of the body's glutathione is made by the liver. Sulfur intake, from protein foods and, perhaps, in the form of supplemental methylsulfonylmethane (MSM) increases the body's glutathione production, as does taking 500 milligrams of N-acetylcysteine (NAC) a day. Taking 250 milligrams of glutathione by mouth each day may be less effective than taking NAC, as glutathione gets digested. It is also more expensive than NAC.

Stevia and Sweet Balance—Healthy Sweeteners!

Stevia is a natural sweetener that is 30 to 100 times sweeter than sugar. It has been used for centuries and is likely to be much safer than sugar or aspartame (sold under the brand names Equal and NutraSweet). Stevia has essentially no calories and is high in several minerals. About 40 percent of Japanese low-calorie products are made with stevia and many other countries permit stevia to be used in food processing.

In addition, stevia inhibits dental cavities. Small amounts go a long way. It tastes good and can be used in drinks, cereals, and so on. Use the liquid form. For sources of what I feel is the best tasting liquid stevia, see Appendix J: Resources. If you want to make your own from scratch, mix the powdered leaves with water and let them stand overnight. You can then cook the mixture down into a concentrated syrup that will keep in the refrigerator for about one week. I prefer the premade form recommended above. It is easy, tastes good, and lasts a long time. Some people prefer a product called Sweet Balance, a powder made from the lo-han fruit that tastes like sugar but is much more healthful.

St. John's Wort—For Depression

St. John's wort, also known as hypericum, is used more than fluoxetine (Prozac) to treat depression in Germany, where about 70 percent of physicians routinely treat with herbal remedies. In an analysis of twenty-three studies on 1,757 depressed patients, 60 percent improved with hypericum, versus 22 percent on placebo. In eight studies comparing hypericum with standard antidepressants such as Prozac, the herb was found to be as effective or more effective. Over 66 million daily doses of hypericum were prescribed in Germany in 1994, where it is used for anxiety, depression, and sleep disorders.

St. John's wort has been used since ancient times as a diuretic and for wound healing, sciatica, and hip pain. It has been used throughout Europe and the Americas. Its name comes from the fact that its flowers bloom around June 24, St. John's day in the Christian calendar, and from its red pigment, which was associated with the blood of St. John the Baptist.

In addition to being an effective antidepressant, St. John's wort has mild antifungal effects when used topically in tincture form or taken orally. It also speeds wound and incision healing and decreases scar formation. Although it was initially thought that St. John's wort acted by inhibiting an enzyme called monoamine oxidase (MAO), new research shows this not to be the case. This is important because MAO inhibitors cannot be combined with other antidepressants. Happily, we have seen no problems with drug interactions, but I would limit the dose to 900 milligrams a day if you are taking it with another antidepressant.

Although its exact mechanism of action is still being actively explored, St. John's wort seems to work by increasing the effectiveness of the brain chemicals serotonin and dopamine, modulating the relationship between the immune system and the mood, and supplying important nutrients such as flavonoids. St. John's wort is safer and better tolerated than Prozac and other antidepressants. Thirty-one percent of patients taking tricyclic antidepressants and 17 percent of those patients taking Prozac stop taking those medications because of side effects, including sexual dysfunction, headache, nausea, anxiety, insomnia, dry mouth, drowsiness, diarrhea, sweating, and tremors. In contrast to this, St. John's wort is almost free of significant side effects at the usual dose of 300 to 600 milligrams three times a day (or one-third in the morning and two-thirds at night). It has been prescribed for millions of people, and I have seen almost no published cases or reports of any serious toxicity. At twice the standard dose, heightened sensitivity to sunlight and/or or ultraviolet light can occur. Adding 200 to 250 milligrams of 5-hydroxytryptophan (5-HTP) a day (take most of it at night) makes St. John's wort even more effective and also helps improve sleep. Do not take it with AIDS medications.

St. John's wort comes in many forms. Be sure to protect it from light, which inactivates the active hypericum, or temperatures over 85°F. It takes approximately six weeks to see its effect.

Elderberry Extract—For the Flu

Elderberry extract can help ease flu symptoms and shorten the duration of the illness. In one study, taking 4 tablespoons a day (2 tablespoons a day for children) for three days was found to significantly improve flu symptoms, and 90 percent of patients were completely well in two to three days, versus six days for the placebo group.

Feverfew—For Headaches

Feverfew, a member of the aster family, is very effective in preventing migraines in some patients, while decreasing their severity in others. Originating in the Balkans, it now grows wild throughout much of North and South America. Its name derives from its history of being used to lower fever.

Traditionally, feverfew has been used for headache, vertigo, fevers, depression, menstrual regulation, and colic. Its use dates back to the writings of the first-century Greek physician Dioscorides. In the Andes, one twig is steeped in a cup of boiling water and drunk once daily. Feverfew has also been applied topically for pain relief.

As with many herbs, the formulation is very important. One vital component for smooth muscle relaxation, parthenolide, a type of compound known as a sesquiterpene lactone, was shown to be absent in extracts made from dry leaves. Several studies have shown feverfew to be effective for decreasing the frequency of migraines in about 70 percent of patients. These studies used either encapsulated freeze-dried leaves containing 40 to 114 milligrams once a day or one large fresh leaf (or three small ones) once a day. Make sure the product you use is standardized to have at least 0.2-percent parthenolide or grow the plant and use the fresh leaves (don't chew the leaves if they cause mouth sores). It takes a few weeks for the effect to begin. Feverfew is best used to prevent, rather than treat, migraines. Although studies of its effectiveness have been done, and no significant side effects have been reported in 300 patients who had taken it for about two and a half years, studies to fully document the safety of long-term use have yet to be done. *Do not* take feverfew if you are pregnant.

Trigger Point Pressure—For Painful Spots

This simple and often overlooked technique can be helpful for treating tender spots. If you push on these spots for thirty to forty-five seconds, applying about twenty to thirty pounds of pressure (for example, with your thumb), they will often be very tender and then the pain will subside. This can often be done in the context of a massage. Although not recommended for dozens of tender areas at one time, it can be very helpful if a few nagging spots remain after treatment.

Glucosamine Sulfate—For Aches and Pains

Glucosamine is a cartilage compound that has been shown, in several controlled studies, to be helpful for osteoarthritis (wear-and-tear arthritis). Although the exact way it works is not certain, it appears to stimulate cartilage production by bone cells. The usual dose is 500 milligrams three times a day. It usually takes two weeks to see *any* effect and six weeks to tell if it will help or not. After six weeks, I would stay on 1,500 milligrams a day until the beneficial effect plateaus, and then drop it to the lowest dose it takes to maintain the effect.

In a head-on study of 200 osteoarthritis patients using 1,500 milligrams a day of either glucosamine sulfate or 1,200 milligrams a day of ibuprofen (Motrin), the Motrin worked better for the first two weeks. After that, the glucosamine was as effective as Motrin. The glucosamine group had significantly fewer side effects than the Motrin group (six versus thirty-five). These side effects were much milder as well.

Another important point is that Motrin and other nonsteroidal anti-inflammatory drugs do not slow down the progression of arthritis, and may actually make the arthritis worse. Glucosamine may actually help to heal the arthritic joint. Benefit often persists after the glucosamine is stopped.

I would use glucosamine *sulfate* (not chloride), as the sulfate may also be helpful in both joint repair and the body's mitochondrial (energy furnace) function.

Pantothenic Acid—For Adrenal Function and Weight Loss

Pantothenic acid is vitamin B_5, and is a major part of coenzyme A. The recommended daily intake (RDI) is 10 milligrams a day. In one study, animals supplemented with pantothenic acid lived about 20 percent longer. Taking anywhere from 100 milligrams of pantothenic acid a day to 500 milligrams three times a day can improve adrenal gland function and allergic runny nose. Taken in the form of 600 milligrams of dexapanthenol at bedtime, it is also very helpful for constipation. Dexapanthenol is available by prescription from Professional Arts Pharmacy. (See Appendix J: Resources.)

A Chinese study suggested that pantothenic acid helps weight loss by decreasing appetite while you're dieting. Patients took 2,000 milligrams of pantothenic acid four times a day while on a 1,000-calorie per day diet. They lost two to six pounds per week without weakness or hunger, and without making ketones, a sign that the body is reacting to what it perceives as starvation. When your desired weight is achieved, cut back to 1,000 to 3,000 milligrams a day.

Essential Fatty Acids—For Many Benefits

Essential fatty acids (EFAs) play an important and yet poorly recognized role in human health. They are involved in many functions, including hormone production, immune function, and the regulation of inflammation, blood flow, and the amount and wateriness of saliva, tears, and other bodily fluids produced. EFAs also are part of the makeup the membranes surrounding every cell in the body.

Most Americans get only about 10 percent of the amount of EFAs they need for optimal well-being. This is despite the fact that the average person's fat intake has increased by about fifty pounds a year in the last century. Unfortunately, food-processing techniques have essentially removed the EFAs from our food supply because oils are expressed at high temperatures and previously healthy vegetable oils are hydrogenated, or saturated, to harden and stabilize them. These processing steps both eliminate the EFAs, and make it difficult for your body to use the EFAs it does get.

Symptoms of EFA deficiency are many and varied, and include fatigue, poor memory, recurrent respiratory infections, gas, bloating, arthralgias (aches and pains), constipation, cracking nails, depression, dry hair and skin, and inadequate saliva, tears, and vaginal lubrication.

Oils and fatty acids are not the same thing. *Fats* usually refer to saturated fats, which are solid at room temperature. *Oils* usually refer to unsaturated fats, which are liquid at room temperature. *Saturated* means that the hooks (bonds) that connect each of the atoms in the fat molecules are all in use, and there is no room for any new atoms to attach. This makes the fat molecules straight and rigid, and thus hard. Unsaturated fats are either monounsaturated or polyunsaturated. Monounsaturated fats have one open hook and polyunsaturated fats have several open hooks where molecules can attach. This makes them more flexible (fluid). If the first open hook (double bond) is six carbon atoms from the end of the fat molecule, it is called an omega-6 fatty acid. Most vegetable oils are omega-6 oils. If the first open hook is 3 carbon atoms from the end, the molecule is an omega-3 fatty acid. Fish oils and flaxseed oil are omega-3 oils.

How your body is able to use the fat depends on whether it is a saturated, omega-3, or omega-6 fatty acid. In many processed foods (for example, margarine) the unsaturated fats are changed from their healthy natural state, in which they are known as cis-fatty acids, to an unnatural unhealthy state, in which they are called trans-fatty acids. These trans-fatty acids can cause heart disease, obesity, immune suppression, and decreased testosterone levels, while worsening fatty acid deficiencies. Despite advertising hype to the contrary, margarine is probably less healthy than butter, and I recommend not using it.

All cells in the body are enclosed in a cell membrane, a balloon-like wall. This wall is made up of fatty acids and a phosphorus molecule, usually choline or serine. This combination is called a *phospholipid*. The type of fat available to your body when it makes cell membranes (saturated versus omega-3 and -6) is critical. Your body likes to use omega-3 and -6 fatty acids because these are more fluid. When these are not available, your body has to use saturated fats. This results in rigid, poorly functioning cellular walls. Cell membranes perform the critical functions of allowing and keeping in water, minerals, and nutrients. In addition, the regulatory hormones and neurotransmitters—molecules that tell the cells what they need to do—function by fitting into receptors located in the cell membranes. Stiff cell walls can make it hard for these functions to occur properly.

EFAs are also critical for making an important class of body chemicals called prostaglandins. These are an important group of hormones that regulate inflammation, pain, bowel function, fluid balance, mood, allergies, and the production of some other hormones. There are three main series of prostaglandins, designated PGE_1, PGE_2, and PGE_3. Series 1 and 3 prostaglandins, which are made from vegetable EFAs and fish oils, decrease inflammation and improve mood. Series 2 prostaglandins, which are produced from animal fats, increase inflammation. To summarize this:

- Linoleic acid (in safflower or corn oil) ⇨ dihomogamma linolenic acid (DGLA, also in primrose and borage oil) ⇨ PGE_1, which decreases inflammation and improves mood. Making PGE_1 also requires vitamin B_6, zinc, and magnesium. The process is inhibited by sugar, alcohol, trans-fatty acids, and saturated fats.

- Arachidonic acid (in animal fats) ⇨ PGE_2, which promotes inflammation and increases the risk of heart disease.
- Alpha-linolenic acid (in flaxseed oil) ⇨ eicosapentaenoic acid (EPA, also in fish oils) ⇨ PGE_3, which is anti-inflammatory and protects against heart disease.

To treat possible essential fatty acid deficiency, I recommend taking the following:

- Flaxseed oil. Take ½ tablespoon (or 4,000 to 5,000 milligrams in capsule form) daily.
  plus
- Cod liver oil or EPA. Take ½ tablespoon (or 5,000 milligrams in capsule form) daily. *Do not* take cod liver oil if you are pregnant or trying to get pregnant, however. EPA can be helpful during pregnancy.
  plus
- Evening primrose oil or borage oil. Take 500 milligrams of either one twice a day.

Take these supplements for three months. If pain improves, which is likely, and dry skin, dry hair, dry mouth and/or dry eyes improve, then you probably had an essential fatty acid deficiency. After three months, you can decrease the above regimen to ½ tablespoon of flaxseed oil or fish oil a day and two to three servings a week of tuna, salmon, or herring. At the same time, decrease your consumption of saturated fats and trans-fatty acids, found in solid fats and processed foods such as margarine, and substitute olive, canola, and/or safflower oil. It is worth buying good brands of oils from a health food store, even though they may be more expensive. Look for a brand that is certified as organic on the label by a third-party source. Healthy oils have a smooth, nutty flavor instead of tasting bland or bitter. It is best if the oil is in an opaque plastic bottle and kept in the refrigerated section of the health food store. When you get it home, keep it in your refrigerator or, if you want to extend its shelf life, your freezer. I would add 1,200 to 2,000 units of vitamin E to any bottle of oil when you open it. This can be done by popping and squeezing the contents of three to five 400-unit vitamin E capsules into the bottle of oil. One highly respected maker of flaxseed oil is Barlean's Organic Oils (see Appendix J: Resources).

Combined with magnesium, evening primrose oil can be *very* helpful for PMS. The recommended dose is six to twelve capsules a day and it takes three months to see the effect. You can then drop to six capsules a day for the week before your period. Over time, you can cut back to the lowest dose that maintains the benefit. Depression that does not respond to St. John's wort or antidepressant medications will sometimes improve with omega-3 fatty acids (flaxseed or fish oils).

A Word of Caution

While herbs are generally safe when used correctly, there are a number of herbs that can cause liver inflammation. Chaparral has caused liver failure. Some other herbs that may cause liver disease include germander, comfrey, mistletoe, skullcap, margosa oil, maté tea, gordolobo, yerba tea, Jin Bu Huan, and pennyroyal. And there are many more. Always follow label instructions. If you have unexplained mild elevation of your liver blood tests (SGOT and SGPT [ALT and AST]), stay off your herbs for three months and then repeat the test.

If you are interested in learning more about herbs in general, two excellent resources are the American Botanical Council and the *Quarterly Review of Natural Medicine*. (See Appendix J: Resources.)

Important Points

- Ginger can be very helpful for pain, nausea, and dizzines.
- Valerian, kava kava, lemon balm, 5-HTP, passionflower, and/or low-dose melatonin can help sleep, and also help anxiety.
- Ginkgo biloba can help memory, depression, and antidepressant-induced sexual dysfunction.
- Enteric-coated peppermint oil helps irritable bowel syndrome (IBS or spastic colon).
- St. John's wort is very helpful for depression.
- Stevia and Sweet Balance are healthy sweeteners that you can use instead of sugar.
- If you have dry eyes, dry mouth, and/or dry skin, take supplemental essential fatty acids.

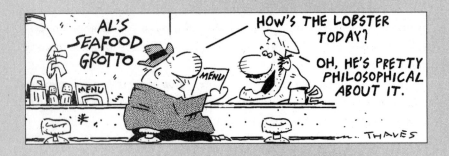

10

Other Areas to Explore

MOST CFIDS/FMS PATIENTS OBTAIN FULL RESO-
lution of, or at least substantial improvement in, their symptoms with the
approaches I have discussed so far. However, some patients still suffer significant disabilities. Several physicians have found success with other treatments. Many of these treatments are worth exploring. In addition, two
areas remain that I hold in high regard and stress with all my patients—exercise (once you are on treatment) and being gentle with yourself.

Food Allergies

I have found that most of my patients' food and other sensitivities resolve
when I treat their underlying yeast overgrowth, parasitic infections, and
underactive adrenal glands. Sometimes food sensitivities persist, however,
and are often hard to isolate or verify because of the diversity of reactions
that people display. Many of these reactions are extremely subtle or are also
symptoms of other conditions. In addition, most people suffer their own
unique combination of symptoms. To further complicate matters, many
people are sensitive to food additives, which are listed on food labels under
a variety of names or are present as integral parts of other additives. One
example is monosodium glutamate (MSG).

Dr. Jeffrey Bland, a well-known nutritional biochemist, has a food product that can be used with an elimination diet to determine food allergies and often helps in bowel detoxification. The product is a powder that supplies necessary nutrients from very low allergy sources, such as rice. During the initial seven to ten days of the elimination diet, it allows you to avoid all "allergic foods." If your symptoms resolve during this time span, you are justified in suspecting that you have food allergies. You can then begin reintroducing the different foods as described below to determine exactly which ones are problems for you. Although Dr. Bland's food product costs about $300, it can help to determine food sensitivities. However, you should not use this approach if you have very severe CFS—for example, if you are bedridden—because you need to strengthen your body as much as possible before you go through the withdrawal phase. For more information on Dr. Bland's powder, contact Metagenics (see Appendix J: Resources).

Unfortunately, I have found the IgG Elisa/EIA test, a blood test used to detect food allergies, not to be very helpful. It is more expensive than elimination diets, and it leaves people with the often incorrect belief that they are sensitive to everything. I have found that most food allergy blood tests are better at making people crazy than at distinguishing true allergies. A recent study done at Bastyr University, an excellent naturopathic school, found that when a single person's blood was sent to a number of laboratories doing IgG Elisa/EIA testing, the labs gave *very* different results on the same blood sample. The patient was found to be allergic to 22 percent versus 76 percent of foods tested, depending on which lab did the test! Even when several tubes of blood from one person—but labeled with different names—were sent to each lab, they still got very different results![1] I sometimes use a blood test called an IGE immuno-linked immunosorbent assay (ELISA) (*not* the IgG or IgG ELISA) that screens for common foods and is more likely to give a false-negative than a false-positive result. In addition, ELISA-ACT allergy testing at Serammune Physicians Laboratories may be more reliable.[2] IgE food allergy testing can be done at Great Smokey Mountain Labs (though I order the test only if the patient agrees to ignore the part of the test that gives IGG results—see page 77). However, the best approaches that I have found for determining what food allergies, if any, are present is the elimination diet.

In an elimination diet, the most common problem foods are eliminated from the diet for two weeks. The foods that seem to cause problems for the most people are milk, wheat, eggs, citrus, monosodium glutamate (MSG), sugar, alcohol, chocolate, and coffee. People with food allergies usually go through withdrawal when they cut out the foods to which they are allergic. They feel worse for the first seven to ten days. But once they get over the hump, they often feel dramatically better. The eliminated food groups are then reintroduced, one every few days, to isolate the specific problem foods. These problem foods are left out of the diet for a few months and then are slowly reintroduced, since the sensitivity will often have decreased. Once reintroduced, the problem foods are initially used only every three to seven days to see how they are tolerated.

Many physicians who practice what is called environmental medicine use sublingual neutralization, among other approaches, and are very skilled at treating food allergies. Although I don't use these approaches, and although they are controversial, I have seen them work wonders for many people. Another excellent technique is the Nambudripad allergy elimination technique (NAET), named after Dr. Devi S. Nambudripad, who developed it (see page 332). It combines acupressure and applied kinesiology (muscle-testing) to look for and treat underlying sensitivities. The wonderful thing about sublingual neutralization and NAET is that there is no need to use an elimination diet and they often eliminate your sensitivity to these foods. They can also be used for severe cases called "multiple chemical sensitivity."

Multiple Chemical Sensitivity Syndrome

NAET practitioners and environmental medicine physicians can be especially helpful for people who have multiple chemical sensitivity (MCS) syndrome. I believe that this syndrome is a subset of chronic fatigue syndrome. In multiple chemical sensitivity syndrome, the body has given up and is reactive to almost everything in the environment. Many CFIDS/FMS patients have multiple allergies and sensitivities to environmental chemicals and medications. However, while this is common, it is not multiple chemical sensitivity syndrome.

Patients with multiple chemical sensitivity syndrome cannot live in a normal house because they can become deathly ill if a new carpet is put in, if the walls are painted or wallpapered, or if pesticide is sprayed. They can become ill just from washing the dishes or reading a book. They can react negatively to any or all of the thousands of chemicals with which we normally come in contact in our day-to-day lives.[3] For patients who have this very extreme problem, I recommend an excellent book by Sherry Rogers, M.D., entitled *Tired or Toxic* (see Appendix I). Dr. Grace Ziem, in Baltimore, Maryland, is also very skilled at treating MCS.

Methylsulfonylmethane (MSM), a natural sulfur compound (*not* sulfa) is very helpful for arthritis, allergies, wound healing, and pain. The recommended dose is 3,000 to 12,000 milligrams a day, and it should be taken with vitamin C to enhance absorption. This is a lot of capsules. A powder form is available, but it tastes awful. If you choose to use a high dose, mix the powder in 1 to 2 ounces of water and drink it down quickly, all at once, followed by a glass of water. A better tasting form is being developed. After six to twelve weeks you can taper down the dose. I used to use 3,000 milligrams a day during hay fever season and 500 to 1,000 milligrams a day other times of the year for general allergies and well-being—until one twenty-minute NAET treatment eliminated my hay fever.

Magnesium sulfate, injected intramuscularly, often helps people with CFIDS/FMS, especially those whose achiness is severe but who get diarrhea from taking magnesium by mouth. A good dose is 2 grams (2,000 milligrams) once a week for four weeks. Administered this way, magnesium sulfate is inexpensive, but it can be a literal pain in the butt. To combat this problem, I like to add a small amount of Novocain to the shot. Some physicians increase the level of magnesium and add the B vitamins, including intramuscular B_{12}, and calcium. Called a Myers cocktail and given intravenously, this combination has produced dramatic benefits, especially for people whose main problems are achiness, asthma, or migraine. (For one recipe for this mix, see Appendix G.)

Nasal Congestion and Sinusitis

If you enjoy relief from your chronic fatigue whenever you take tetracycline, and if the other infections discussed in Chapter 4 do not seem to be your problem, you may have chronic sinusitis. Dr. Alexander C. Chester III, a physician practicing in Washington, D.C., has been a strong advocate of checking for nasal congestion and sinusitis as a cause of chronic fatigue. He has found that many patients improve significantly when they observe a regimen to combat sinusitis. This includes people who never even suspected that they had nasal problems.[4] Fatigue as a result of nasal problems used to be more recognized in medicine. Its importance is being rediscovered.

The treatment trial that Dr. Chester recommends for nasal congestion and sinusitis includes the following:

- 500 milligrams of the antibiotic Keflex four times a day for one week. If there is no improvement in your symptoms, switch to 100 milligrams of Doxycycline (also sold as Doryx, Monodox, Vibramycin, and Vibra-Tabs) twice a day for one week. Both Keflex and doxycycline are prescription antibiotics. Although Dr. Chester begins with Keflex, I prefer to begin with doxycycline.
- A 0.1-percent xylometazoline spray three times a day for three days. This is a prescription nasal spray.
- 60 milligrams of pseudoephedrine (in Sudafed and other over-the-counter medications) four times a day, or 120 milligrams of sustained-release Sudafed twice a day for two weeks. This is a decongestant. Be aware that it can cause shakiness or heart palpitations in some people.
- Inhaling steam for twenty minutes three times a day for two weeks to open your nasal passages. To do this, boil water in a pot on the stove or fill your bathroom sink with steaming water. Then lean over the water, with a towel draped over your head, and inhale the steam. Be careful not to burn yourself. Better yet, use a nasal steamer (see Appendix J: Resources for suppliers of these products).
- Sleeping for at least eight hours each night.
- Consuming no beer, wine, or milk products.

I also recommend following the regimen for treating infections described on page 65. If you find your sinus symptoms improving with these regimens, you should consider using Breathe Right nasal strips to keep your nostrils open. Sometimes, nasal or sinus surgery is needed. For patients with chronic sinusitis, I also strongly recommend the book *Sinus Survival* by Robert S. Ivker (Tarcher/Putnam, 2000; see Appendix I: Recommended Reading).

Medications

Many medications can cause fatigue as a side effect. If you are on a medication and your fatigue has been worse since you started taking it, talk to your physician about alternative measures or about just stopping it.

Interestingly, a blood pressure–raising enzyme called angiotensin-converting enzyme (ACE) has been found to be elevated in CFIDS/FMS patients.[5] Despite this, their blood pressure may still be low, due, for example, to underactive adrenal glands. According to some physicians, CFIDS/FMS symptoms and depression have improved in a few patients who were given the ACE inhibitor captopril (Capoten) for hypertension. Other doctors have found that some CFIDS/FMS patients improved with nimodipine (Nimotop) or amlodipine (Norvasc), calcium-channel blockers that relax the blood vessels to allow more blood and oxygen to get to the brain and heart.[6] If your blood pressure is high, you might consider a trial of Nimotop or, if that is too expensive, Norvasc, followed by a trial of hydralazine (Apresoline) and then a trial of quinapril (Accupril), for two weeks each, to see which feels the best to you. More importantly, if you have CFIDS/FMS and high blood pressure, you are at high risk of having sleep apnea.

Researchers are also studying treatment with high doses of intravenous gamma globulin and ampligen, both of which are immune-function enhancers. These treatments cost many thousands of dollars per year, and I do not think that most patients need them. I do find, though, that weekly intramuscular injections of 4 cc of gamma globulin (Gammar) for four weeks sometimes help patients with recurrent infections. These shots, luckily, are not as expensive. The Gammar has been difficult, but not impossible, to find since the Gulf War, however.

The Goldstein Protocol

Dr. Jay Goldstein, a well-known researcher working on brain chemistry and CFIDS/FMS, has come up with a list of recommended treatments that may be helpful. Because the agents he uses act directly on the disordered blood flow in the brain, Dr. Goldstein finds that patients generally know what effect each medication will have within one hour—and even within minutes for some agents.[7] (For information about some Goldstein Protocol treatments, see Appendix E: Treatment Protocol Checklist for Chronic Fatigue and Fibromyalgia.) His book, *Treatment Options in Chronic Fatigue Syndrone* (Haworth Press, 1995) gives a more detailed description of his protocol.

Chiari Malformations and Cervical Stenosis

Mike Rosner, M.D., a wonderful neurosurgeon, has reported seeing some patients with a diagnosis of CFIDS/FMS who improved with surgical treatment. He found that two unusual malformations of the skull or spinal canal could compress the brain and/or spinal cord, causing symptoms that mimicked those of CFIDS/FMS. When the compression was surgically released, patients with these malformations sometimes improved.

The Chiari I malformation (CMI) is a condition in which the back of the skull is underdeveloped, compressing the back of the brain, which is called the *cerebellar tonsils*. These tonsils are then squeezed out of the opening at the base of the skull, called the *foramen magnum*. This is called *tonsillar herniation*. The cerebellar tonsils are also squeezed against the brain stem. CMI is defined as occurring when these structures are pushed out of the bottom of the skull through the foramen magnum by at least 3 to 5 millimeters (0.12 to 0.2 inch). As with FMS/CFS, CMI can be genetic. There are also situations in which the brain stem is compressed without tonsillar herniation.

In cervical stenosis, the spinal cord is compressed because the spinal tube is unusually narrow. Nerve signals leave the brain via the spinal cord to travel the rest of the body. This critical nerve bundle passes through and is protected by the spinal canal, a kind of protective bony tube in the neck. If the spinal canal is narrowed, whether genetically, by arthritis, or for any other reason, this is called cervical stenosis. This can compress the spinal cord, again causing symptoms that mimic those of CFIDS/FMS.

While it is not known how common these problems are, it is a current topic of research. Early data suggests, first, that CMI and CS are not much more common in people with CFIDS/FMS than in healthy people, based on magnetic resonance imaging (MRI) scans as read by most radiologists. Second, the kinds of changes seen in neurologic tests done during physical examinations of people with CMI or CS are *much* more common in CFIDS/FMS patients than in healthy patients (75 percent versus 10 percent). About 90 percent of the neurologic changes could, however, be explained by changes on the (technically normal) MRI.

Because of these two seemingly opposite findings, some people may use this study to suggest that CMI and CS are rare *or* common in people CFIDS/FMS! As often happens, this study raises as many questions as it answers.

Let me put this in perspective. In disc disease, x-rays and MRIs by themselves are not very reliable in making the diagnosis. The same problem occurs with CMI and CS. Given fifty spine MRIs of patients with and without disc disease, radiologists cannot reliably tell which group of patients has severe pain and which group is healthy and pain-free. Indeed, if you lie and say the healthy patients have severe back pain, the MRI report will usually be read as showing several areas of disc disease. This is not to put down radiologists. The radiologists I've had the honor of knowing and working with have been superb. It simply shows the limits of our technology.

Like disc disease, the diagnosis of CMI and CS needs to be made by a combination of MRI, symptoms, and physical exam findings that all match up. Unfortunately, many of the symptoms of CFIDS/FMS are similar to CMI/CS symptoms, making it harder to tell if CMI/CS is rare in CFIDS/FMS patients or suggesting that they all have CMI/CS. Since over 85 percent of CFIDS/FMS patients improve without surgery, I suspect it's the former.

Unlike disc disease, which tends to be very overread on MRIs (that is, it is often seen when, in fact, there is no problem from disc disease), it seems that CMI/CS are very underread on MRIs. In a study by Dan Malone, M.D., a wonderful University of Wisconsin rheumatologist, 271 chronic pain patients were evaluated neurologically. Of these, 144 showed changes that lead Dr. Malone to recommend an MRI for CMI/CS using a special, more sensitive, MRI procedure. Eighty-eight of these had the MRIs. Only 1 was read as positive for CMI and 7 were read as having significant CS. In contrast, when Dr. Malone and another neurosurgeon read 79 of these MRIs, they felt 63 of 79 patients had significant CS or CMI. Thirty-nine of the 63 patients were evaluated by a neurosurgeon, 23 had surgery, and another 11 had surgery recommended but had not yet undergone surgery when the study was presented.

In another study, of 22 FMS patients operated on (I don't know if they were part of the 23 patients above), 81 percent had less pain, 75 percent less brain fog, and 20 percent less fatigue after surgery. These results persisted when the patients were checked at least six months after surgery. This suggests that CMI and CS are underdiagnosed—that is, most cases are missed—when radiologists use standard CMI/CS diagnostic criteria.

As research and clinical experience show that over 85 percent of patients improve with nonsurgical therapies, I suspect that either the symptoms of most CFIDS/FMS patients are not caused by CMI/CS, or that because the MRI test shows normal-sized bony structures in most CFIDS/

FMS patients yet neurologic examination suggests CMI or CS, it could be that there is swelling of the brain or spinal cord tissue causing the compression, despite a normal-sized skull or spinal canal. This could occur with infections and/or hormonal or nutritional deficiencies, and would account for all the above findings. It may be analogous to carpal tunnel syndrome—a result of nerve compression that improves with thyroid or B_6. Spinal cord compression could then be aggravated by whiplash injury or other head and neck injuries, or if the head is bent backward during surgical intubation for an extended period. These same triggers could cause FMS/CFIDS by a host of other mechanisms, however, and usually resolve without surgery. This is why some experts recommend a thorough neurological examination and (if indicated by exam) a screening MRI scan of the cervical spine and brain in all patients with FMS *who do not respond to conventional medical therapy.*

As noted above, CMI and CS are checked for with a neurologic exam of the brain and an MRI of the brain and cervical (neck) spine. Unfortunately, as with most tests, significant abnormalities in people with CFIDS/FMS will often be read as normal if not done and/or interpreted in specific ways. Although the exam for CMI and CS is complex, there are some screening tests that can simplify things. Here are some examples:

- You have *very* active knee reflexes (present in most CFIDS/FMS patients) *and* the reflex gets even more active if checked with your head extended backward on the neck, so your head is looking up at the ceiling.
- You have a lot of trouble with the hand-flip exam: With the palms of your hands down in front of you (parallel to the ground, with one hand on top of the other and touching), repeatedly quickly turn the top hand over back and forth. This means the upper palm, alternating with the back of the upper hand, will be touching the back of the bottom hand. Flip the top hand back and forth around five to ten times.
- Cold sensation to touch diminishes markedly as a cold object moves from your face to your neck to midchest—for example, while your skin is touched with a cool spoon or other metal object. The spoon should not slide down, but six or so areas should be touched for one to two seconds each.

If two of these three tests are positive, I would recommend a referral to Dr. Rosner and order an MRI if the patient does not get better with my medical therapy. Not everyone with a positive MRI has symptoms. It makes sense to me to treat this without surgery before spending thousands of dollars on MRIs and even more on surgery, with its attendant risks.

There are also some other very helpful tests suggested in these scenarios that you can do yourself:

- Almost all CMI/CS patients have intense pain at the base of the skull that radiates to the head and neck. This is also very common in people who have CFIDS/FMS but not CMI/CS. In CMI/CS, though, it is more likely to be much worse when the head is tilted all the way back for thirty seconds while sitting, so that your head is facing the ceiling. In this position, it is also likely to be worse when coughing. In addition, if you have nystagmus (the eyes, while wide-open, involuntarily flit back and forth or in a circular motion) when the head is tilted back, this also suggests CMI/CS. Have someone watch your eyes while this is tested for.

- Most people with CMI or CS also have neurally mediated hypotention (NMH), with a positive tilt table test. The NMH also improves with surgery. Interestingly, around 30 percent to 40 percent of CMI and CS patients also have sleep apnea, despite not being overweight.

- If you can do a fairly quick tandem walk for fifty feet, according to Dr. Rosner, you probably do not have CMI. The tandem walk test is similar to the test for drunk drivers, except that you put your heel just in front of the toes of the other foot with each step you take. Try to walk a twenty-five- to fifty-foot straight line doing this.

- While sitting, lift one foot three to six inches off the ground. Have someone push down on the top of your thigh with one hand, trying to push the foot back down, while you resist strongly for a few seconds (don't have your partner push down hard enough to hurt). You can also do the pushing yourself. If the foot can be pushed down *easily*, it's suspicious for CS. However, similar results can be seen with generalized weakness in FMS.

- About 50 percent of people with CMI and CS patients have no gag reflex. Use a spoon, pen (not the point), or similar object, to test your gag reflex. Put the object all the way into the back of the throat and move it against the right and left wall to test for gagging.

- Dr. Rosner reports that about 50 percent of his patients have a positive Romberg test. With your feet together, stand up straight, close your eyes, and hold your arms straight out in front of your body with the palms up for about fifteen to twenty-five seconds. Have someone watch you. If there is a *lot* of swaying from side to side, the Romberg test is positive.

If treatment for CFIDS/FMS fails to help you and you have a positive MRI for CMI/CS, I would seek out a doctor who has a *lot* of experience in treating CMI/CS in people with CFIDS/FMS. Otherwise, you run the risk of having the CMI/CS diagnosis missed or having surgery that is not effective because it does not remove enough bone to fully relieve the compression of the brain tissue. (See Appendix J: Resources for information on how to contact Dr. Rosner and the NFRA, a wonderful educational group that advocates CMI/CS surgery.)

Seasonal Affective Disorder

If your fatigue is a problem mainly from October to May, is less pronounced on sunny days, and is associated with increased sleep, weight gain, and carbohydrate craving during the winter, you may suffer from sunlight deprivation. This malady is known as seasonal affective disorder (SAD), or the winter blues.

SAD is treatable with a light box, which is available by mail order (see Appendix J: Resources). Use a 10,000-lux box positioned at a 45-degree angle in relation to your face and about eighteen inches away. Spend thirty to forty-five minutes in front of the box every morning from September through May. Add a half-hour at night if necessary. Experiment to find the best times of the day and session lengths for you. You do not have to sit still in front of the box, but can do table work such as reading, writing, or cutting vegetables.

If you have trouble waking up in the morning, attach a bright (about 250 lux) bedside lamp to a timer and program it to turn on two hours before your alarm is set to go off. Portable light visors are also available by mail order. Most patients find that it takes one to six weeks of light treatment to see any results.

Serotonin deficiency has also been put forward as a possible cause of SAD. Serotonin is a neurotransmitter that is connected in particular with the process of sleep. Medications that raise the serotonin level, such as fluoxetine (Prozac), have been shown to be effective against SAD.[8]

Exercise

Exercise is very important for your sense of well-being. People with CFIDS/FMS often find that when they exercise, they feel exhausted the next day, because their bodies do not produce enough energy. Because of this, they begin a cycle in which they feel that they are unable to exercise, they do not exercise, they become further deconditioned from the lack of exercise, and they feel even more tired so that they cannot exercise. Pushing exercise to the point of exhaustion is not healthy. But the good news is that as you treat your CFIDS/FMS problems, your postexercise exhaustion will change to a "good tired" for a couple of hours after exercising, and then to a good feeling the next day.

As your health starts to improve, slowly add exercise to your regime. Begin with something gentle, such as walking or swimming. If you feel exhausted the next day, you probably pushed too hard and should take it easier the next time. Soon, you will find your ability and stamina normalizing. Give yourself time to build up slowly, though. You may be severely deconditioned from years of not exercising.

I recommend walking as your primary exercise during the initial stages of your recovery. Walking conditions the heart and muscles and is easy on the joints and ligaments. When you walk outdoors, you can also enjoy the fresh air. Although getting fresh air may seem like a silly point, it is important. Fresh air is good for the lungs and clears the mind. Cold wind, however, causes fibromyalgia symptoms to flare. When the weather is chilly, walk around your local mall. Some malls even host walking clubs.

Wait until six to eight weeks into your treatment regimen. Then begin at your current level of exercise or start taking a five-minute walk each day. You can increase the walk by three minutes every three to seven days as you are able—that is, if you feel "good tired" after the exercise and better the next day. When you get to an hour a day, you can increase the intensity of your exercise, perhaps switching to or adding bicycle riding, using a stairmaster, or hiking. If you feel "bad tired" and wiped out the next day, you did too much. If this happens, don't work out for a few days, decrease the workout by 15 to 20 percent, and move up more slowly. Remember, the idea of *no pain, no gain* is stupid!

Many CFS patients feel a sense of powerlessness and an inability to defend themselves. Although the idea of practicing a martial art may seem impossible right now, you may be pleasantly surprised at your ability when your symptoms resolve. Research the different martial arts that are currently popular and check your Yellow Pages for the closest training center.

Detoxification

Many excellent practitioners use detoxification techniques very effectively. For more information on this, I would read Dr. Majid Ali's book, *The Canary and Chronic Fatigue* (IPM Press, 1994). Many toxic substances, such as mercury from dental fillings, monosodium glutamate (MSG), pesticides, and others too numerous to list, can contribute to CFIDS/FMS.

Yoga and Meditation

Yoga, meditation, and other approaches to quieting and resting the mind while accessing your spirit/deep psyche can be very helpful. A recent study, in fact by Arthur Hartz, M.D., Ph.D., asked people to list the therapies they were using for CFIDS/FMS. They then checked two years later to see how the patients were doing. Dr. Hartz was shocked to find that yoga appeared to help the CFIDS/FMS patients more than anything else—despite their not even considering yoga when they began the study.

Yoga is the art of moving your body's energy and connection with the wholeness of all that is. This energy has many names: God, soul, the collective unconscious, even "Feel the Force, Luke," in *Star Wars*. There are many approaches to meditation and yoga and inner connection, most of which are wonderful. There are a few approaches that may not be healthy, however. As a general guideline, if it hurts, ease back until it's comfortable and let your teacher know. Also, look for a practice or discipline that teaches you to love everyone and everything, especially yourself (there are no enemies), and that we are all equal, albeit different. Finally, look for a teacher who recognizes that once you have learned what you need, you don't need a teacher anymore. The power to grow and connect with the divine is in you and in everyone; you are not dependent on a particular individual to maintain your connection.

Be Gentle with Yourself

People who develop severe chronic fatigue states are often type-A individuals who were overachievers before becoming ill. As they begin to recover, they tend to want to make up for lost time by trying to get everything done that they could not finish while ill. *Do not do this!*

When you first begin recovering, you should reserve the energy that is slowly returning for activities that make you feel good. Most of the things that you have left undone can remain undone. Many probably do not ever need to be done.

As you start feeling better, take your time adding new activities and returning fulfilling old ones to your life. Do just those things that you really want to do. Do not go "shoulding" (should do this, should do that) on yourself.

Although you likely view your illness as an enemy, you should let it become your ally. Many people with CFIDS have been caught in role entrapment. Role-entrapped people were taught that they have to be the perfect spouse or the perfect parent or the perfect employee. The superwoman complex is a good example. CFIDS can be your body's way of getting out of the roles in which you are trapped. Most of us have so bought into society's expectations of us that we have taken them on as our own. What we fail to recognize is that because of its tremendous rate of acceleration, our current society is an aberration. There has been no other stable society during the last three thousand–plus years, nor are there many others presently on the planet, in which "normal" change occurred so rapidly. Despite all our modern conveniences and laborsaving devices, which were supposed to give us more free time, most people find that they are running ever faster. Whereas one parent used to be home to take care of the children while the other parent worked, both—even when both parents are in the same household—now often must work to maintain the family's standard of living.

Because our whole society is trapped in roles, this chaos may seem normal. *It is not.* It is abnormal. Although some people thrive on it, more people every day are becoming burned out. I suspect that the physical processes that make up CFS and fibromyalgia are manifestations of this— and that we are just beginning to see the tip of the iceberg.

As you get well, you will need to reclaim your own natural speed and pace of life. This may mean a somewhat lower standard of living, but you may have been living with that for several years now anyway. On the plus side, it may also mean that your children will have an improved parent and that your life will be more fulfilling. Many people live their lives like hamsters running faster and faster on the exercise wheels in their cage while going *nowhere*. Give yourself permission to step off the wheel! These are important points. Let's discuss them further in the next chapter!

Important Points

- Check for food sensitivities, then temporarily remove suspect foods from your diet or eliminate them with desensitization techniques such as NAET.
- Treat nasal congestion or sinusitis by treating underlying yeast. If it persists, add the antibiotic Keflex or doxycycline, xylometazoline nasal spray, the decongestant Sudafed, steam treatments, and sleep.
- Ask your doctor for alternatives to medications that have fatigue as a side effect.
- Treat high blood pressure with Nimotop, Apresoline, or Accupril. If you feel worse between September and April, consider the possibility of seasonal affective disorder.
- Patients have benefited from gamma-globulin shots, kutapressin shots, intravenous nutritional support, and a variety of treatments developed by Dr. Jay Goldstein.
- If you have hyperactive knee reflexes, your symptoms get much worse when you look up at the ceiling, and you don't respond to the other treatments in this book, consider evaluation for Chiari malformation and cervical stenosis.
- When you can, begin an exercise program. Walking or warm-water swimming are excellent for beginners.
- Get plenty of fresh air.
- *Do not* try to make up for lost time as you start to feel better.

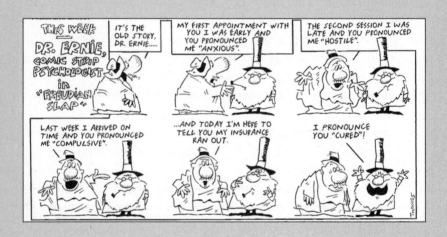

11

Am I Crazy?

IN MEDICINE, WE HAVE A BAD HABIT. IF A DOCTOR cannot figure out what is wrong with a patient, the doctor brands that patient a turkey. Imagine calling an electrician because your lights do not work. The electrician checks all your wiring, can't find the problem, and says, "You're crazy. There's nothing wrong with your lights." You flip the switches and they still do not work, but the electrician just says, "I've looked. There's no problem here," and walks out the door. This is analogous to what many CFS patients experience. I apologize for the medical profession's calling you crazy just because we cannot determine the cause of your problem. It is inappropriate and cruel.

What you have is a very real and physical illness. And, like most other physical processes—such as diabetes, heart disease, cancer, and ulcers—it has an associated psychological component. As is true for any disease, when you treat the physical component, you must also treat the underlying psychological issues. If you do not, the disease will simply manifest itself in another way.

It might also help you to understand that you may sometimes mistake uncomfortable feelings such as disappointment or sadness for fatigue. Try to be aware of when you do this. There is no such thing as an inappropriate feeling. You have the right to feel whatever you feel.

Does this mean that you are crazy? No. It simply means that, like all human beings, you have emotional issues to deal with as part of your growth process. In my practice, I frequently see CFS patients who seem to be caught on the horns of a dilemma emotionally. These patients find themselves in situations in which they are unable to make a choice between two or more alternatives—for example, between working and having children, or between staying with or leaving their spouse. These conflicts come in an infinite variety. Defending yourself against *acknowledging* a conflict can sap your energy.

Unfortunately, some patients also become so frustrated by being told their CFS is "all in their head" that they are in a Catch-22. They feel that if they acknowledge that they also have emotional issues (the way everyone does), they are validating the doctors who say that their illness is all emotional. That patients in the active group in our study improved dramatically and the placebo group did not also proves that this is a real, physical disease. If it was "all in your head" the placebo group would have improved as much as the active group. This means that anyone who says it's all in your head is unscientific! Give yourself permission to be human. You are no more and no less crazy than anyone else.

In my experience, when people start to feel better physically, they find it easier to deal with their emotional issues. The issues are often holdovers from the past and are now easier to resolve. Actually, however, you do not have to resolve every conflict. If you have something that you cannot settle at your current level of growth, you might find it helpful to simply hold the conflict in your awareness instead of suppressing it. Tell yourself, "Yes, I have these two areas that are in conflict and I cannot reconcile them now." The tension of holding those opposites and the conflict in your awareness will result in psychological growth, the same way that exercising helps a muscle to grow. Many people find that after a while, a solution comes from a new perspective.

A large percentage of CFS patients are type-A overachievers who were driven by having low self-esteem as children. In the first part of their lives, these patients needed to overachieve for their growth and self-image. Although not the easiest method, CFS helps them slow down long enough to reclaim themselves. For many, a period of deep rest is essential. CFS actually serves many patients well. Part of getting well is "lightening up." The old Zen image of worry being an old man carrying a load of feathers that he thinks are rocks often fits perfectly. Many of the worries we carry around sort themselves out as soon as we let go of them. Although things may not always work out the way we would like them to (CFS patients are often "control freaks"), they usually work out for the best. Because of this, it helps to have (or reclaim) a sense of humor.

I am a firm believer in psychological counseling. Counseling is helpful to anybody who is growing. People who are emotionally or intellectually brain-dead and living by a "social cookbook" instead of thinking for themselves may never need counseling. People who are growing, however, frequently come across areas that are difficult and with which it is usual and natural to need help.

Although many CFS patients feel depressed because of their illness, only a small minority have depression as the cause of their fatigue.[1] The depression caused by CFS is often simply frustration. Fatigue patients usually have a lot of interests and are frustrated by their lack of energy. If a patient has depression causing fatigue, that patient probably has few interests. The stress of CFIDS/FMS can itself cause depression. When combined with other treatments, the new antidepressants—such as sertraline (Zoloft), fluoxetine (Prozac), paroxetine (Paxil), nefazodone (Serzone), and venlafaxine (Effexor)—often act as energizers even in the absence of depression. If you use one of these medications, start with a low dose—for example, 10 milligrams of Paxil—and slowly raise it as needed. It takes six weeks to feel the full effect. If the effect decreases over time, take buspirone (Buspar) an antianxiety agent, or increase the antidepressant dose to restore the effectiveness. Although in many ways, depression and CFS are opposites—for example, cortisol levels are high in depression and low in CFS—low serotonin levels are seen in both diseases. Zoloft, Prozac, Paxil, Serzone, and Effexor raise serotonin levels, even when depression is not a factor.

If you are depressed, taking natural Armour Thyroid (not Synthroid) and the nutritional supplements discussed in Chapter 2, can be helpful. In addition, taking 300 to 600 milligrams of St. John's wort in the morning and 600 to 900 milligrams at night and/or 200 to 800 milligrams of S-adenosylmethionine (SAM-e) twice a day can be very helpful. The St. John's wort and SAM-e take about six weeks and ten days, respectively, to see their effect. Be sure to get a good brand of SAM-e, such as Nature Made.

Whether or not you are depressed, you may consider some type of therapist for emotional support and guidance. Be careful who you choose, however. Many therapists have never dealt with their own problems and simply work out their personal conflicts and issues on their patients. Others have worked through their issues and are excellent with patients. Make sure *psychotherapist* is one word—not two! Talk to your friends and relatives to find somebody who is good. Your physician is an excellent resource. There are many good therapeutic approaches, but my own personal bias is for a therapist who takes a transpersonal psychology or Jungian approach. I have found one physician, Brugh Joy, M.D., to be extraordinarily skilled at helping people to understand their deep psyches. (See Appendix J: Resources.) Dr. Joy runs workshops in the mountains of Arizona. I cannot recommend these workshops too strongly. They demand a lot of work, are somewhat expensive, and last approximately twelve days each. They are more effective than a year of regular counseling. For beginners, I recommend the Foundation workshop. Do not attend Dr. Joy's workshops for the purpose of treating your chronic fatigue, however. Go to learn to accept and understand more fully who you really are.

By using your chronic fatigue as a springboard for personal growth, you can find your CFS turning into a blessing. I found this to be the case for me. My CFS gave me a firsthand understanding of the problem and a powerful incentive to learn how to overcome it. It also has led me into wonderful areas of growth.

The Mind-Body Connection

I feel that *all* illnesses have a psychological component. Although someone may have a bacterial infection such as *Helicobacter pylori* or excess acid causing his or her ulcer, it helps if I can remove the three telephones from the highly stressed executive's ears while treating the infections and excess acid.

I find that I, and most people with CFIDS/FMS, are mega-type-A overachievers. As a group, our sensitivity and intuitive abilities are high. We had low self-esteem as children and tended to seek approval, often from someone who simply was not going to give it. This, combined with our sensitivity to the feelings of others, caused us to avoid conflict and to try to meet other people's needs—at the expense of our own. Many of us closed off our feelings (and our empathic nature) for a while because we were too young to handle their intensity. Because of our approval-seeking and low self-esteem, we often drove ourselves to being the best at what we did, or to try to be all things to all people. Not being able to say no (because we wanted to avoid conflict or loss of approval) led us to feel as though we could not defend our emotional boundaries, and left us feeling drained. We responded to fatigue by redoubling our efforts, instead of resting, as our bodies tried to tell us to do. As we depleted our energy reserves—sometimes while feeling great on an adrenaline "high"—we encountered the physical trigger to our disease, whether it was an infection, an injury, childbirth, or something else. This, combined with physical problems such as yeast overgrowth or hormonal deficiencies and, often, a genetic tendency to the disease, set the process in motion.

What can we do about it? First, we can recognize that all this helped us to grow and achieve. One of the fun parts of working with people with CFIDS/FMS is that they are very intelligent and inquisitive. People with diabetes, high blood pressure, or even cancer don't usually come in having done a computer search on their illness! CFIDS/FMS patients often have. It is great to work with patients who can teach me, as well as my teaching them.

CFIDS/FMS forces us to take care of our needs first. After all, you don't have much of a choice when taking a shower uses up all of your energy for the day. Taking care of yourself first is an important lesson for you to learn and to continue, even when you get well. Start by easing up on yourself. It's okay to recognize that you tend to be a perfectionist and a bit controlling. But we also beat up on ourselves by feeling that we're never quite good enough. I find it very helpful to begin with the following prescription:

- No blame.
- No fault.
- No guilt.
- No judgment.
- No comparing yourself with other people.
- No expectations.

This applies to *yourself* and *others*. It is okay to feel anything you feel. Whatever you feel is totally valid. Own your feelings as *your* feelings, however, and recognize that they may not have much to do with the person they are directed at. Feel the feelings, then let go of them. Don't blame the person you're feeling them toward. Don't feel guilty or blame yourself (or others) for *anything*—this includes not feeling guilty when you catch yourself blaming someone else!

In the beginning, you may catch yourself blaming, finding fault, judging, or laying a guilt trip on yourself and/or other people hundreds of times a day. This is normal. When you catch yourself doing it—even if it's three days later—just drop it in mid-thought. Don't beat yourself up for it. Just recognize that it's an old pattern that you have decided to change. Over the next few weeks, it will happen less and less. Eventually, it will be uncommon. Even then, when you catch yourself blaming, feeling guilty, making comparisons between yourself and others (or comparing two other people), simply gently let go of it—without blame. In a few weeks, your whole view of reality will change.

What happened? When you were judging others, you were in truth judging yourself and projecting it outward. These judgments were often views and expectations that had been placed on you by others, such as your parents, school, religious institutions, or society. Most likely, this happened early in your life and you internalized it. By letting go of blame, fault, comparisons, guilt, and judgment on others, you stop judging yourself. Hence the truism, "Judge not, lest ye be judged" (having been a good Jewish lad, I get to know these lines). When you release these old expectations/programs, that's when the fun can begin.

Once you have done this, use your feelings (not your brain) to figure out what *you* want. Although our minds are wonderful tools, they are too subject to outside childhood programming to know what we want. Your feelings know, though. If something *feels* good from a centered place when you picture or do it—I suspect it's what your inner self (whether you call it your *psyche*, soul, or whatever) really wants to do. If it feels bad, you don't want to do it, no matter how much your brain is saying you should. Stop "shoulding" on yourself!

As you start feeling better with treatment, use your energy to do the things that *feel* good. You've managed to survive not doing most of the things that feel bad for years, without being arrested or thrown out on the street. Let those things stay undone. Pace yourself as you add in the new things that feel good and check with your feelings frequently. Don't make up for lost time!

One day, a friend of mine, Jeffrey Maitland, Ph.D., sent me an article entitled "Stone Agers in the Fast Lane." I was really ticked off because he beat me to the punch. On the other hand, I knew he was brilliant because he had independently come to the same conclusions I had! I think you'll enjoy the article. It is reproduced in Appendix F.

Remember: While you're doing the treatments discussed in this book:

- No blame.
- No fault.
- No guilt.
- No judgment.
- No comparing yourself with other people.
- No expectations.

Then, continually shift your thoughts and actions to things that *feel* good. Let go of thoughts and stop doing things that feel bad. Then allow space and time in your mind and life for what you want to manifest. The result of doing this is the joy that comes with connecting with your deeper, inner being and being who you truly are!

Important Points

- CFS and fibromyalgia are physical processes with physical causes. However, like other illnesses, they have psychological components that must be treated also.
- CFS patients both with and without depression have been helped by the new generation of antidepressants, such as Zoloft, Prozac, Paxil, Serzone, and Effexor.
- Consider therapy for emotional support and guidance.
- Get into a "centered space," then constantly shift your attention and actions to things that (in that centered space) feel good!

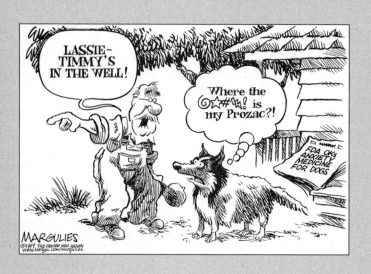

CHAPTER **12**

Finding a Physician

HAVING DEVELOPED AN EFFECTIVE TREATMENT
protocol for fibromyalgia and chronic fatigue syndrome over the last twenty
years, and having proven it to be effective in two studies—one a well-done
randomized, double-blind, placebo-controlled trial—my colleagues and I
have now turned to our goal of making effective treatment available to the
over 50 million people worldwide who suffer from these illnesses. Your
doctor should be willing to order the blood tests you need to be evaluated
properly and to be treated using our protocol. If not, your physician may
be willing to read this chapter plus Appendix A: For Physicians, and to run
the tests listed on page 206. If he or she is not willing, for whatever reason,
you can go on our website and obtain laboratory requisitions for the blood
tests (see Appendix J: Resources). Thus, obtaining the tests that you are entitled to should no longer be a problem. If your insurance does not cover
the cost of the testing, it is a good idea to call different laboratories to see
what they charge, as the price can vary markedly. You may be able to ne-
gotiate a discount (especially in a doctor's office) if you are willing to pay
for the tests at the time of service.

The next job is for you to be able to obtain the treatment you need. A
thorough consultation for CFIDS/FMS takes three to four hours, even if
the physician has treated many patients with these illnesses and is very
good at what he or she does. Hopefully, your doctor will have the time and

expertise needed to properly evaluate and take care of you. If not, there is a teaching tool available on the From Fatigued To Fantastic website that can help. (See Appendix J: Resources.) The printout will supply the following, which will make things much easier for you and your doctor:

- A complete medical record (except, of course, for the physical examination—which is usually unremarkable for people with CFIDS/FMS).
- A list of probable factors contributing to the illness in *your specific case.*
- Natural remedies (again, based on your specific case) that can help you to begin a major part of treatment on your own.
- A list of prescription treatments, in order of priority.
- Detailed information sheets on your different diagnoses and treatments, as well as a flow chart to simplify your application of our protocol.

In essence, your treatment program printout will be like a book written specifically for your case. This is important because CFIDS/FMS is not a single illness—it is, rather, a combination of dozens of underlying problems, which vary from person to person. With the program in hand, you will be able to begin your own effective treatment protocol and give your doctor the information he or she needs to guide and treat you effectively as well.

There are many approaches that you can take to find a physician to help you with your illness. The best place to begin is with your family physician. Although most physicians are too busy to read this whole book, your physician may be willing to read the studies (Appendix B) and/or Appendix A: For Physicians and to run the lab tests listed on page 206. If these stimulate your physician's interest, he or she may then read the whole book. Even if your physician is unwilling or unable to spend the time necessary to read any of the book, you can ask him or her to run the lab tests as discussed above. If your doctor won't even order the tests, you can get a lab requisition form on our website, and then do the extensive computer program on our website. You can also interpret the results yourself using the explanations beginning on page 311 and then then talk to your physician about trying the recommended treatments.

In your search for a doctor, you will discover that physicians tend to fall into three categories:

1. *Simply not interested.* Try another physician.

2. *Skeptical but willing to explore new possibilities.* Offer this physician a copy of our recent placebo-controlled study and Appendix A, as discussed above, or the whole book, if he or she prefers. Be persistent, yet gracious, in encouraging the physician to give the treatments a try. Most of the treatments are benign if used in the ways that I recommend. Although the physician initially may be uncomfortable with using Cortef, encourage him or her to give you a trial prescription. Current evidence suggests that it is reasonably safe in the dosages that I suggest. I was also uncomfortable with Cortef until I read the studies and the book on it. (For a complete discussion of cortisol and my reference sources, see page 30. For a complete discussion of DHEA and my reference sources, see page 41.)

3. *Willing to work with you.* Wonderful. You can concentrate on getting well rather than on convincing your physician to treat you.

If your physician is simply not interested in learning about CFIDS/FMS, or if he or she is skeptical though open but you want someone familiar with CFIDS/FMS who wants to work with you, look at Appendix J: Resources to find doctors who fit into that category. In addition, our website (www.endfatigue.com) has a list of over 700 health-care practitioners who treat people with CFIDS/FMS. Also check with your local support groups. I strongly recommend joining the Chronic Fatigue and Immune Dysfunction Syndrome Association of America and the Fibromyalgia Network (again, see Appendix J: Resources). These are two of the best patient support groups I have ever come across. They can put you in touch with your local support groups, which can refer you to physicians in your area. In addition, the more members they have, the more effectively they can function as your advocates.

Your Insurance Plays a Role

The type of health insurance you have may also play a role in your selection of a physician. Although some health maintenance organizations (HMOs) are excellent and very interested in their patients' well-being, some seem to be interested only in making money. When the latter is the case, the HMO may readily approve of tests and treatments that are clear-cut and lifesaving but, unfortunately, may drag its feet on allowing new treatment approaches, claiming that these are experimental. There are, indeed, few readily accepted tests for chronic fatigue syndrome and fibromyalgia. If, however, you have any of the symptoms listed in Table 12.1, you can push for, and are legally entitled to have, the appropriate tests, listed beside the symptoms. The main tests to push for are those listed as most important on page 206 in Appendix A. Although the tests listed as helpful offer valuable information, they are less likely to be useful in the hands of a disinterested physician. Except for the stool testing, which I would do at the Parasitology Center or at The Great Smokies Diagnostic Laboratory (see Appendix J: Resources), or tests for CMV, HHV-6, mycoplasma/chlamydia infections (see page 84) or the ISAC Panel for clotting/bleeding disorders (see page 91) the tests can be effectively done anywhere. Again, you should review the results with pages 310 to 312 in front of you. Otherwise, your physician may dismiss levels that are problematic and contribute to your CFS as "within normal limits."

If your physician is *capitated*—that is, if he or she is paid a set monthly fee by the insurance carrier for every patient on their panel, whether a patient is seen or not—that physician may lose money on every test ordered. This creates a perverse incentive for the physician to not do anything—and to hope that sick people go away. If your insurance company pays physicians a *fee for service* payment based on the care provided—you stand the best chance of getting the help you need.

When talking to your physician, be courteous but firm in your requests. Most physicians are very compassionate and want to help their patients. Don't be hostile when you ask your doctor to try the treatment approach outlined in this book. At the same time, though, you must stand up for your needs. Give your doctor a copy of the double-blind, placebo-controlled study we did (see page 229) and ask if he or she would like a copy of this book. Doing the educational program on our website will help a willing doctor to treat you properly, and make it much easier to get the help you need.

As medicine becomes more competitive, groups of patients might be able to interest physicians in their cases. CFIDS/FMS support groups in an area can discuss which physicians seem the most interested, competent, and caring. A physician who is paid a fee for service or who has a family member or personal experience with CFS or fibromyalgia will likely be much more interested, since capitated physicians and physicians connected with HMOs would be committing financial suicide by seeking out sick patients. Representatives of the patient group can then approach the selected physician, in person or by letter, to see if the physician would be willing to treat the group members using the desired treatment approach. Let the physician know how many patients in the group would be interested in seeing him or her.

Dealing with Your Insurance Company

If your insurance company does not give you a choice of physicians, and your physician has no interest in running the tests that you need, you may have to file an appeal with the insurance company and with the state insurance commissioner. Unfortunately, you may also need to find legal assistance. Again, remember that you are *not* requesting the tests for *diagnosis* of CFS or Fibromyalgia. The tests are in response to your symptoms (see Table 12.1). If your physician still refuses to do the testing, make sure that he or she has recorded *all* your symptoms in your chart, has described how incapacitating they are, and has noted his or her refusal to order the tests, despite your strong requests. Then ask for copies of the progress notes in your chart that document these points. With these notes in hand, you may be able to receive reimbursement from your insurance company (on appeal) if you must pay to have the tests done by a *nonparticipating* physician. Getting into a hostile fight with a close-minded physician is not worth your while. Simply take the necessary steps to protect your rights.

Fighting your physician or insurance company is not a good use of your precious energy. In the long run, you will do better grouping together with other CFIDS patients to find physicians who will work with you. Remember, CFIDS, fibromyalgia, and other chronic fatigue states are now treatable illnesses. You will do best using your energy to find a physician who wants to work with you to help you move beyond your disease.

Table 12.1. Tests for Symptoms

If you have any of these symptoms:	You have the right to have these tests done:
Fatigue, abdominal discomfort, confusion	Complete blood count (CBC) and erythrocyte sedimentation rate (ESR) and differential
Fatigue, abdominal discomfort, confusion, recurrent infections	Chemistry (for example, chemistry 16) and magnesium
Anemia	Iron (Fe), total iron binding capacity (TIBC), and ferritin (all three iron studies are necessary)
Fatigue, constipation or diarrhea, achiness, confusion, cold intolerance, sweating, palpitations	Thyroid studies including free or total T_3, free T_4, and thyroid-stimulating hormone (TSH) (all three tests are necessary)
Anemia, confusion, poor memory, fatigue, or paresthesia (numbness or tingling in the fingers)	Vitamin B_{12}
Malabsorption (for example, bowel distention or gas) or anemia	Folic acid
Increased thirst or urination	$HgbA_1C$ (diabetes screen) or glycosylated hemoglobin
Chronic diarrhea or abdominal cramps, gas, bloating, or other gastrointestinal complaints	Stool for ova and parasites, with antigen testing for amoeba, giardia, Cryptosporidium, and Clostridium difficile
Chronic muscle aches or joint aches	Creatine phosphokinase (CPK), antinuclear antibody (ANA), latex fixation (rheumatoid factor)
Fatigue, recurrent infections	Human immunodeficiency virus (HIV)
Vaginitis, confusion, rash	Rapid plasma reagin (RPR) (syphilis test)
Fatigue, achiness, joint pains, confusion, or poor memory	Lyme disease (necessary only in certain regions)
Runny nose, recurrent respiratory infections, nasal congestion, rashes, wheezing	Allergy testing and immunoglobulin E (IgE)
Under- or overactive thyroid (often helpful in interpreting the significance of borderline results)	Thyroid antibodies
Irregular or absent periods or hot flashes (check for menopause)	Follicle-stimulating hormone (FSH), luteinizing hormone (LH), estradiol level
Decreased libido (in male or female), decreased erections	Testosterone and free testosterone
Abnormal body-hair growth, fatigue, or infertility	Dehydroepiandrosterone-sulfate (DHEA-S)
Fatigue, hypotension, or recurrent infections	Cortrosyn stimulation test (for adrenal insufficiency) or morning cortisol
Fatigue with snoring, overweight, high blood pressure or periods of apnea	Sleep study
Chronic sinusitis	Sinus computed tomography (CT) scan
Fever and sweats	HHV-6, Mycoplasma, Chlamydia PCR Tests

Important Points

- If your physician is not willing to treat you for CFIDS, find one who is. Check our website or ask your friends and family for recommendations. Other good resources are local support groups, health food stores, and other health related workers (for example, chiropractors and pharmacists).
- Check your health insurance regarding your rights in selecting a physician, having testing done, and getting treatment.
- Consider banding together with other CFIDS patients to interest a physician.

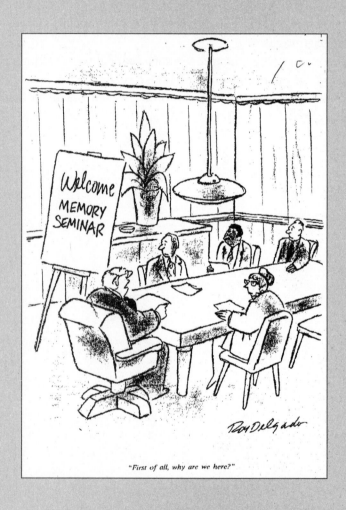

"First of all, why are we here?"

Conclusion

OLD MINDSETS ARE OFTEN DIFFICULT TO CHANGE. It took many years for chronic fatigue syndrome and Fibromyalgia to be recognized as real and physical processes. As time goes on and more physicians become aware of these illnesses, patients will no longer have to accept being labeled as crazy because of the medical profession's ignorance.

We are entering the next stage.

Chronic fatigue syndrome and fibromyalgia are treatable. This simple fact needs to be demonstrated and reported over and over again to become accepted by physicians. The controlled study that I recently completed on my treatment approach should help. There are plans to replicate the study at several medical centers in England, and perhaps in Australia, as well. Over time, more physicians will learn how to treat chronic fatigue and how to encourage and support their fatigue patients. Others, sadly, will continue to keep their heads stuck in the sand. It is all right to ignore these doctors who ignore you. You will be better off spending your energy tending to and taking responsibility for your physical and emotional needs so that you can attain and then maintain optimum health. This is especially true as there are more and more doctors learning to effectively treat CFIDS/FMS.

Because your illness may have been treated as being "all in your head" for so long, do not fall into the trap of ignoring your emotional and psychological needs. Many CFS patients were overachievers in an effort to compensate for childhood low self-esteem. *Love yourself* for having had that low self-esteem, *love yourself* for having been an overachiever, then let go of both these experiences. Take the *shoulds* placed on you by your family, yourself and society—you *should* be a mother, you *should* be a lawyer, you *should* do this, you *should* be that—and drop them. Love yourself for having had them, then love yourself for letting go of them. Although CFS is devastating, even this dark cloud has a silver lining. It has taught you what you do not have to do and has given you space to explore who you truly are. It has also taught you to stop "shoulding" on yourself! You have earned the right to be yourself.

As you start feeling better, slowly add activities to your life that make you *feel* good. If you add something that makes you *feel* poorly, stop doing it. Joseph Campbell, a world-renowned teacher of the mythology of and paths for personal growth in many diverse cultures, was asked how people can stay true to themselves. Put succinctly, his advice was to "follow your bliss." Perhaps a *should* led you to become an accountant, doctor, or lawyer, but your bliss truly lies in being an artist, poet, or dancer. Perhaps the opposite is true. If you do what makes you *feel* happy and excited, you will get yourself on the right track. Whatever you do, however, *do not try to make up for lost time.* The few lingering symptoms of your illness will effectively let you know when you are pushing too hard. Recognize that your illness may have been a valuable teacher.

As your chronic fatigue resolves and you begin to feel well again, let your friends, the media, and former physicians (most CFIDS/FMS patients have seen quite a few!) know. Because no single expensive drug exists for the treatment of CFIDS/FMS, millions of pharmaceutical dollars are not spent on publicity. As you get well, that part—letting other fatigue patients know that an end to the tunnel does exist—is up to you!

A

For Physicians

THE MEDICAL MANAGEMENT OF CHRONIC FATIGUE syndrome (CFS) and fibromyalgia is, in many ways, fairly straightforward. Because the lab testing needs to be done and interpreted somewhat differently than for other conditions, I recommend reading this entire book. If time does not allow this, I recommend reading my initial study on CFS treatment, published in the Winter 1995 issue of the *Journal of Musculoskeletal Pain* and our recently completed randomized, placebo-controlled study (see Appendix B). This will help you understand the rationale behind my approach and will give you a good overview of what occurs in CFS. To help you to take care of these complex patients in the time you have available, patients can complete an educational program on our website (see Appendix J: Resources), which will allow them to print out a complete medical record (except, of course, for the physical exam) with a treatment protocol and information sheets tailored to that patient's case. If you are willing to use a significant part of this protocol, we will be happy to add your name to the free referral list on our website.

Effective Treatment of Chronic Fatigue Syndrome and Fibromyalgia

Chronic fatigue syndrome (CFIDS) and fibromyalgia (FMS) are two common names for a spectrum of common disabling illnesses. It is estimated that FMS alone affects 3 to 6 million Americans, causing more disability than rheumatoid arthritis.[1] Fortunately, much progress has been made in the last five years. Although we still have much to learn, effective treatment is now available for the large majority of patients with these illnesses.[2]

Why Have These Diseases Been So Confusing?

CFIDS/FMS represents a syndrome—a spectrum of processes with a common end point. Because it affects major "control systems" in the body, there are myriad symptoms that initially do not seem to be related. Recent research has implicated hypothalamic and mitochondrial dysfunction.[3] These explain the large number of symptoms and why most patients have a similar set of complaints.

How Do I Make a Diagnosis?

The clinical and research criteria for diagnosing CFIDS and FMS are given on pages 229 and 258, respectively. These criteria are useful for research and for confirming the diagnosis. Although the FMS criteria require a tender point exam that takes a good bit of time to master, this adds little clinically and will likely be eliminated in the future. Instead of focusing on the tender point exam, you may want to begin by asking a patient if he or she has the following symptoms:

- Severe fatigue lasting over four months.
- Feeling worse (often described as feeling as if he or she was "hit by a truck") the day after exercise.
- Diffuse, often migratory, achiness.
- Disordered sleep. (Ask if your patient is getting seven to eight hours of uninterrupted sleep a night).

- Brain fog (difficulty with word finding and substitution, poor short-term memory and poor concentration).
- Bowel dysfunction. Many people diagnosed with irritable bowel syndrome (IBS) or spastic colon have CFIDS/FMS.
- Recurrent infections and/or chemical/medication sensitivities.

Give your patient this list of symptoms. If an individual looks at you with an amazed look of "How did you know?" he or she likely has CFIDS/FMS.

The Causes of CFIDS/FMS

It is my belief, and that of many other workers in this area, that (1) CFIDS and FMS represent a common outcome for many different processes and that (2) FMS and CFIDS are often the same disease.

Current research and clinical experience show that these patients have a mix of disordered sleep, hormonal deficiencies (often with "normal" laboratory test results), low body temperature, and autonomic dysfunction (for example, low blood pressure, and neurally mediated hypotension [NMH]). This mix makes sense when you recognize that the hypothalamus is the major control center for all four of these functions.

Although still controversial, a large body of research also strongly suggests mitochondrial dysfunction as a unifying theory in CFIDS/FMS. In several genetic mitochondrial diseases, severe hypothalamic damage is seen (possibly because the hypothalamus has high energy needs).[4] The mitochondrial dysfunction, combined with secondary hypothalamic suppression, can cause the poor function seen in tissues with high energy needs. This includes dysfunction of the immune system, liver (with medication/chemical sensitivities secondary to decreased ability to detoxify), gastrointestinal tract, muscles, and central nervous system (CNS) (brain fog and decreased neurotransmitters).

Evaluating and Treating CFIDS/FMS

There are many approaches to evaluating this disease. The diagnosis of CFIDS/FMS itself requires little testing. The evaluation of the symptoms, however, which allow for effective treatment, usually requires extensive testing. Although many tests (for example, immune system testing) are interesting, I stick to tests that will affect treatment. A thorough and systematic approach works best. Following is a discussion of areas to look at.

HORMONAL DYSFUNCTION

This can have several major sources, including hypothalamic dysfunction and autoimmune processes (for example, thyroiditis), as well as other causes. Our current norms and testing often miss important deficiencies. For example, increased hormone binding to carrier proteins is often present in CFIDS/FMS. Because of this, *total* hormone (for example, testosterone) levels are often normal while the *active* hormone levels are low. Also, many blood tests use two *standard deviations* to define blood test norms. This means you have to be in the lowest or highest 2 to 3 percent of the population to be abnormal. Other tests use late signs of deficiency (for example, anemia or life threatening hypotension) to define an abnormal lab value. These ranges are inadequate in CFIDS/FMS. You should aim for the midrange of normal.

Thyroid Function

Suboptimal thyroid function is very common and very important. Because thyroid-binding globulin function and conversion of T_4 to T_3 may be altered if you have CFIDS/FMS, it is important to check a free (or total) T_3 and a free T_4 (*not* T_7 or T_3RU). I discussed hypothyroidism with Dr. Janet Travell, the world's leading authority on muscle disorders, at her ninety-fourth birthday party. Dr. Travell was an emeritus professor of medicine at George Washington Medical School and was the White House physician for Presidents Kennedy and Johnson. She felt that it was important to treat *all* chronic myalgic patients with thyroid hormone replacement if their T_3 or T_4 blood levels were below even the fiftieth percentile of normal. She was right. Many CFIDS/FMS patients also have difficulty in converting T_4 (which is fairly inactive) to T_3 (the active hormone). Blood levels (even a T_3 level because of T_3 being intracellular and conversion to reverse T_3) can miss this problem. Synthroid has only inactive (storage form) T_4, while Armour Thyroid has both inactive T_4 and active T_3. Many clinicians will give an empiric trial of Synthroid, 25 to 150 micrograms (mcg) every morning (qam), or Armour Thyroid, ½ to 2 grains (gr) qam. I am more likely to try an empiric trial of thyroid-hormone therapy if one or more of the following is true:

- The patient has fibromyalgia, and/or
- The patient's oral temperatures are generally less than 98.2°F, and/or
- The patient has symptoms and signs suggestive of hypothyroidism, and/or
- The patient's TSH test result is less than 0.95 or greater than 3.0, and/or
- The patient's T_3 or T_4 are below the fiftieth percentile of normal.

As physicians, we are trained to interpret a low-normal TSH—that is, 0.5 to 0.95—as a confirmation of euthyroidism. The rules, however, are different with CFIDS/FMS. In this setting, hypothalamic hypothyroidism is common and the patient's TSH can be low, normal, or high.[5] This is why I recommend an empiric therapeutic trial of thyroid-hormone treatment if the TSH and T_4 are both low normal. Also, if subclinical hypothyroidism is missed, the patient's fibromyalgia simply will not resolve. The inadequacy of thyroid testing is further suggested by studies that show:

- That most patients with suspected thyroid problems have normal blood studies.[6]
- That when these patients with symptoms of hypothyroidism and normal labs are treated with thyroid (Synthroid in an average dose of 120 mcg every day [qd]) a large marjority improve sigificantly.[7]

In addition, I would add the following:

- If the patient does not respond to Synthroid, switch to Armour Thyroid, and vice versa. For every 50 mcg of Synthroid, have the patient take ½ gr (30 mg) of Armour Thyroid. If the free or total T_3 result is low or low normal, begin with Armour Thyroid, which has both T_3 and T_4, instead of Synthroid, which has only T_4. I usually recommend beginning with Armour Thyroid.
- Adjust the thyroid dose according to how the patient *feels* and also to keep oral temperatures greater than 98°F, as long as the T_3 or T_4 tests do

not show *hyper*thyroidism. *Do not* use TSH to monitor thyroid replacement. Because of the hypothalamic suppression, it may be low despite inadequate hormonal dosing.

- Make sure that the patient does not take any iron supplements within six hours or calcium within two hours of the morning thyroid dose or the thyroid hormone will not be absorbed. Have the patient take the iron between 2:00 and 6:00 P.M.—on an empty stomach and away from any hormone treatments.

- Thyroid supplementation can increase a patient's cortisol metabolism and unmask a case of subclinical adrenal insufficiency. If the patient feels worse on low-dose thyroid replacement, the patient may have adrenal (or thiamine) insufficiency.

Remember that every patient is an individual and will respond differently to medications.

Adrenal Insufficiency

The hypothalamic-pituitary-adrenal (HPA) axis does not function well in CFIDS/FMS.[8] Dr. William Jefferies, a professor of medicine at the University of Virginia Medical School and previously a professor at Case Western University School of Medicine is the world's leading clinical expert on subclinical adrenal insufficiency. His book *Safe Uses of Cortisol* discusses the history of this disease and its treatment.[9] Because early researchers used massive doses of cortisol (not knowing the physiologic dose), their patients developed severe complications. What is not common knowledge is that these side effects are *not* seen with physiologic dosing of Cortef (that is, up to 20 milligrams [mg] a day).[10] Twenty mg of hydrocortisone (Cortef) is ≅ 4 to 5 mg of prednisone.

To put it in perspective, if the early thyroid researchers had given ten times the physiologic dose of thyroid hormone (for exmaple, 1,000 to 2,000 mcg qd instead of 100 to 200 mcg), a situation analogous to early adrenal research, many people would have had severe complications. Thyroid hormone would be viewed as very dangerous and we would only be treating hypothyroid patients on the verge of myxedema and coma. In adrenal insufficiency, this is what occurs now. Many hypoadrenal patients are only treated when they are ready to go into Addisonian crisis. Research and clinical experience shows that this approach misses many hypoadrenal patients.[11]

Symptoms of an underactive adrenal include weakness, hypotension, dizziness, sugar craving, and recurrent infections—all of which are common in CFIDS/FMS. I evaluate CFIDS/FMS patients' adrenal function with a cortrosyn stimulation test. The test *must* be begun between 7:00 and 9:00 A.M. The patient should be NPO and have no caffeine for twenty-four hours before the test. Check a baseline cortisol level and then give ACTH (Cortrosyn) 25 units or 1 unit IM (current data suggests the 1 unit Cortrosyn test is more reliable) and recheck cortisol levels at one-half hour and at one hour. Although a baseline of 6 mcg/dl is often considered "normal," most healthy people run approximately 16 to 24 mcg/dl at 8:00 A.M.

My treatment guidelines are that if the baseline cortisol is less than 16 mcg/dl *or* the cortisol level does not increase by at least 7 mcg/dl at thirty minutes *and* 11 mcg/dl at one hour, or does not double by one hour and is less than 35 mcg/dl, I treat with a therapeutic trial of 5 to 15 mg Cortef in the morning, 2.5 to 10 mg at lunchtime and 0 to 2.5 mg at 4:00 P.M. (maximum of 20 mg a day). Most patients find 5 to 7½ mg qam plus 2½ to 5 mg at noon to be optimal (the equivalent of 1½ to 3 mg prednisone qd). Cortef is much more effective than prednisone in CFIDS/FMS.

After keeping the patient on the initial dose for two to four weeks, adjust the dose up to a maximum of 20 mg daily or, if no benefit has been evident, taper it off. Adjust the Cortef to the lowest dose that feels the best. Give most of the Cortef in the morning and at lunchtime. I often tell my patients to take the last dose, 2.5 to 5 mg, no later than 4:00 P.M. Otherwise, the Cortef may keep the patient up at night.

After nine to eighteen months, taper the Cortef off over a period of one to four months. If the other physiologic stresses, such as infections or fibromyalgia, have been eliminated, the patient's adrenal function may be adequate or normalized. If symptoms recur off the cortef, continue treatment with the lowest optimal dose.

Improvement is often dramatic and is usually seen within two to four weeks. The Cortef should be doubled during periods of acute stress and raised even higher during periods of severe stress such as surgery. Consider also giving the patient 1,000 mg of calcium and 400 international units (IU) of vitamin D daily with the Cortef.

There are different approaches to treatment and more is *not* better. High dose Cortisol taken at night will worsen already disrupted sleep patterns. A recent study by Strauss published in the *Journal of the American Medical Association* gave too high a dose (about 25 to 35 mg a day) and too much at night—severely disrupting patients' sleep (p ≤ .02). Although he did not treat the sleep disorder, most patients felt somewhat better on treatment. A small percentage of the patients had significantly decreased post-treatment Cortrosyn tests, without complications, and he, I believe *in*correctly, recommends against using Cortef in CFIDS/FMS.[12] Our study did not show adrenal suppression using lower Cortef dosing.[13] Dr. Jefferies, with thousands of patient-years' experience in using low-dose Cortef, recommends an empiric trial of Cortef in *all* patients with severe, unexplained fatigue.[14] Our research and clinical experience suggests this is the best approach.

DHEA

Dehydroepiandrosterone (DHEA) is a major adrenal hormone that has recently been getting a lot of attention in the press. Although its function has not yet been determined, it plays an important role in people's sense of well-being.[15] Like any hormone, it is best kept near the midrange of optimal. I suspect that too high or too low a level can cause problems. I use the middle of normal range for a twenty-nine-year-old, keeping the DHEA-sulfate (DHEA-S) level at 150 to 180 mcg/dl in females and 350 to 480 mcg/dl in males.

The majority of CFIDS/FMS patients have suboptimal DHEA-S levels, and the benefit of treatment is often dramatic. Most females need 10 to 25 mg a day and most males 25 to 50 mg a day. Adjust to the dose that feels best, as long as the DHEA-S level stays under 200 mcg/dl in females and 480 mcg/dl in males.

Interestingly, as patients improve, their bodies begin to make DHEA on their own and the DHEA-S level can shoot up. If the level goes too high, the patient can get acne or darkening of the facial hair. Because of this, it is reasonable to initially check the DHEA-S level every two months in a female or every three to four months in a male. Although the body's DHEA-S level is fairly stable throughout the day, which is why I check the DHEA-sulfate level as opposed to the more variable DHEA level, the DHEA-S level does show significant peaks and troughs when DHEA is taken by mouth. I recommend either prescribing timed-release DHEA (available at General Nutritional Centers) or using two to three times a day (bid–tid) dosing and check blood levels two to four hours after taking a dose of DHEA. When the DHEA-S level rises over 200 mcg/dl in a female or 450 mcg/dl in a male, start to taper the dose.

Do not be surprised if a patient's gray hair turns back to its original color in six to eighteen months. This is one reason DHEA got the name "the fountain of youth hormone."

Low Estrogen and Testosterone

Although we are trained to diagnose menopause by cessation of periods, hot flashes and elevated FSH and LH, these are late findings. Estrogen deficiency often begins many years before, and may coincide with the onset of fibromyalgia.[16] To compound the problem, research done by Dr. Phillip Sarrel at Yale shows that 60 percent of women who have a hysterectomy (even with the ovaries left in) will go into menopause within six months to two years.[17] The same may apply to woman who have had a tubal ligation. This is not something we were taught in our medical training, and has major implications for younger women who have had hysterectomies or tubal ligations!

In her excellent book on estrogen and testosterone deficiency, Dr. Elizabeth Vliet gives a well referenced, in-depth foundation for evaluation and treatment of these problems.[18] To summarize, the initial symptoms of estrogen deficiency are poor sleep, poor libido, brain fog, achiness, PMS, and decreased neurotransmitter function. Dr. Vliet feels that estradiol levels at midcycle should be at least 100 pg/ml. If a woman's CFIDS/FMS symptoms are worse at ovulation and the ten days before her period, then a trial of estrogen is warranted. Dr. Vliet prefers to use a high-estrogen OCP such as Ovcon-35 in women in their thirties and forties. Side effects (bleeding, fluid retention, and so on) are common for the first three to four months. If these are poorly tolerated, or the woman is older than forty-five years of age, it is reasonable to use natural 17-B-estradiol instead (for example, Estrace or Climara patches). Although the Premarin company has a wonderful marketing department, their conjugated *horse* estrogens can flare fibromyalgia.

The usual dose of Climara is one 0.05- to 0.1-mg patch a week and the usual dose of Estrace is ½ to 2 mg a day, adjusted to what feels best to the patient. In the absence of a hysterectomy, progesterone should be added to prevent uterine cancer. Natural progesterone (available from most pharmacies as Prometrium 100 mg), is better tolerated than Provera. The dose is 100 mg at bedtime (qhs), instead of Provera 2.5 mg, or 200 mg a day for ten to fourteen days a month, instead of Provera 10 mg.

Testosterone Deficiency

Testosterone deficiency is important in both males and females. It is important to check a *free* (not total) testosterone level. If the age-adjusted *free* testosterone is low or low-normal, a trial of treatment is often very helpful. Seventy percent of my male CFIDS/FMS patients and many of my female patients have low (in the lowest quintile) free testosterone levels (and normal total testosterone levels). Be sure the free testosterone normal range is "age-adjusted" using ten-year age groups (for example, twenty to thirty years old). It is meaningless to have a normal range that includes eighty-year-olds if the patient is twenty-eight. If the result is below normal, and possibly even in the lowest 20 percent of the normal range, I would consider a trial of testosterone.

For men, the standard dose is about 100 to 125 mg by intramuscular injection (IM) every seven to ten days. It can also be given as 200 mg each two weeks, but this can result in peak levels (right after the shot) that are too high, and levels that go too low for a few days before the next shot. Adding the testosterone patches on day nine through fourteen (when getting the shot every fourteen days) can avoid the levels going too low. I feel that giving the shot weekly is much better, however. I use Delatestryl 200 mg/cc and give ½ or ⁹⁄₁₀ cc every seven to ten days. Unfortunately, the skin patches alone are not adequate for the job. Although I've avoided using testosterone tablets in men, testosterone cream (100 mg/gm in PLO Gel) 25 to 100 mg bid (available from Ron's Pharmacy; see Appendix J: Resources) can be very effective. I will sometimes wait until after a man has been on the shots for eight weeks so he can tell what the optimal effect is. The problem (for men) with taking tablets instead of transdermal creams is that oral testosterone goes to the liver first. The higher dose in men (versus women) can sometimes raise cholesterol levels (cholesterol is produced by the liver). Avoiding other possible side effects by taking the transdermal hormone daily, instead of getting high and low levels by taking it IM every week or two, may be another benefit of the transdermal creams. The benefits of treatment (it takes six to eight weeks to see the effect) are often dramatic. Androderm gel (25 and 50 mg/5 cc) is also now available in most pharmacies, but is much more expensive than compounded testosterone.

For women, the treatment is easier. Natural micronized testosterone (and natural estrogen and progesterone) are available through most compounding pharmacies. Belmar pharmacy and Cape Drugs are two of many that do mail-order prescriptions. (See Appendix J: Resources.) The usual dose is 2 mg one to two times a day by mouth (po) or transdermally (4mg/gm cream). If the patient needs estrogen or progesterone, these hormones can be combined in the same capsule for a lower cost.

I check *free* testosterone blood levels (in men and women) six to eight weeks after starting therapy (in men, before their eight-week shot) and adjust the dosing accordingly. Blood levels are not reliable, however, if the patient is taking synthetic methyltestosterone instead of natural testosterone. In addition, blood levels for oral or transdermal dosing peak at about two to three hours and are back to baseline by five hours, so the blood level should be checked two to three hours after oral or transdermal dosing.

In women, if acne, intense dreams, or darkening of facial hair occurs (as can occur with DHEA as well), the dose is too high and should be decreased (these are usually reversible). These side effects can also be caused by estrogen being too low, relative to the testosterone level and may be avoided in women by supplementing both together. In men, acne suggests the dose is too high. It is important to monitor levels because (as in body builders who abuse testosterone by taking many times the recommended physiologic dose) elevated levels can cause elevated blood counts, liver inflammation, decreased sperm counts with infertility (also usually reversible) and elevated cholesterols with increased risk of heart disease. Because of this, in *men,* I would monitor a CBC, cholesterols, and liver enzymes intermittently. Testosterone supplementation can also cause elevated thyroid hormone levels in those taking thyroid supplements. If the patient is on thyroid supplements, I would recheck thyroid hormone levels after six to twelve weeks or sooner if they get palpitations or anxious or hyper feelings. Raising a low testosterone level has been shown repeatedly to lower cholesterol, decrease angina and depression, and improve diabetes. Unfortunately, our training mostly focused on the effects of abusing testosterone with pharmacologic and illicit dosing.

DISORDERED SLEEP

A foundation of CFIDS/FMS is the sleep disorder.[19] Many patients can only sleep three to five hours a night with multiple wakings. Even more problematic is the loss of deep stage 3 and 4 "restorative" sleep. Using medications that increase *deep* restorative sleep, so that the patient gets seven to nine hours of solid sleep without waking or hangover, is critical. Start with a very low dose. The next-day sedation that most patients experience often resolves in two to three weeks. If it does not, have the patient take the medication earlier in the evening—for example, at around 9:00 P.M. so that it wears off earlier the next day, or switch to shorter acting agents such as Ambien, Sonata, and/or Xanax.

I do *not* recommend most addictive sleeping pills. Most addictive sleep remedies, except for clonazepam (Klonopin) and alprazolam (Xanax), actually *decrease* the time that is spent in deep sleep and can worsen fibromyalgia.

The medications that I do recommend include the following:

- Zolpidem (Ambien), 5 or 10 mg. Use 5 to 20 mg qhs. This medication is a newer agent with fewer side effects than the other medications. It is very helpful for most patients and is my first choice among the sleep medications. Although only to be used for one week in routine insomnia, experience shows that extended use is appropriate in CFIDS/FMS. Patients can take an extra 5 to 10 mg in the middle of the night if they wake.
- cyclobenzaprine (Flexeril), 10 mg, and/or carisprodol (Soma), 350 mg. Use ½ to 2 tablets qhs. Both medications are often very sedating. Use one of these first if myalgias are a major problem.
- Trazodone (Desyrel), 50 mg. Use ½ to 6 tablets qhs. Use this medication first if anxiety is a major problem. Warn patients to call immediately if priapism occurs.
- Amitriptyline (Elavil), 10 mg. Use ½ to 5 tablets qhs. This drug causes weight gain and can worsen NMH.
- Natural remedies. I have designed a sleep formula containing valerian root, melatonin, lemon balm, passionflower, kava kava and 5-HTP.[20] Dr. Teitelbaum's Sleep formula is available through my office. (See Appendix J: Resources.)
- Doxylamine (Unisom for Sleep), 25 mg qhs.

For patients with disabling muscle aches or anxiety, respectively, I recommend Klonopin or Xanax. Begin with 0.25 mg qhs and slowly adjust the dose upward as needed as the next-day sedation diminishes.

Some patients will sleep well with 5 mg of Ambien and others will require all of the above combined. Because the malfunctioning hypothalamus controls sleep and the muscle pain also interferes with sleep, it is often necessary and appropriate to use multiple sleep aids. Because of next-day sedation and possibly slow liver clearance, CFIDS/FMS patients do better with combining low doses of several medications than with a high dose of one.

Although less common, two other sleep disturbances must be considered and, if present, treated. The first is sleep apnea. This should especially be suspected if the patient snores and is overweight and hypertensive. If two of these conditions are present and the patient does not improve with our treatment, I would consider a sleep apnea study. I would get preapproval from the patient's insurance company, as the test usually costs $1,500 to $2,000. Sleep apnea is treated with weight loss and nasal C-pap. A sleep study will also detect restless leg syndrome (RLS or PLMs), which is also more common in fibromyalgia.[21] (Yunus, 1996). Asking the patient if the bed sheets are scattered about when he or she awakes and/or if the patient kicks his or her spouse during the night will often let you know RLS is present. It is treated with Ambien, Klonopin, and/or Sinemet 10/100, and by keeping ferritin levels over 50.

Autonomic Dysfunction

Low blood pressure and dizziness, increased thirst, polyuria, cold extremities, and night sweats are a few of the symptoms that reflect autonomic dysfunction in CFIDS/FMS. A recent study at Johns Hopkins Hospital showed that a majority of CFIDS patients had neurally mediated hypotension (NMH) on tilt table testing.[22] This means that CFIDS/FMS patients can severely drop their blood pressure with standing or minimal exertion. If the patient has a low BP or dizziness or a positive tilt table test, a treatment trial is appropriate. I predominantly use clinical history and the "poor man's tilt table test" (free instead of $1,800), which consists of having the patient stand while leaning against the wall for ten minutes. If this aggravates symptoms, the test is positive. Treatment consists of markedly increasing salt and water intake. In children, fludrocortisone (Florinef), 1/10-mg tablets, 1 to 2 qd, can be helpful. Begin with ¼ tablet a day and increase by ¼ tablet a day each three to seven days. Increasing more quickly can cause headache. The most responsive patients need 0.1 milligram a day, although Dr. Rowe (a pediatrician and the primary Johns Hopkins Hospital NMH researcher) notes that 0.2 milligram a day is sometimes needed. As Florinef can cause potassium loss, have the patient increase potassium intake (for example, one banana and 12-ounce V-8 juice a day) and check potassium levels every six to twelve weeks. It takes six weeks on the full dose to see the effects of treatment. Younger patients often respond the best. Florinef helped only 14 percent of CFIDS patients in a recent study, versus 10 percent of placebo patients. Fluoxetine (Prozac), sertraline (Zoloft), ephedrine (*not* pseudoephedrine), and dextroamphetamine (Dexedrine) are clinically much more effective in treating NMH in CFIDS patients, and I rarely use Florinef in anyone over eighteen years old.

IMMUNE DYSFUNCTION AND INFECTIONS

Although not as severe as AIDS, and not progressive, marked immune dysfunction is part of the process (CFIDS stands for chronic fatigue and immune dysfunction syndrome). Because of this, some of the opportunistic infections seen in AIDS are present in CFIDS/FMS. These include chronic URIs and sinusitis, bowel infections (for example, parasites and fungal overgrowth as in AIDS—often with agents that are nonpathogenic in healthy people), UTIs, and chronic, low-grade prostatitis. These need to be treated.

Chronic sinusitis responds poorly to antibiotics. Conservative measures (for example, saline nasal rinsing, avoiding milk products, and so on) are more appropriate. These are discussed briefly in my book, and at length in the wonderful book *Sinus Survival* written by Dr. Robert Ivker (Tarcher/ Putnam, 2000).[23] Avoiding antibiotics also decreases the risk of secondary fungal overgrowth in the sinuses and GI tract.

Bowel infections with alterations of normal bacterial flora, fungal overgrowth, and parasitic infections (parasites are seen in one-sixth of my patients) are the norm in this disease. This is reflected by the patient's bowel symptoms. Because of the lack of a definitive test for yeast overgrowth, there is little research published in this area and treatment is controversial. Treatment is empiric, and based on the patient's history.

A history of frequent yeast vaginitis, frequent antibiotic use (especially tetracycline for acne), onchomycosis, or gas, bloating, diarrhea or constipation, in my experience with over 1,000 CFIDS/FMS patients, warrants an empiric therapeutic trial. Many CFIDS/FMS patients who failed other therapies for spastic colon have responded dramatically to anti-infectious treatments. This was also shown in our 1995 study.[24]

Treatment consists of nystatin, two 500,000-IU tablets po bid or tid (start slowly) for five months. The patient's symptoms, especially fibromyalgia pain, may flare initially as the yeast die off. Therefore, begin with one 500,000-unit tablet of nystatin once a day and increase by one tablet every one to three days, as tolerated, up to two tablets tid. After four weeks on the nystatin, add 200 mg of fluconazole (Diflucan) or itraconazole (Sporanox) qd for six weeks. Mild liver enzyme elevations are sometimes seen with Diflucan and Sporanox, but taking lipoic acid, 200 mg/d, seems to markedly decrease this side effect. The other major side effect of both Diflucan and Sporanox is the price—a six-week course can cost more than six hundred dollars. If symptoms *recur* after the first six weeks on Diflucan or Sporanox, I recommend repeating the 200 milligrams per day for another six weeks. If no benefit is derived from the first course, I do not recommend repeating it. Have your patient stay on the nystatin for a total of five to eight months. I recommend patients be on nystatin while they are taking Sporanox or Diflucan to avoid development of resistant organisms.

Sporanox must be taken with food (it needs stomach acid) to be properly absorbed. Acid blockers such as ranitidine (Zantac) and Maalox will prevent its absorption. Diflucan does not require stomach acid for proper absorption. *Do not use Seldane, Hismanal, or Propulsid with Diflucan or Sporanox, as the combination can cause fatal arrhythmias.* Claritin can be used. Mevacor family medications can also cause problems when taken with Sporanox or Diflucan. Sweets must also be avoided, since they seem to stimulate yeast growth. One cup of yogurt with live and active yogurt cultures eaten daily is helpful. Refrigerated acidophilus bacteria, 4 billion units per day, also can help to restore normal bowel flora.

Parasitic infections, often with "nonpathogenic" or normally self-limiting organisms (again, as seen in AIDS patients) are common. Stool samples can be sent to your local lab for antigenic and chemical testing for giardia, cryptosporidium, and especially clostridium difficile (which was present in approximately 22 percent of our CFIDS study patients versus approximately 1 percent of the healthy populace). I would send the O&P test, however, to Great Smokies Diagnostic Laboratory or the Parasitology Center. (See Appendix J: Resources.) Sending the O&P to most other labs is a waste of money. Most labs will report stool O&P's as being negative, even if parasites are present. If the patient has parasites (even if nonpathogenic) treat them. If he or she uses well water, I would recommend a water filter that eliminates parasites (most do not) such as the Multi-Pure filter. (See Appendix J: Resources.)

In patients with low-grade fevers (anything over 98.6°F in CFIDS/

FMS patients), occult infections (for example, chlamydia and mycoplasma incognitus) are being found. Empiric therapy with doxycycline 100 mg tid for six months to two years (while on nystatin) can be very helpful. Recent research is showing that HHV-6, CMV, and EBV are also commonly active in CFIDS/FMS.

NUTRITIONAL DEFICIENCIES

CFIDS and FMS patients are often nutritionally deficient. This occurs because of (1) malabsorption from bowel infections, (2) increased needs because of the illness, and (3) inadequate diet. Early evidence suggests that defects in membrane function may also play a role.

Although space does not allow a detailed discussion of mitochondrial dysfunction here, the B-vitamins (including B_{12}), magnesium, iron, sulfur, coenzyme Q_{10}, malic acid, and aspartates, and other minerals are critical.[25] These nutrients (and others) are also critical for many other processes. Although blood testing is not reliable or necessary for most nutrients (a 20-cent-a-day vitamin will cover these), checking for some nutrient deficiencies (that is, B_{12}, Fe, TIBC, and ferritin levels) is very important.

I would treat CFIDS/FMS patients with:

1. A good multivitamin (most are not). Specifically, I would use Berocca Plus, 1 qd, or Natrol's "My Favorite Multiple—Take One." I have developed a powdered formula (the From Fatigued To Fantastic powder formula) that replaces fifteen to thirty tablets of other supplements a day. (See Appendix J: Resources.) Whenever I make a product, I ask the company producing it to donate my share of any profits to charity, and I never take money from any company whose products I recommend.
2. Magnesium with malic acid. This is critical and the brand is important. I would use Fibrocare, 2 tid (use less if diarrhea develops). This is included in the From Fatigued To Fantastic powder formula.
3. If the iron percent saturation is under 22 percent *or* the ferritin is under 40 mg/ml (check both!), give iron. I recommend Chromagen LA, 1 qd for four to six months. It should be taken on an empty stomach. Food decreases absorption by over 60 percent. It should *not* be taken within six hours of thyroid (and possibly other hormones), as it blocks thyroid absorption.

4. If B_{12} is under 540 pg/ml, I recommend B_{12} injections, 3,000 micrograms IM three times a week times for twelve weeks, then as needed (prn). Recent reports on CFIDS are showing absent or near-absent CSF B_{12} levels with low normal serum B_{12} levels (Regland, B).[26] Metabolic evidence of B_{12} deficiency is seen even at levels of 540 pg/ml or more (Lindenbaum, 1994).[27] Severe neuropsychiatric changes are seen from B_{12} deficiency even at levels of 300 pg/ml (Lindenbaum, 1988) (a level over 209 is technically normal).[28] As an editorial in *The New England Journal of Medicine* notes, the old-time doctors may have been right about giving B_{12} shots (Beck, 1988).[29] Compounding pharmacies can make B_{12} at 3,000 mcg/cc concentrations. I use hydroxycobalmin.

5. Coenzyme Q_{10}, 100 to 200 mg a day. This is often helpful.

6. K-Mg aspartate. This is very helpful in fatigue states.[30] The dose is 500 milligrams, 2 bid for three months (then stop). Most brands may not work as they are not chemically fully reacted (Hicks, 1964).[31] General Nutrition Centers' house brand appears to be an effective product.

7. The patient should avoid sugar, caffeine, and excess alcohol (warn him or her that there may be a seven- to ten-day withdrawal period when coming off the sugar and caffeine).

Final Thoughts

Many illnesses are associated with various psychological profiles. For example, a "helpless/hopeless" attitude is associated with cervical cancer and hostility with ASCVD. In CFIDS/FMS, a common profile is a "megatype-A" overachiever who, because of childhood low self esteem, overachieves to get approval. They tend to be perfectionistic and tend to have difficulties protecting their boundaries—that is, they say yes to requests when they feel like saying no. Instead of responding to their bodies' signal of fatigue by resting, they redouble their efforts. Taking time to rest, and getting and staying out of abusive work environments (even after they feel better on treatment!) is critical. As they start to feel better, they need to be instructed to take it slow, and not to go back to the level of over functioning that made them sick in the first place. They especially need to be instructed *not* to make up for lost time.

In treating well over 1,000 CFIDS/FMS patients, a treatment protocol has now evolved that offers effective therapy for the 6 million Americans unnecessarily crippled with CFIDS/FMS. Our initial pilot study and our follow-up randomized trial show that over 85 percent of patients improved with treatment (Teitelbaum, Bird, 1995 and 2000) (see Appendix B).[32] A replicative, multicenter placebo-controlled study is being developed in England as well. These very ill patients require time and compassion—as well as an organized treatment approach. I think you'll be as thrilled as we've been, though, to watch these previously crippled patients become healthy!

Studies of Effective Treatment Modalities for Chronic Fatigue and Fibromyalgia

Study #1: published as the lead article in the Journal of Chronic Fatigue Syndrome *Vol. 8, No. 2, 2001.*

Effective Treatment of Chronic Fatigue Syndrome and Fibromyalgia—a Randomized, Double-Blind, Placebo-Controlled, Intent to Treat Study

Jacob E. Teitelbaum, MD[*1]; Barbara Bird, M.T.,C.L.S.*[*];
Robert M. Greenfield, MD*[1]; Alan Weiss, MD*[1]; Larry Muenz, Ph.D*[2];
Laurie Gould, BS*[*3]

[*Annapolis Research Center For Effective FMS/CFIDS Therapies, 466 Forelands Rd., Annapolis, MD 21401; 1) Anne Arundel Medical Center, Annapolis, MD; 2) Gaithersburg, MD; 3) USDA, Beltsville, MD]

No outside funding. Multivitamins supplied by Twinlab; Synthroid by Knoll; Fibrocare and Valerian Rest by To Your Health; Sporanox by Janssen; Oxytocin and DHEA by Belmar Pharmacy; Prozac by DISTA; Zoloft by Roerig; Paxil by SKB; Chromagen by Savage Labs; Serzone by Bristol-Myers Squibb; and Flagyl by Searle.

ABSTRACT. Background: Hypothalamic dysfunction has been suggested in Fibromyalgia (FMS) and Chronic Fatigue Syndrome (CFS). This dysfunction may result in disordered sleep, subclinical hormonal deficiencies, and immunologic changes. Our previously published open trial showed that patients usually improve by using a protocol which treats all the above processes simultaneously. The current study examines this protocol using a randomized, double-blind design with an intent to treat analysis.

Methods: Seventy-two FMS patients (thirty-eight active: thirty-four placebo; sixty-nine also met CFS criteria) received all active or all placebo therapies as a unified intervention. Patients were treated, as indicated by symptoms and/or lab testing, for: (1) subclinical thyroid, gonadal, and/or adrenal insufficiency, (2) disordered sleep, (3) suspected NMH, (4) opportunistic infections, and (5) suspected nutritional deficiencies.

Results: At the final visit, sixteen active patients were "much better," fourteen "better," two "same," zero "worse," and one "much worse" versus three, nine, eleven, six, and four, respectively, in the placebo group (p<.0001, Cochran-Mantel-Haenszel trend test). Significant improvement in the FMS Impact Questionnaire (FIQ) scores (decreasing from 54.8 to 33.2 versus 51.4 to 47.7) and Analog scores (improving from 176.1 to 310.3 versus 177.1 to 211.9) (both with p<.0001 by random effects regression), and Tender Point Index (TPI) (31.7 to 15.5 versus 35.0 to 32.3, p<.0001 by baseline adjusted linear model) were seen. Long-term follow-up (mean 1.9 years) of the active group showed continuing and increasing improvement over time, despite patients being able to wean off most treatments.

Conclusions: Significantly greater benefits were seen in the active group than in the placebo group for all primary outcomes. Using an integrated treatment approach, effective treatment is now available for FMS/CFS.

Introduction

Fibromyalgia (FMS), which currently affects an estimated 3 to 6 million Americans (1, 2), and Chronic Fatigue Syndrome (CFS) are two illnesses which often coexist. Severe persistent fatigue, diffuse migratory pain, cognitive dysfunction, and disordered sleep are common symptoms that patients often report in these overlapping syndromes. Current research suggests that many triggers can initiate a cascade of events, causing hypothalamic—target gland axis dysfunction (3, 4) and associated loss of normal circadian cycling of cortisol secretion (5). Hypothalamic dysfunction may result in some of the changes reported in FMS and/or CFS. These include:

1. Disordered sleep (6, 7) with associated pain (8). Disordered sleep (as well as hormonal and other changes) may cause immune dysfunction—e.g., Natural Killer Cell dysfunction (9), decreased proliferative responses (10) and opportunistic infections (6, 11).

2. Hormonal deficiencies and hypothalamic-pituitary-target gland axis dysfunction (3, 4, 6, 12). These can also contribute to the neurotransmitter changes seen in FMS (13). And

3. Autonomic dysfunction—including Neurally Mediated Hypotension (NMH) (14, 15). Macro and micro nutrient deficiencies have also been shown by some authors (16–19). In our initial pilot study (20), we explored the side effects, dosing and effectiveness of simultaneously treating the above problems. We found that simultaneously treating these resulted in significant clinical improvement. Which mix of treatments were needed, however, varied from patient to patient.

    Although a concept that is sometimes uncomfortable and foreign to traditional styles of thinking, the need for multiple interventions can occur when an illness affects a critical control center (such as the hypothalamus) which impacts the multiple systems noted above. Unfortunately, we have not yet found a single treatment that reverses hypothalamic dysfunction directly. Thus, this situation is different from illnesses that affect a single target organ and which can be treated with a single intervention. For example, pituitary dysfunction itself often requires treatment with several hormones. This effect is multiplied in hypothalamic dysfunction, which affects several critical systems in addition to the pituitary gland. We therefore hypothesized that an integrated treatment approach based on simultaneously treating the above problems (even if a modest degree of suspicion that would usually not be treated is present) will be clinically beneficial in CFS and FMS. Subgroup analysis was done to assess the effect of antidepressant therapy. Our current study tests the efficacy of this therapeutic approach and the above hypothesis using a randomized, double-blind, placebo-controlled protocol with an intent-to-treat analysis in an outpatient setting.

Materials and Methods

INCLUSION CRITERIA

Seventy-two patients with FMS who met entry criteria were entered into the study between November 1995 and November 1997. All but three (all in the active group) also met the 1994 Center For Disease Control (CDC) criteria for CFS (21). Patients were recruited by word of mouth, patient support groups, and media reports regarding our research center. All patients were required to meet 1990 American College of Rheumatology (ACR) criteria for FMS (22). Patients were not considered study candidates if major intercurrent illnesses (e.g., active cancer, multiple sclerosis, poorly controlled Diabetes, Emphysema, or Lupus) were present that could cause their symptoms. In addition, patients were excluded if: they were overtly hypothyroid (i.e., low T4 and elevated Thyroid Stimulating Hormone [TSH]) or hyperthyroid (i.e., high T4 and low TSH). Creatinine >1.9 mg/dL (168umoL/L), AST >60 u/L (1.00 ukat/L), glucose > 200 mg/dL (11.1mmol/L), Hematocrit (HCT) < .34 or Erythrocyte Sedimentation Rate (ESR) >45mm/h were present. Patients were not excluded for depression, anxiety or sleep disorders.

Patients discontinued any previous treatments when able (except thyroid hormones, estrogen and progesterone) that were part of the study protocol. Patients were allowed to continue or begin active treatment upon completing the study and to participate in any other interventions on their own that were not part of the study protocol. Patients received a thorough history, physical exam and lab testing including a Complete Blood Count (CBC), Chem 18, serum magnesium, ESR, Urinalysis with micro, B12, Folate, Total T3, Free T4 or Free T7 index, TSH, HgbA$_1$C, Cortrosyn (25 unit) Stimulation test, DHEA-Sulphate, IgE and stool O & P's. Follicle Stimulating Hormone (FSH), Luteinizing Hormone (LH) and estradiol levels were checked in females. Free Testosterone levels and stool tests for Clostridium difficile toxin were checked in a subset of the patients. Detailed informed consent was obtained from each patient.

PATIENT POPULATION

Patient demographics at study entry are described in Table 1. Mean age at entry was 44.6 years (std. dev. 8.1, range 23–61). Sixty-six of 72 patients

(92%) were female, and mean reported duration of CFS was 8.3 years (std. dev. 6.5, range 0.5–34 years). Average number of physicians consulted before coming to this clinic was 7.7 (range 0–100). Placebo patients were four years older, on average, than active-treatment patients (p = 0.037 by t-test), but there were no other significant demographic differences. The two treatment groups had no significant, or nearly significant, differences in mean entry values of the outcome measures, including the individual components of the Analog Total. With a possible range of 0–500, entry visit mean Analog Total was 176.5 (std. dev. 64.1, range 20–355) and, with a possible range of 0–80, the entry visit mean Fibromyalgia Impact Questionnaire score was 53.2 (std. dev. 9.6, range 30.4–74.6). Seventy-two patients met entry criteria and began treatment. Thirty-eight patients were randomized to the active intervention and 34 to the placebo intervention. The treatment protocol described below was completed by 32 patients in each group. The remaining 8 (6 active, 2 placebo) dropped out between visits 1 and 3. For some outcomes and visits, missing data yield sample sizes below 72 but, unless indicated, reported results concern the intention-to-treat sample. Participants gave written informed consent at the time of the initial examination and were informed of the double-blind, placebo-controlled nature of the study. The protocol is consistent with the principles of the Declaration of Helsinki.

RANDOMIZATION AND BLINDING

Treatment was assigned in randomized blocks of six (B.B.). Patients then chose a date convenient for them to begin the study. Midway through the study, our statistician (L.M.), using the random number facility in SAS, generated the remaining code to maintain an equal number of active and placebo patients. Codes were kept away from the clinic in areas not accessible to patients or to the treating physician. Decisions as to whether the patients met entry criteria and their treatment prescriptions were made by the treating physician (J.E.T.), who was blinded to the patients' assignment and allocation sequence.

When possible, medications and identically appearing placebos were obtained from the companies making them. When not available, placebos were made by the pharmacist to approximate the medications' appearance. The treating physician did not have access to the medications. Containers of medications were labeled with various codes, with the code sheet accessible only to the pharmacist and the person responsible for dispensing medication (B.B.).

Outcome Measures

Four outcome measures were used. The primary outcome measures were the initial versus the final visit scores:

1. Overall response—At the final visit the patients were asked whether they felt much worse, worse, same, better or much better after completing the protocol.
2. Visual Analog (well-being) Scale (VAS) of 0–100 for 5 questions (obtained at each visit):
   A. How is your energy? 0 (near dead)–100 (excellent)
   B. How is your sleep? 0 (poor sleep)–100 (excellent, uninterrupted sleep)
   C. How is your mental clarity? 0 (severe "brain fog")–100 (normal healthy)
   D. How bad is your achiness? 0 (very severe, painful)–100 (no problem)
   E. How is your overall sense of well being? 0 (horrible)–100 (great)

3. FIQ or Fibromyalgia Impact Questionnaire (disability index)—described previously (23) (obtained at each visit).
4. Tender Point Index (TPI)—This value is calculated by multiplying the number of positive tender points (TP—out of 18) by their degree of tenderness (1= TP painful, 2= grimaces, withdrawal or involuntary jerk on TP palpation, 3= markedly withdraws on palpation, 4= patient refuses to allow a TP to be examined because of the severity of the pain) (maximum score of 72). Five patients had their TPI checked 3 times (each 1 hour apart) at the initial visit, with TPI scores showing good intra-visit consistency. The TPI was assessed at the initial and final visits.

After the study was completed, overall response, Analog and FIQ scores were checked on all available patients (who opted to stay on treatment) to assess for tachyphylaxis and/or continuing improvement and the patient's ability to maintain their improvement after tapering off most of the treatments.

TREATMENT

It has been suggested that, in Myofascial Pain Syndrome (MPS), tissue needs for various hormones and nutrients are often greater than can be supplied by low-normal blood levels (24). Our initial study suggests that this also occurs in FMS (20). The symptom checklists we used (25), and a detailed discussion of our overall diagnostic and treatment protocols and the rationale behind them have been discussed and published previously (20, 25, 26). The protocol has also been integrated into a computerized algorithm (27). The specific (and less extensive) treatment protocol we used in this study is described in Table 2. Each patient received either all active or all placebo treatments as a unified intervention. How many active patients received each treatment and how decisions were made on which treatments to use in each individual patient is also described in Table 2.

SAMPLE SIZE AND POWER

With a two-sided t-test, power 80% and type I error 5%, sample sizes of 38 and 34 allow detection of a standardized effect of 0.67, which is considered moderate. At the last visit, this effect corresponds to about 73 points and 11 points for the Analog Total and FIQ scales respectively—effects that we judged to be clinically significant.

STATISTICAL METHODS

Analog score totals and the FIQ, both of which were measured repeatedly, were compared between placebo and active treatment groups by two regression models, one for post-baseline trends in scores (random effects regression in SAS PROC MIXED, with time defined by visit number) and one for time to a 30% improvement over baseline scores, (i.e., a reduction for the FIQ and an increase for the Analog Total). Not all subjects had such changes, so the latter is a possibly-censored outcome and was analyzed by the Cox proportional hazards regression SAS PROC PHREG and by non-parametric Kaplan-Meier estimates implemented in SAS PROC

LIFETEST, with time defined by elapsed days since study entry. Two random effects regression models were considered, one with treatment main effect only and one with both main effect and treatment by time interaction; the main effect estimates average post-baseline differences while the interaction assesses how rapidly treatment group means diverge. Stepdown likelihood ratio tests were used to select the best regression models. The Tender Point Index was recorded only at baseline and completion, and was analyzed by linear regression with baseline value as a covariate. The Cochran-Mantel-Haenszel test was used to compare treatments regarding the categorical Patient=s Summary. $P < 0.05$ was considered significant and statistical tests are two-sided, but without multiple comparison adjustments.

Timing of Visits and Duration of Follow-up

Excluding a several-month time-period during which follow-up visits were unavailable, time trends in all analyses were based on elapsed days since study entry. Visits were scheduled one month apart and the median interval between consecutive visits was 31 days (26 and 37 days are the 25th and 75th percentile). The interval was nearly constant over the full period of follow-up. Subjects were followed for a median duration of 101 days and 96 days in active and placebo groups, respectively (25th percentiles: 88 and 89 days, 75th percentiles: 124 and 106 days).

Results

Analog Total and FIQ Scores

Means and standard deviations by visit are in Table 3. Figures 1a and 1b show both observed means and average predicted values from a random effect regression model, the latter only for visits 2 and later since baseline scores are predictors in the model. After adjustment for baseline score and age, the best model for Analog Total (Figure 1a) has only a significant main effect of the treatment (estimated effect 72, 95% Cl (37, 108), $p < 0.0001$ for a test of no difference). Mean Analog Total increases rapidly from visits 1 to 2 in the actively treated group and more slowly thereafter. After visit 2, there is a similar rate of improvement in the placebo group but not the early rapid increase seen in the actively treated group. The between-treatment difference of mean Analog Total scores was significant by visit 2 (two-sided p-value 0.005 by t test) and roughly constant thereafter. Also adjusting for baseline score and age, the best model for FIQ (Figure 1b) shows a significant main effect of treatment (estimated effect—11, 95% CI [-16, -6], p < 0.0001 for a test of no difference). Mean FIQ declines slowly in the placebo group and more rapidly in the actively treated group with a significant difference seen by the third visit (two-sided p-value 0.0012 for t-test of no difference at visit 3). At the final visit, significant improvement in the FIQ (decreasing from 54.8 to 33.2 vs. 51.4 to 47.7) and Analog scores (improving from 176.1 to 310.3 vs. 177.1 to 211.9) (p ≤ 0.0005 by unadjusted t-test comparing final scores and p < 0.0001 by random effects regression incorporating repeated measures for both FIQ and Analog) are seen.

By treatment group, Kaplan-Meier curves of the time to 30% improvement in the two outcomes are seen in Figures 2a and 2b. Exact event times were interpolated between visits to identify when a 30% change was first seen. Events occurring after 100 days past baseline were truncated because of the small remaining sample size. For the Analog Total, 30/35 active group patients (86%, median time 22 days) improved by 30% while on study compared to 19/34 (56%, median time 70 days) of placebo group patients. Again, the time to 30% improvement is substantially and significantly shorter in the active group (log-rank test p-value 0.0006, Cox model p-value 0.0013 after adjustment for age and baseline Analog Total). For the FIQ 25/36 active group subjects achieved this improvement while on the study (69%, interpolated median time 58 days) compared to 11/34 placebo group subjects (34%, median time 101 days); the time to 30% improvement is substantially and significantly shorter in the active group (log-rank p-value 0.003, Cox model p-value 0.007 after adjustment for age and baseline FIQ).

Impact of Anti-Depressants on Study Outcomes

At some time during the study, Serotonin Uptake Inhibitors (SSRI's), Amitriptyline and Cyclobenzaprine were used by 76, 26, and 26 percent of the active group subjects and 74, 32, and 32 percent of the placebo group subjects. To address the possible impact of the non-randomized use of antidepressants on evidence of an overall treatment effect, random effects regressions tested the effect of the primary, randomized treatment adjusting for baseline score, visit, age, and the time-varying use of an SSRI, Amitriptyline, or Cyclobenzaprine. Antidepressant use was coded as three time-dependent covariates, each taking value 0 (no use or use stopped on that visit) or 1 (antidepressant prescribed or still in use) one visit before the Analog Total or FIQ outcome. In the placebo group, the antidepressants were shams so, for these subjects, a test of antidepressant effect compares a sham product to no product.

The regression models showed that SSRIs significantly decrease the FIQ (estimated 5.2 points improvement in sham or true SSRI users, p-value 0.029 for a test of zero effect) with no significant difference in the impact of the SSRI according to whether it was true or sham (p-value 0.55 for the interaction of treatment by SSRI). There were no other significant antidepressant effects in either treatment group on either Analog Total or FIQ. Furthermore, in models that adjusted for use of the three antide-pressants, tests of the effect of the randomized treatment on the two pri-mary outcomes remained highly significant (p < 0.0001 for both Analog Total and FIQ). Thus, these analyses identified a single significant effect of antidepressants with little impact on the primary comparisons of the active and placebo treatments.

TENDER POINT INDEX AND PATIENT OVERALL RESPONSE

At the last visit, the mean TPI (Figure 3) was significantly lower in the ac-tively treated group (p < .0001 by t-test). A regression analysis showed that TPI score at the final visit was significantly related only to treatment and TPI score at entry and not to age or number of visits. At each TPI entry score, actively treated patients had mean adjusted scores 15.1 points lower than placebo patients (p < .0001).

The distribution of patients overall response scores are in Figure 4 and Table 3 for 66 of 72 patients including all 64 patients who completed the study. Scores were significantly better among actively treated patients: p < .0001 by Cochran-Mantel-Haenszel trend test. If the ratings are assigned values from −2 (much worse) to +2 (much better), with zero for "same," mean scores were 1.33 (SD = 0.85) in the actively treated group and 0.03 (SD = 1.16) in the placebo group (p < .0001 by t-test). Overall response scores were missing for 6 patients, of which 5 were in the actively treated group (mean final Analog Total score of 214) and 1 was in the placebo group (final Analog Total score of 260). There is no evidence that the end-of-study summary was biased by the missing values.

Patients Meeting CFS Criteria
and Patients Completing the Study

Conclusions for these patient subgroups (n = 69 and n = 64) were qualitatively the same as for the 72 patients in the intention-to-treat sample. For 69 patients in the intention-to-treat sample who met CFS criteria, random effects regression analyses for Analog Total and FIQ scores yielded estimated treatment effects of 71.5 and -11.4 points (p < .0001 for both), which are similar to findings for the 72 intention-to-treat patients. Results for the 64 patients that completed the study, including both effect sizes and p-values, were also similar to those for the 72 patients (details omitted).

Drop Outs

One patient in each group dropped out because of side effects and one in each group dropped out with no reason given. One active patient dropped out because "there were too many pills" and three active patients dropped out because they were "too busy" to be in the study (two of these because of new, severe illnesses in a family member).

Adverse Events

By treatment group and body system, numbers of reported adverse events are given in Table 4. Patients were asked if they had complaints, but possible responses were not suggested. There were no significant differences between the treatment groups regarding any adverse event category although 7/38 active recipients compared to 2/34 placebo recipients reported a dermatological event (one-sided p = 0.10 by Fisher's exact test).

Pre and Post Study Cortrosyn Testing

Toward the end of the study 7 active patients given cortisol (and 13 given cortisol placebo) had post study Cortrosyn stimulation tests done. In the 7 active patients, average cortisol levels increased or stayed the same after treatment. Average cortisol levels (mcg/dL) pre, ½ hour and 1 hour post cortrosyn Intra-Muscularly (I.M.) were 14, 23, and 26 before treatment and 17, 23, and 26 after treatment. These results suggest that adrenal suppression did not occur with the low doses of cortisone used in the study.

Post Study Follow-Up

We were able to obtain follow-up data on 41 patients who chose to continue active treatment (many with their primary physicians) after the study. This data was obtained an average of 1.9 years after beginning active treatment. One had died (Melanoma). In the other 40, Analog and FIQ scores improved from 185 to 351 and 51.5 to 28.2 in those originally in the active group (180 to 308 and 51.4 to 36 in the total group). Of 38 patients for which "overall response" scores were available, 23 were "much better," 10 "better," 4 "same," 0 "worse," and 1 "much worse." The above includes 11 patients (10 from the placebo, 1 from the original active group) who were unable to get part of the treatment because of the medications' cost or because their primary care physician was unwilling to prescribe it.

Discussion

There are times that an illness occurs as a cascading series of events, where each dysfunction may trigger several others. We believe that this pathophysiology occurs in CFS/FMS. While these syndromes can be somewhat improved by treating a single underlying process, our pilot (20) and current studies suggest that treatment is more effective when all of the processes are treated simultaneously as an integrated whole.

Immune dysfunctions have been suggested in CFS (9, 10). In this current study, Clostridium difficile testing was positive in 11 out of 53 of the CFS/FMS patients we tested (20.7%), vs. a 2% prevalence in a healthy population (36). This may reflect both the host defense against opportunistic infections and the need for (often recurrent) antibiotics. Treating the various bowel infections frequently resolved severe gastrointestinal symptoms, often previously diagnosed as Irritable Bowel Syndrome, that had been present for years.

Non-restorative sleep is also suspected in FMS/CFS. Hypothalamic dysfunction can cause insomnia (6), which may be especially disruptive to slow-wave sleep. In healthy subjects, short-term sleep deprivation causes diminished cognitive function, decreased oral temperature and increased pain sensitivity. Experimental disruption of deep (slow-wave) sleep results in myalgias and fatigue (7). Clinical studies in FMS show that measures of pain and fatigue correlate with patients' assessment of sleep quality and improve with medications (e.g., amitriptyline and cyclobenzaprine) that restore stage 3 and stage 4 sleep (6). Sleep deprivation is immunosuppressive in animal models (6, 11) and may cause the decreased growth hormone levels seen in FMS patients (6).

Unfortunately, most hypnotic sleep aids currently in use decrease deep stages of sleep. Zolpidem (Ambien), however, maintains deep (stage 3 and 4) sleep (37). Because zolpidem is short acting, and because of the severity of the disordered sleep, it may be necessary to add other sleep treatments (e.g., trazodone, clonazepam, and carisprodol—often in combination). These treatments are adjusted so that the patient gets 7–8 hours of uninterrupted sleep without waking or next day sedation.

Autonomic dysfunction (e.g., Neurally Mediated Hypotension or NMH) is also common in CFS (15, 38), and may be ameliorated by increasing salt and water intake. Fludrocortisone (Florinef), may occasionally also improve NMH.

Some physicians may be uncomfortable with a study: 1) that uses multiple interventions adjusted for each patient and 2) that treats patients based on symptoms despite lab values being within the normal range. When possible, we prefer approaches without these difficulties. When not possible, it is important to remember that neither of these concerns has any significant impact on the scientific or clinical validity of the study data. It is, however, helpful to explore the rationale for using this approach in FMS/CFS.

Chronic unrelieved stress or distress (e.g., infectious, metabolic, situational, etc.) may "blunt" the stress response and its various axes and result in hypothalamic suppression. This may cause the cascade effect discussed in the introduction, and FMS/CFS may therefore effect multiple systems throughout the body. Each of these may then require simultaneous treatment. We believe that this mitigates the bias toward testing each individual treatment separately. It is helpful to remember that this bias comes from our having been trained in a period when a reductionistic approach was fashionable—and not because this approach holds any greater scientific validity.

Why then, would one treat for a process if the blood test is "normal"? Unlike primary organ failure, where the deficits eventually become marked, alterations in the patients' regulatory system can cause multiple marginal deficiencies, which, in the aggregate, may cause severe dysfunction. Much of our hormonal testing is based on primary gland failure and may not have been validated in conditions where blunting of the hypothalamic axes or peripheral resistance to hormone activity (4, 39, 40) may occur. To use thyroid testing as one example, the TSH level, which is the only thyroid test that some physicians check in these illnesses, has been shown to have a blunted response to Thyrotropin Releasing Hormone (TRH) stimulation in FMS (4). Recent research suggests that normal thyroid lab tests are also often seen in the presence of multiple symptoms common in hypothyroidism (41), and that subclinical hypothyroidism is highly prevalent in some subgroups (e.g., elderly woman) with a concomitant increase in significant morbidity (42). In fact, in a Health Maintenance Organization HMO, when thyroid blood testing was ordered (*i.e., even where it was likely that the ordering physician strongly suspected a thyroid disorder*), only 3.2% (~2 Standard Deviation [SD]) of the tests showed overt hypothyroidism (43). The problem with using a lab standard of 2 SD, is that even though it's statistically useful, it may not be clinically appropriate. As Professor A.J. Padilla, of Einstein College of Medicine, notes, some disorders occur "in continuity" without a clear defining line between health and illness. "Physicians and normal persons tend to derive comfort from the ability to classify things based on objective criteria. In the case of disorders in continuity, this requires the establishment of arbitrary cutoffs to separate the well from the ill . . . This results in a trade off between sensitivity . . . and specificity." He notes four methodologies for defining this cutoff. Using 2 SD appears to be the least sensitive by far (one option is the top 10% [vs. 2½%] of the population) (44)! This also suggests that our current lab norms, while possibly specific, may not be adequately sensitive and will miss many patients who might benefit from treatment. As has often been the case in medicine's history (e.g., diagnosing Angina based on symptoms before stress testing was available), physicians may need to rely on clinical information (e.g., weight gain, fatigue, myalgias, slow ankle reflex relaxation phase, etc. for hypothyroidism) to treat patients while waiting for the confirmatory technology to be developed and tested. Indeed, the importance of this concept is further supported by newer data that suggests that *most* patients who are clinically hypothyroid may have normal thyroid blood tests (45) and, when treated with thyroxine, have significant clinical improvement (46)! Indeed, when following thyroid therapy, thought-provoking work by Fraser, et al., suggests the possibility that "biochemical tests of thyroid function are of little, if any, value clinically" and that following clinical signs and symptoms may be more reliable (47).

While recognizing our natural resistance to multiple treatments of perhaps subtle deficiencies, we also recognized the need to test, in a randomized, placebo-controlled trial, the clinical experience of many physicians who effectively treat these syndromes using the above approach. Despite these misgivings, the possible limitation of our tests' sensitivity, the relative safety of low dose hormonal supplementation (34, 35), and the marked improvement in the severe debilitation experienced by many patients speak in favor of our moving beyond this resistance.

There are several other limitations to our study. Because inclusion criteria selected only adult FMS patients without other major intercurrent illnesses and only CFS patients who also had FMS, our results may not be generalizable to secondary FMS (e.g., patients who also have Lupus or Rheumatoid Arthritis), a pediatric population, or to CFS patients without FMS. We have found that these smaller subsets of patients usually improve with our treatment protocol, but have a higher incidence of treatment failures. We do not recommend that this protocol be used in patients with multiple sclerosis.

A second limitation was our inability to get exactly identical placebos for some study medications. Also, in any placebo-controlled study using psychoactive drugs, unblinding may occur because of the side effects of these medications. That there was no significant difference in the number of patients experiencing side effects between the two groups, however, suggests that unblinding did not occur. The treating physician did not have access to the medications during the study. In addition, at the final visit only 5 patients thought that they could tell if they were on active or placebo based on the medications' appearance or side effects. Of these, two guessed correctly and three incorrectly suggesting that blinding was effective.

A third concern is whether the benefit seen in our study was predominantly caused by SSRI and/or tricyclic use. Several other controlled studies have shown benefit with using tricyclics (e.g., amitriptyline or cyclobenzaprine) (48). Unfortunately the benefit is often modest and may wane after 6 months (31). A report by Goldenberg, et al. showed that Fluoxetine and Amitriptyline (individually or combined) for 6 weeks, were much more effective than placebo (32) Other controlled studies using SSRI's alone, however, did not show them to be of significant benefit relative to placebo (49, 50, 51). In our study, analysis of the data suggests that SSRI's and/or tricyclics were not significantly more effective than placebo and p values remained $\leq$ .0001 when our data was adjusted to exclude the effect of these agents.

A fourth limitation is the lack of objective measures to monitor the effectiveness of treatment. The impact of FMS/CFS may, however, be reasonably estimated by subjective symptoms. Thus, the patient's symptom assessment can be used as a reliable method to measure the treatments' effectiveness. Though no consensus yet exists on what the best outcome measures are for use in FMS/CFS studies, the FIQ has been validated (23) and the VAS, TPI and patient overall responses are also commonly used (52).

A fifth concern relates to whether the treatments' effectiveness might diminish over time. Although not blinded, our follow-up of patients an average of 1.9 years after beginning treatment showed that effectiveness of the active group's treatment increased over time and that this benefit persisted even after some or most of the treatment was (as per our protocol) terminated.

We hope this study will be helpful to physicians, patients and researchers studying FMS/CFS. Over time, treatment hopefully will be improved, markedly simplified and better understood. An independent, randomized, multi-center, replicative study of our findings is currently being developed. In the interim, this treatment protocol offers effective treatment for patients suffering with FMS/CFS.

ACKNOWLEDGEMENTS

We would like to thank Amy Podd of A.P. Business Solutions, Mary Groom and David He for their superb technical support.

We would like to dedicate this study to the memory of Janet Travell, M.D., whose pioneering work in the treatment of Myofascial Pain Syndrome forms the foundation of our treatment protocol.

REFERENCES

1. Goldenberg DL. Fibromyalgia Syndrome—An Emerging but Controversial Condition. JAMA 1987; 257: 2782–2787.

2. Wolfe F, Ross K, Anderson J, Russell IJ, Hebert L. The Prevalence & Characteristics of Fibromyalgia in the General Population. Arthritis & Rheumatism 1995 Jan; 38 (1): 19–28.

3. Demitrack MA, Dale JK, Straus SE, Laue L, Listwak SJ, Kruesi MJP, et al. Evidence for Impaired Activation of the Hypothalamic-Pituitary-Adrenal Axis in Patients with Chronic Fatigue Syndrome. J Clin Endocrinol Metab 1991; 73: 1224–1234.

4. Neeck G, Riedel W. Thyroid Function in Patients With Fibromyalgia Syndrome. J Rheumatol 1992; 19: 1120–1122.

5. McCain GA, Tilbe KS. Diurnal Hormone Variation in Fibromyalgia Syndrome: A Comparison With Rheumatoid Arthritis. J Rheumatol 1989; 16 Suppl 19: 154–157.

6. Pillemer S, Bradley LA, Crofford LJ, Moldofsky H, Chrousos GP. The Neuroscience and Endocrinology of FMS–[An NIH] Conference Summary. Arthritis & Rheumatism Nov 1997; 40 (11): 1928–1939.

7. Drewes AM, Nielson KD, Taagholt SJ, Bjerregaard K, Svendson L, Gade J. Slow Wave Sleep in FMS [Abstract]. J. Musculoskeletal Pain 1995; 3 Suppl 1: 29.

8. Older SA, Battafarano DF, Danning CL, Ward JA, Grady EP, Derman S. Delta Wave Sleep Interruption and FMS in Healthy Patients [Abstract]. J. Musculoskeletal Pain 1995; 3 Suppl 1: 159.

9. Barker E, Fujimura SF, Fadem MB, Landay AL, Levy JA. Immunologic Abnormalities Associated with Chronic Fatigue Syndrome. Clin Infect Dis 1994; 18 Suppl 1: S136–S141.

10. Straus SE, Fritz S, Dale JK, Gould B, Strober W. Lymphocyte Phenotype & Function in the Chronic Fatigue Syndrome. J Clin Immunol 1993; 13 (1): 30–40.

11. Everson CA. Sustained Sleep Deprivation Impairs Host Defense. Am J Physiol 1993; 265 (Regulatory Integrative Comp. Physiol 34); R1148–R1154.

12. Griep EN, Boersma JW, de Kloet ER. Altered Reactivity of the Hypothalamic-Pituitary-Adrenal Axis in the Primary Fibromyalgia Syndrome. J Rheumatol 1993; 20: 469–474.

13. Hammond CB. Menopause and Hormone Replacement Therapy: An Overview. Obstet Gynecol 1996; 87 Supplement: 2S–15S.

14. Rowe PC, Bou-Holaigah I, Kan JS, Calkins H. Is NMH an Unrecognized Cause of Chronic Fatigue? Lancet 1995; 345: 623–624.

15. Bou-Holaigah I, Rowe PC, Kan J, Calkins H. The Relationship Between NMH and the CFS. JAMA 1995; 274: 961–967.

16. Cox IM, Campbell MJ, Dowson D. Red Blood Cell Magnesium & Chronic Fatigue Syndrome. Lancet 1991; 337: 757–760.

17. Romano TJ, Stiller JW. Magnesium Deficiency in Fibromyalgia Syndrome. J Nutr Med 1994; 4: 165–167.

18. Evengard B, Nilsson CG, Astrom G, Lindh G, Lindqvist L, Olin R, et al. Cerebral Spinal Fluid Vitamin B12 Deficiency in Chronic Fatigue

Syndrome [Abstract]; Proceedings of The American Association for Chronic Fatigue Syndrome Research Conference; 1996 Oct 13–14; San Francisco, California.

19. Regland B, et al. Increased Concentrations of Homocysteine in the Cerebrospinal Fluid in Patients With Fibromyalgia and Chronic Fatigue Syndrome. Scandinavian Journal of Rheumatology 1997, 26: 301.

20. Teitelbaum J, Bird B. Effective Treatment of Severe Chronic Fatigue: A Report of a Series of 64 Patients. J Musculoskeletal Pain 1995; 3 (4): 91–110.

21. Fukuda K, Straus SE, Hickie I, Sharpe MC, Dobbins JG, Komaroff A, et al. The Chronic Fatigue Syndrome: A Comprehensive Approach to its Definition & Study. Ann Intern Med 1994; 121: 953–959.

22. Wolfe F, Smythe HA, Yunus MB, Bennett RM, Bombardier C, Goldenberg DL, et al. The American College of Rheumatology 1990 Criteria for the Classification of Fibromyalgia—Report of the Multicenter Criteria Committee; Arthritis & Rheumatism 1990 Feb; 33 (2): 160–172.

23. Burckhardt CS, Clark SR, Bennett RM. The Fibromyalgia Impact Questionnaire: Development and Validation. J of Rheumatology 1991; 18: 728–734.

24. Travell JG, Simons DG. The Trigger Point Manual- Volume 1. Baltimore (MD): Williams & Wilkins; 1983.

25. Teitelbaum J. From Fatigued To Fantastic!. 2nd ed. Garden City Park (NY); Avery Press; 1996.

26. Teitelbaum J. From Fatigued To Fantastic Newsletter. Annapolis (MD); Deva Press; 1997–1999.

27. *www.endfatigue.com.*

28. Zhdanova IV, Wurtman RJ, Lynch HJ, et al. Sleep Inducing Effects of Low Doses of Melatonin Ingested in the Evening. Clin Pharmacol Ther 1995; 57: 552–558.

29. Dressing H, et al. Insomnia: Are Valerian/Melissa Combinations of Equal Value to Benzodiazepine? Therapiewoche 1992; 42: 726–736.

30. Bennett RM, Gatter RA, Campbell SM, Andrews RP, Clark SR, Scarola JA. A Comparison of Cyclobenzaprine & Placebo in the Management of Fibrositis—A Double-Blind Controlled Study. A & R Primary Care Review 1990 July-Aug; 2 Suppl 4: 16–24.

31. Carette S, Bell MJ, Reynolds WJ, et al. Comparison of Amitriptyline, Cyclobenzaprine & Placebo in the Treatment of Fibromyalgia—A

Randomized, Double-Blind Clinical Trial. Arthritis and Rheumatism 1994: 37: 32–40.

32. Goldenberg D, Mayskiy M, Mossey R, Ruthazer R, Schmid C. A Randomized, Double-Blind Crossover Trial of Fluoxetine and Amitriptyline in the Treatment of FMS. Arthritis and Rheumatism 1996; 39 Suppl 11: 1852–1859.

33. Lindenbaum J, Rosenberg IH, Wilson PWF, Stabler SP, Allen RH. Prevalence of Cobalmin Deficiency in the Elderly Framingham Population. Am J Clin Nutr 1994; 60: 2–11.

34. Jefferies WM. Low-dosage Glucocorticoid Therapy. Arch Intern Med 1967; 119: 265–278.

35. Jefferies WM. Safe Uses of Cortisol. 2nd ed. Springfield (Illinois): Charles C. Thomas; 1996.

36. Wainstein MA, Resnick MI. Managing Nosocomial Infection With C. Difficile. IM Nov 1995: 15–22.

37. Merlotti L, Roehrs T, Koshorek G, Zorick F, Lamphere J, Roth T. The Dose Effects of Zolpidem on the Sleep of Healthy Normals. J Clin Psychopharmacol 1989; 9 (1): 9–14.

38. Freeman R, Komaroff AL. Does the Chronic Fatigue Syndrome Involve the Autonomic Nervous System? The American Journal of Medicine 1997 April; 102: 357–363.

39. Lowe JC, Garrison RL, Reichman AJ, Yellin J, Thompson M, Kaufman D. Effectiveness and Safety of T3 Therapy for Euthyroid Fibromyalgia: A Double-Blind, Placebo-Controlled Response Driven Crossover Study. Clinical Bulletin of Myofascial Therapy 1997: 2 (2/3): 31–58

40. Lowe JC, Reichman AJ, Yellin J. The Process of Change During T3 Treatment for Euthyroid Fibromyalgia: A Double-Blind, Placebo-Controlled, Crossover Study. Clinical Bulletin of Myofascial Therapy 1997; 2 (2/3): 91–124

41. Canaris GJ, Manowitz NR, Mayor G, Ridgway EC. The Colorado Thyroid Disease Prevalence Study. Archives of Internal Medicine; 2000 Feb 28; 160: 526–534.

42. Hak AE, Pols HAP, Visser TJ, Drexhage HA, Hofman A, Witteman JCM. Subclinical Hypothyroidism is a Risk Factor For Atherosclerosis & M.I. in Elderly Women. Ann Intern Med 2000; 132: 270–278.

43. Nordyke RA, Reppun TS, Madanay LD, Woods JC, Goldstein AP, Miyamoto LA. Alternative Sequences of Thyrotropin and Free Thy-

roxine Assays for Routine Thyroid Function Testing. Arch Intern Med 1998; 158: 266–272.

44. Padilla AJ. Who Has Diabetes? Cortlandt Forum, 2000 Feb; p110–111.

45. Skinner GRB, Thomas R, Taylor M, Bolt S, Krett S, Wright A, et al. Thyroxine Should be Tried in Clinically Hypothyroid but Biochemically Euthyroid Patients. BMJ 14 June 1997; Volume 314.

46. Skinner GRB, Holmes D, Ahmad A, Davies JA, Benitez J. Clinical Response to Thyroxine Sodium in Clinically Hypothyroid Biochemically Euthyroid Patients. J Nutritional And Environmental Medicine 2000; 20: 115–124.

47. Fraser WD, Biggart EM, O'Reilly DJO, Gray HW, McKillop JH, Thomson JA. Are Biochemical Tests of Thyroid Function of Any Value in Monitoring Patients Receiving Thyroxine Replacement? Br Med J 1986 Sept; 293: 808–810.

48. Goldenberg D, Fibromyalgia Syndrome a Decade Later. Arch Intern Med 1999; 159: 777–785.

49. Wolfe F, Cathey MA, Hawley DJ. A Double-Blind Placebo Controlled Trial of Fluoxetine in Fibromyalgia. Scand J Rheumatol 1994: 23: 255–259.

50. Norregaard J, Volkmann H, Danneskiold-Samsoe B. A Randomized Controlled Trial of Citalopram in the Treatment of Fibromylagia. Pain 1995: 61: 445–449.

51. Vercoulen JH, Swanink CM, Zitman FG, Vreden SG, Hoofs MP, Fennis JF, et al. Randomized, Double-Blind, Placebo-controlled Study of Fluoxetine in Chronic Fatigue Syndrome. Lancet 1996 Mar 30; 347(9005): 858–861.

52. Goldenberg D. Treatment of Fibromyalgia Syndrome. Rheumatic Disease Clinics of North America 1989 Feb; 15(1): 61–71.

Table 1. Patient demographics		
Variable	**Active**	**Placebo**
Age in Years—Average (Range)	42.7 (28–58)	46.7 (23–61)
Sex- Percentage—Female	92%	91%
Length of Fatigue in Years—Average (Range)	7.1 (.5-18)	9.7 (1-34)
Onset— Percentage—Gradual	42	35
# of Doctors Seen Previously For Symptoms		
Average (Range)	6.3 (0–20)	9.2 (1–100)
Standard Deviation	4.8	16.7

Table 2. Treatment protocol
Patients received all active or all placebo treatments as a single intervention.

Table 2a. Medicines that all patients received

For Sleep:

A	Melatonin 3/10 mg P.O. QHS (28) and
B	Valerian 180 mg/Melissa 90 mg combination (Valerian Rest by To Your Health), 1–2 tablets P.O. QHS (29)

Plus the below treatments as needed to result in 7–8 hours of solid sleep without waking or next-day sedation. Mixing of a low dose of several medications was used instead of a high dose of a single agent in order to decrease next-day sedation.

A	Zolpidem (Ambien) 10 mg, ½–1½ P.O. QHS and/or
B	Trazodone (Desyrel) 25–200 mg P.O. QHS and/or
C	Cyclobenzaprine (Flexeril) 10 mg, ½–2 P.O. QHS (30,31) and/or
D	Carisprodol (Soma) 350 mg, ½–1 P.O. QHS and/or
E	Amitriptyline (Elavil) 10 mg, ½–5 P.O. QHS (31,32) and/or
F	Clonazepam (Klonopin) ½ mg, ½–8 tablets P.O. QHS

For nutritional support (these two supplements are used long-term):

A	Daily One Cap Multivitamin (Twinlab), 1 tablet P.O. QAM
B	Magnesium with malic acid (Fibrocare by To Your Health) , 2 tablets p.o. Tid

Table 2b. Treatments that were individualized based on test results or clinical history:

Treatment	If
Ferrous Fumarate (Chromagen) 1 P.O. QD between 2 and 6 PM on an empty stomach.	Ferritin ≤ 40ng/mL (ug/L) or iron % saturation ≤ 22%.
B₁₂ 1000mcg/cc, 1cc I.M. 1-3 x a week for 12 doses then PRN or B₁₂ 1000mcg SL QD (if patient was unable to obtain injections).	B₁₂ level < 540 pg/mL (398pmoL/L) (18, 19, 33).
Levothyroxine (Synthroid) 25mcg, 1–4 QAM or dessicated thyroid (Armour) 30 mg ½–3 tablets QAM (adjust to a clinically optimal dose based on relief of symptoms while keeping the free T4 within normal range).	If TSH > 2.5 or < .9U/mL and/or total T3 is < 95ng/dL (1.5nmoL/L) and/or free T4 is < 1.0ng/dL (13pmoL/L) and patient has ≥ 3 of the following symptoms: weight gain, oral temp < 98.3, dry skin, thin hair, constipation, achiness, and/or cold intolerance.
Cortisol (Cortef) 5 mg, 1–3 tabs QAM, ½–1½ tabs at noon and ½ tab at 4PM, using lowest clinically optimal dose (usual dose 5–12½ mg/day- up to 20–25 mg/d) (34,35).	Cortrosyn stimulation test with cortisol baseline ≤ 12ug/dL, (331nmoL/L) and/or ½ hour increases < 7ug/dL (193nmoL/L), or 1 hour increase < 11ug/dL (303nmoL/L) with a 1 hour cortisol level < 28 ug/dL (773nmoL/L) or HgbA₁C < 5.1% and/or patient has ≥ 3 of the following: sugar craving, shakiness relieved by eating, dizziness, moodiness, recurrent infections that persist longer than expected, high stress at illness onset or low B/P.
DHEA 5–50 mcg P.O QD (decrease the dose if acne or darkening of facial hair in females) occurs.	DHEA-Sulphate (mcg/dl) (x.02714=umoL/L)

In Males			In Females		
DHEA-Sulphate		RX (mg/d)	DHEA-Sulphate		RX (mg/d)
umoL/L	mcg/L		umoL/L	mcg/L	
0 – 2.7	0 – 100	50	0 – 0.8	0 – 30	25
2.8 – 5.4	101 – 200	40	0.9 – 2.2	31 – 80	20
5.5 – 7.6	201 – 280	25	2.3 – 3.0	81 – 110	10
7.7 – 8.7	281 – 320	10	3.1 – 3.8	111 – 114	5

Treatment	If
Testosterone Enanthate (Delatestryl) 100 mg I.M. QWK (in males) or natural Testosterone 2 mg P.O. QD or BID in females.	Free testosterone in lowest quintile for age.
Estrogen replacement (in females) offered to patient (26): if < 40 Y.O.—Ovcon 35, if > 40 Y.O. or side effects on Ovcon, Estradiol ½–2 mg QD or Triestrogen (10% Estradiol, 10% Estrone, 80% Estriol) 1¼– 5 mg/d P.O. on day 1–25 of cycle and (if uterus present) natural progesterone 100 mg P.O. qhs or 200 mg P.O. qhs day 16–25 of cycle.	Estradiol < 75pg/mL (275pmoL/L) and/or FSH & LH > 10 ml.U./mL (I.U./L) and/or irregular periods, hot flashes, inadequate vaginal lubrication, low libido, flaring of FMS symptoms before periods or S/P TAH or tubal ligation.

Oxytocin 10 units P.O. QD	Severe cold hands /feet and pallor.
Fludrocortisone (Florinef) .1 mg/d (and increase dietary salt, water & potassium) beginning at ¼ tab/day & increasing by ¼ a tab Q 3–7 days	B/P < 100/60, or orthostatic dizziness or FMS symptoms worsened by standing against wall for 10 minutes.
Sertraline (Zoloft) 50 mg, ½–2 QHS OR Paroxetine (Paxil) 20 mg, ½–2 QAM OR Fluoxetine (Prozac) 20 mg, 1–2 QAM OR Nefazodone (Serzone) 100 mg B.I.D.	If NMH symptoms above, depression or persistent severe pain.
Nystatin 500,000 units 2 P.O. T.I.D. x 3–5 months plus, in more severe cases, Itraconazole (Sporanox) 100 mg 2 P.O. QD with food x 6–12 weeks (begin 4 weeks after Nystatin begun). Do not take Seldane, Hismanal, Propulsid or antacids with Itraconazole.	If stool microscopic exam showed higher than normal fungal levels or symptoms suggesting fungal overgrowth (e.g., thrush, recurrent yeast vaginitis or antibiotic use, onchomycosis)—by questionnaire (25).
Metronidazole (Flagyl) 250 mg P.O. QID x 10 days. or 750 mg P.O. TID x 10 days followed by iodoquinol (Yodoxin) 650 mg P.O. TID.	If stool was positive for Clostridium difficile, or if other Metronidazole (Flagyl) sensitive parasites were present.
Doxycycline 100 mg P.O. B.I.D. x 6 weeks.	Recurrent body temperatures > 98.6° F.

Table 2C. Number of Patients on Each Treatment (at Some Time During the Study) Out of 38 Active Patients	
Treatment	**# of Patients on Treatment**
Daily One Multivitamin	38
Valerian Rest	38
Magnesium/Malic Acid (Fibrocare)	38
Melatonin 3/10 mg	38
Chromagen (iron)	24
Vitamin B_{12}	30
SSRI (Sertraline, Paroxetine, Fluoxetine, Nefazodone)	29
Amitriptyline (Elavil)	10
Cyclobenzaprine (Flexeril)	10
Desyrel	24
Ambien	23
Klonopin	8
Soma	22
Synthroid	18
Armour Thyroid	15
Cortef	29
DHEA	24
Florinef	19
Oxytocin	15
Estrace	7
Triestrogen	6
Progesterone	9
Testosterone	12
Nystatin	35
Sporanox	27
Flagyl	10
Doxycycline	4

Table 3. Summary of FMS treatment outcomes among 72 patients

Analog scales, totals, by visit

Active				Placebo			p-value	
time	n	mean	std.dev	n	mean	std. dev.		
1	37	176.1	70.3	34	177.1	57.6	.95 (1)	
2	35	249.7	88.0	32	187.5	87.3		
3	32	264.1	115.2	31	189.2	93.4		
4	27	295.7	90.0	28	221.3	99.5	<.0001(2)	
Last	38	310.3	111.3	34	211.9	103.7	.0002 (1)	< .0001 (3)

FIQ scale, by visit

Active				Placebo			p-value	
time	n	mean	std.dev	n	mean	std. dev.		
1	38	54.8	10.3	34	51.4	8.4	.14 (1)	
2	36	45.1	15.1	33	48.3	14.1		
3	33	38.0	17.7	31	51.5	14.0		
4	27	37.0	15.5	28	44.4	15.3	<.0001(2)	
Last	38	33.2	18.2	34	47.7	15.5	.0005 (1)	< .0001 (3)

TPI

Active				Placebo			p-value	
time	n	mean	std.dev	n	mean	std. dev.		
1	38	31.7	10.5	34	35.0	10.6	.19 (1)	
Last	32	15.5	9.5	30	32.3	11.4	<.0001 (1)	<0.0001(3)

Patient's overall response

	much better	better	same	worse	much worse	p-value
Active	16	14	2	0	1	<.0001 (4)
Placebo	3	9	11	6	4	

(1) t-test comparing treatment groups, without baseline adjustment

(2) treatment main effect in a repeated measures random effects regression model based on data from visit 1 to visit 4, adjusting for entry value and age

(3) treatment effect in a regression adjusting for entry value in patients who completed the study

(4) Cochran-Mantel-Haenszel trend test

Table 4. Side effects		
Side Effect Categories	Active N=38 (Number of patients with side effects)	Placebo N=34 (Number of patients with side effects)
Dermatological	7	2
Psychological	12	8
Gastrointestinal	9	11
Autonomic Dysfunction	6	3
Sleep Changes	3	3
Miscellaneous	9	5
Total number of patients in *group* to report any side effect.	24	22

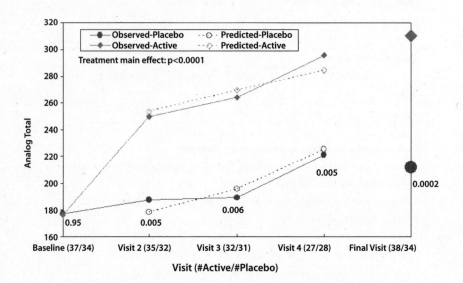

FIGURE 1A: *Observed and predicted well-being (Analog) index score means by group-per visit (with t-test p-values at each visit labeled)*

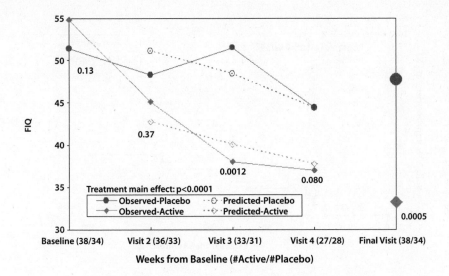

FIGURE 1B: *Observed and predicted disability index (FIQ) means by group - per visit (with t-test p-values at each visit labeled)*

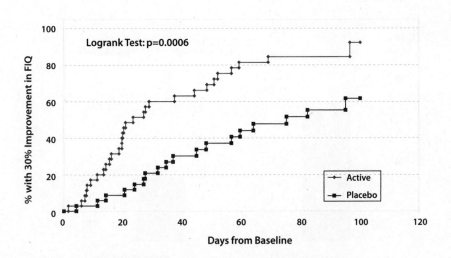

FIGURE 2A: *Kaplan-Meier Estimates of Time to 30% Improvement in Analog Total Stratified by Treatment Group (N=72)*

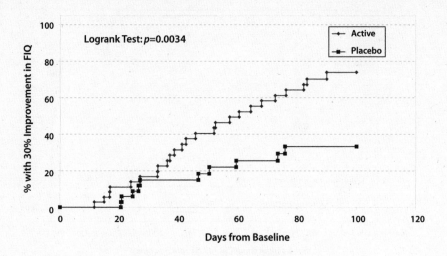

FIGURE 2B: *Kaplan-Meier Estimates of Time to 30% Improvement in FIQ Stratified by Treatment Group (N=72)*

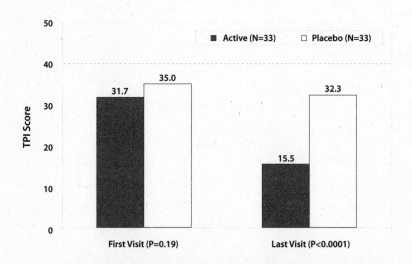

FIGURE 3: *Tender Point Index average scores by group for first and final visit (N=72)*

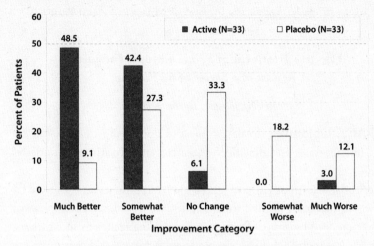

FIGURE 4: *Patient self-report of improvement at final visit (Cochran Mantel-Haenszel trend test: p < 0.0001)*

Study #2: published in the Journal of Musculoskeletal Pain
Vol. 3, No. 4, 1995.

Effective Treatment of Severe Chronic Fatigue: A Report of a Series of 64 Patients

Jacob Teitelbaum, Barbara Bird

ABSTRACT. Objectives: To determine the underlying causes of severe chronic fatigue states and the effect of concurrently treating the underlying etiologies.

Methods: Sixty-four patients with a median of three years of severe fatigue, which markedly limited their activity, were studied. These patients were characterized by a mix of symptoms including recurrent sore throats, swollen glands, increased thirst, sleeplessness, achiness, and poor memory and concentration without apparent cause. They presented in our office during 1991–1993 and were selected by consecutive sampling. The patients were assessed and treated for the processes noted below.

As fatigue is purely subjective, the patient determined if they showed worsening, no significant change, significant but incomplete improvement, or much improvement [that is, fatigue no longer a problem].

Results: 46 patients had at least three or more contributing problems. Fibromyalgia was present in 44 patients. Overt or subclinical hypothyroidism and hypoadrenalism were suspected in thirty and 40 patients respectively. Superinfections associated with immune dysfunction [e.g., bowel parasites or yeast overgrowth] were suspected in thirty cases. Improvement with micronutrient supplementation was noted.

Depression, anxiety/hyperventilation and situational stresses were considered to be the primary processes in four, four, and three patients respectively.

Treatment resulted in complete resolution of fatigue in 57 percent and significant but incomplete improvement in 39 percent of the patients. Improvement was seen at a median time of seven weeks.

Conclusions: Severe chronic fatigue states are multifactorial processes that, in many patients, respond well to treatment.

KEYWORDS. Fatigue, fibromyalgia, adrenal insufficiency, hypothyroidism, chronic fatigue syndrome

Introduction

Severe chronic fatigue states [SCFS] are common. Chronic fatigue syndrome [CFS], representing a small subset of SCFS, is rare. A recent report by Price et al.[1] suggests that only one in 13,535 people [or approximately 20,000 patients in the United States] meet strict Center for Disease Control [CDC] criteria for CFS. By CDC estimates, the prevalence is even lower, at 2 to 7 per 100,000.[2] The prevalence of persistent, often disabling, fatigue has been estimated to be much higher—often up to six million patients for fibromyalgia alone.[3] Unfortunately, despite having sought help for many years, people suffering from severe fatigue often receive little benefit from treatment. This paper reports on an approach to the evaluation and treatment of severe chronic fatigue states which we have found to be effective.

A key factor in helping patients with chronic fatigue was the realization that a combination of interrelated problems was usually occurring. Patients often improved dramatically and quickly when all the underlying problems were treated simultaneously. If only one problem was treated, or if the problems were not treated simultaneously, often the patient's improvement was only partial. In our current study, we examined sixty-four patients with chronic and severe fatigue to define the multiple underlying causes and to assess the efficacy of treating all the discovered problems.

Materials and Methods

The study population consisted of fifty-six females and eight males, ages twenty to seventy-seven years [average age forty-five years] whose major complaint was severe chronic fatigue of at least two month's duration which the patients felt significantly limited their activity. These patients were characterized by a mix of symptoms including recurrent upper respiratory infections [URls], sore throats, swollen glands, increased thirst, achiness, poor sleep, and poor memory and concentration. We defined these patients as having a severe chronic fatigue state.

These patients presented in our office from 1991 to 1993. Most of these patients had been through numerous evaluations and/or treatments without relief before entering our trial. The median duration of their fatigue was three years (average two years; range two months to twenty-five years). Patients were given a thorough history and physical examination. Complete blood count (CBC), automated chemistry profile (Chem 19), erythrocyte sedimentation rate (ESR), urinalysis (UA), B_{12}, serum iron, total iron binding capacity (TIBC), ferritin, glycosylated hemoglobin, thyroid functions and cortrosyn stimulation testing were done. In refractory cases, we checked for stool ova/parasites [O&P], giardia and cryptosporidium [tested in nineteen patients]. Special attention was given to checking for:

1. Subclinical hypothyroidism—for the reasons noted in the discussion, if the free thyroxine (FT_4) index was low normal and signs and symptoms suggestive of hypothyroidism were present (for example, constipation, cold intolerance, low temperature, delayed ankle tendon relaxation phase, and so on), a low-dose Synthroid trial (25 to 50 micrograms) was considered (especially if fibromyalgia was present). If the thyroid stimulating hormone (TSH) was over 4 or less than 0.8 (with a low normal FT_4 index), this also weighed in favor of treatment. The free FT_4 and ultrasensitive TSH assays are microparticle enzyme immunoassays for the quantitative determination of free thyroxine and human thyroid stimulating hormone in human serum as measured on Abbotts IMX.

2. Decreased Adrenal Function—A cortrosyn stimulation test was performed at 8:00 am. Fasting baseline, thirty- and sixty-minute serum cortisol levels were checked after a 25-unit dose of cortrosyn [ACTH] intramuscularly. The test was considered positive for a low baseline if the cortisol was less than 6 mcg/dL. As our experience grew, we found patients often benefitted dramatically from treatment even if the baseline was as high as 11 mcg/dL. Therefore, we expanded our definition of low baseline to include patients with cortisol levels of up to 11 mcg/dL. These patients received a trial of treatment if they failed to respond fully to other treatment. If a patient showed low adrenal reserve (that is, not doubling at one hour or not increasing by 7 mcg/dL at one-half hour and 11 mcg/dL by one hour), the patient was also treated. Although Jefferies[4,5] felt that most patients needed qid (four times daily) dosing of Cortef [for example, 5 milligrams of Cortef qid], we found that most of those with low reserve did well with 5 mil-

ligrams Cortef po (orally) qam (each morning), and, if needed, 2.5 to 5 milligrams at lunchtime. Those with low baselines were more likely to need 5 to 7.5 milligrams tid (three times daily) or qid. Those who don't respond to lower dosing should receive a trial of qid dosing [giving only 2.5 milligrams qhs (at bedtime)]. The cortisol assay is a homogeneous enzyme immunoassay for the quantitation of total cortisol in serum. The reagents are from Cedia Microgenics Corporation and run on the Technicon R.A.

3. Fibromyalgia—Diagnosis was made by the 1990 American College of Rheumatology tender point criteria. Amitriptyline (10 to 50 milligrams), cyclobenzaprine (5 to 20 milligrams), or Trazodone (25 to 75 milligrams) qhs were used to treat disordered sleep in most fibromyalgia patients (see Table 3). We use the terms fibrositis and fibromyalgia interchangeably.

4. Chronic infections:

   A. Bacterial—Urinary tract infection (UTI), chronic sinusitis, or other infections were checked for by history and urinalysis. Most of these had been treated by other physicians before the patient's arrival in our office.

   B. Bowel parasites—Toward the end of our study, we tested patients refractory to other treatment for bowel parasites. The yield with routine O&P is low even if parasites are present. Because of this we used a purged stool specimen and had the slides read by our lab supervisor and a technologist experienced in looking for stool parasites. Antigen tests for giardia and cryptosporidium were also done. We now test all our chronic fatigue patients for bowel parasites. The objective of the stool purge was to secure a watery, "explosive" sample.[6] We feel this gives far better reliability than numerous random samples. Patients are instructed to drink 1½ ounces of Fleet Phospho-Soda and to collect the watery stool specimens in the three vials containing the preservative sodium acetate-acidic acid-formalin (SAF). We use Meridian Diagnostic Para Pak SAF System and Para Pak Concentration Kit and trichrome stain for differentiation of internal structure of intestinal parasites.

   C. Fungal infections—History was taken for risk factors suggestive of possible fungal overgrowth, for example frequent antibiotic use, recurrent vaginal or skin fungal infections, and so on. If this raised a high index of suspicion or the stool microscopic examination was suggestive of fungal overgrowth, a trial of 1 million units of nystatin po qid was given over four to six months. We are currently finding that 200 milligrams of itraconazole (taken with food) po qd (daily) for three to four weeks followed by 100 milligrams qd for one to four months in combination with 500,000 units of nystatin po qid (while on itraconazole) to be more effective. Fluconazole may also be helpful in these patients. Nizoral may aggravate the often subtle adrenal insufficiency frequently seen in patients with chronic fatigue.[7]

5. Depression, anxiety or hyperventilation—These were treated with tricyclic or selective serotonin reuptake inhibitors (SSRIs, for example, Prozac) family of antidepressants if the symptoms were felt to have preceded the fatigue, as opposed to being caused by it. Patients who presented with an ongoing diagnosis of depression without other factors contributing to their fatigue were excluded from the study.

6. Possible micronutrient deficiencies—all patients were placed on a B complex (25 milligrams) vitamin with minerals (such as Berocca Plus or Twin Lab Daily One Caps). Many were placed on two to six tablets of magnesium chloride (Slow Mag) per day (less if diarrhea occurred). Low iron and B_{12} were tested for and treated when present.

We felt that treating coexisting problems simultaneously would improve the effectiveness of treatment. Unfortunately this made it difficult to assess the degree of effectiveness of each individual treatment.

As the patient's symptoms in severe chronic fatigue states are predominately subjective, the determination of degree of improvement after any given treatment was made by the patient. This was complicated, at times, by several treatments being given concurrently.

The experimental nature of parts of the treatment was reviewed with the patient and informed consent was obtained.

Results

As shown in Table 1, thirty-seven of sixty-four patients had almost complete resolution of their fatigue and twenty-five of sixty-four showed significant, but incomplete, improvement. Two out of sixty-four patients had no significant improvement. Improvement was often rapid, at times occurring within a few days. Median length of symptoms before treatment was three years and median time to initial improvement was 1¾ months (that is, at the first follow-up visit). Patients did at times have temporary exacerbations during their treatment course. Improvement was, however, usually sustained (most patients have remained in follow-up for over one year). Only seven patients had a single underlying contributing diagnosis. Most had three or four underlying problems (see Table 1). Table 2 shows the number of patients felt to have each of the different underlying diagnoses and their response to treatment. Table 3 gives a more detailed breakdown of patient characteristics, contributing diagnoses, and responses to treatment.

Table 1. Clinical Characteristics of the Treatment Group and the Effect of Treatment	
Number of patients	**64**
Male	8
Female	56
Ages	
Range	20–77 years old
Average	45 years old
Duration symptoms present	
Range	2 months to 25 years
Median	3 years
Average	2 years
Time until initial improvement was seen with treatment	
Range	4 days to 15 months
Average	3 months
Median	1.75 months [that is, first follow-up visit]
Number of contributing diagnoses per patient	**Number of patients**
1	7
2	11
3	23
4	13
5	9
6	0
7	1
Degree of improvement (out of 64 patients)	**Number of patients**
Much improved [that is, fatigue no longer a significant problem]	37
Moderate improvement [significant improvement but fatigue is still a problem]	25
No significant improvement	2

Table 2. Number of Patients with Each Suspected Diagnosis and Response to Treatment				
Suspected Diagnosis	**Number of Patients**	**Improved with Treatment**	**No Clear Improvement with Rx**	**No Rx or Follow Up**
A. Fibromyalgia	44	37	4	3
B. Low Thyroid				
1. By low T_7/high TSH	12	11	1	
2. By symptom/ exam only	18	14	3	1
C. Underactive Adrenal [Hypo-cortisolism]:				
1. Low adrenal baseline [i.e., 8 A.M. Cortisol 0–5.9 mcg/dL]	7	5	2	
2. 8 A.M. Cortisol 6–11 mcg/dL	16	11	3	2
3. Low adrenal reserve	16	15	1	
D. Fungal Overgrowth	23	14	7	2
E Possible Low B_{12}				
1. <300 PG/ml	7	7		
2. 301–540 PG/ml	19	17	1	1
F. Bowel Parasites: [in 19 pts. checked]				
Cryptosporidium	3	0	3	
Entameba	2	2		
Visceral Larva Migrans	1	1		
Tapeworm	1	1		
G. Depression				
primary	4	4		
secondary	4	4		
Anxiety/hyper-ventilation	4	3	1	

Note: Severe situational stress was felt to be the primary process in 3 patients and a secondary process in 5. Ferritins of 0 to 20 ng/ml and 21 to 40 ng/ml were seen in 7 and 6 patients, respectively. The effect of iron supplementation was not separately monitored.

Table 3. Review of Individual Patient Data

Age	M/F	Hypothyroid Dx	Efct	Hypoadrenal* Dx	Efct	Fibrositis Dx	Efct TR=TRAGER	B12 Level pg/ml	Efct	Yeast Suspct. DX	Efct
53	M	+	+	8.6	+						
27	F			+	+			348	+	+	No Rx
45	F										
33	F					+	—	540	+		
45	F	+	+	4.8		—		+	No Rx		
40	F	sc	+	5.7	++	+	+	484	+		
47	M			7.6	+	+	+ TR			+	— S.E.
42	F	sc	+	+	+	+	+				
44	F			7	++		TR				
44	F									+	+
51	F	sc	+	+	++	+	+ TR				
53	F	+	+								
38	F					+	—	270	+		
53	F	+	+			+	+ TR				
33	F	sc	+			+	— S.E.W. Rx			+	+
37	F	sc	+	4.7	+	+	+			+	+
40	F	sc	+			+	+	440	+	+	+
50	F	sc	+	4	+	+	No Rx				
50						+	+ TR	300	+		
59	F										
34	F	+	+	3	—	+	+			+	+
30	F					+	+	294	+	+	+
41	F					+	+ TR				
26	M	sc	+	+	+	+	+				
55	F			1	++	+	+ TR				
73	F	+	+					220	+		
43	F			+	++	+	+				
42	F	+	+	+	±			524	+	+	—
31	F	sc	+	11	+	+	+	400	+	+	No Rx
29	F	sc	+	8	+	+	No Rx				
21	F	sc	±	+	+	+	+ TR				
51	F	sc	+	9	+	+	+			+	+
57	F	sc	+								

O & P	E F C T	Depressed Anxious Hyper-Ventilatory	Ferritin	Symptoms present x mo/yrs	Time until improvement	Much better	Mod. better	No sig. change
				few months	1 month		+	
				2½ years	6 weeks		+	
		work stress		1 year	115 months left	+		
				>1 year	4-6 months	+		
				app. 10 years	1 year	+		
				1 year	7 weeks	+		
				3½ years	2½ months	+		
		stress		9 months	3 months		+	
		stress		N/A	1 month	+		
				1 year	3 months	+		
				app. 4 months	2 months	+		
				2 months	<2 months		+	
		S.L.E.	28	5 years	1 year 2 months with B_{12}		+	
				1½ years	2 months		+	
				10 years	weeks	+		
				years	6 weeks	+		
				app. 2–3months	2 months	+		
			29	N/A	6 weeks	+		
				4 years	N/A	+		
				years	without improvement			+
—				>6 years	months	+		
				2 years	1 month		+	
				>4 years	1 month	+		
				3 years	2 months		+	
		HV	23	years intermittent	2 months	+		
		depressed		months	<1 week	+		
				months	1-2 months	+		
			5	8–10 years	4 months		+	
		depressed	20	5 years	2 months		+	
				10 years	4-6 months	+		
				years	4 months		+	
		stress		1½ years	N/A		+	
		depressed		years	4 months		+	

Age	M/F	Hypothyroid Dx/Efct		Hypoadrenal* Dx/Efct		Fibrositis Dx/Efct TR=TRAGER		B12 Level pg/ml	Efct	Yeast Suspct. DX/Efct	
67	F	SC	No Rx	9	No Rx	+	+				
20	F	SC	+	+	+			260	+		
51	F			11	+	+	+	247	+		
33	F	+	+					219	+		
57	F	+	+	+	+	+	+				
48	F			6	-	+	+	359	+	+	—
51	F					+	+	425	No Rx	+	+
40	F					+	+			+	±
39	F					+	+			+	+
49	M			6	—			323	—		
67	M										
58	F			+	++	+	—				
59	M					+	+	513	+	+	+
35	F			TR +		+	+ TR	340	+	+	—
34	F	SC	—	+	+	+	+				
39	F	SC	—	+	+	+	+				
45	F			11	+	+	+				
34	F	+	+			+	+				
45	F			10	++	+	+ TR	425	+	+	+
40	F			2	+			340	+		
74	F					+	+	380	+		
77	M			8	+						
63	M			6	+						
46	F	+	+	+	++			328	+	+	±
44	F					+	+	371	+	+	—
45	F					+	+	387	+		
43	F			10	No Rx	+	++ TR				
42	F	SC	+	+	+	+	+	454	+		
41	F	+	—	+	+					+	+
31	F			+	+	+	+	206	+		
36	F									+	+

*Hypoadrenalism—If based on a low baseline cortisol, the baseline cortisol [in mcg/dl] is noted. A [+] indicates an inadequate adrenal reserve [see Methods]. EFCT = Effect of treatment. A [+] means the patient improved with treatment. A [—] means no improvement with treatment. SC = Subclinical. DX means patient had this diagnosis if [+] is in the column. CS = Cryptosporidium. VLM = Visceral larva migrans. Ferritin is in ng/ml.

O E & F P C T	Depressed Anxious Hyper-Ventilatory	Ferritin	Symptoms present x mo/yrs	Time until improvement	Much better	Mod. better	No sig. change
			4–5 years	2 months	+		
			months	1–2 months	+		
	depressed	21	>4 years	4 months	+		
		20	1 year	2 months		+	
			years inter.	4 months	+		
	anxious		> 20 years	5 months	+		
CS —	anxious depressed		30 years	1 week after Sporanox		+	
			6 years	6 weeks	+		
CS —	depressed		7 years	7 months		+	
	depressed		years	N/A			+
	depressed		6 years	10 months	+		
			many years	2 months	+		
			5–6 years	3 months		+	
			4 years	2 months		+	
			N/A	N/A		+	
			years	2 months		+	
VLM+	stress		1 year	6 weeks		+	
			1-2 years	1 month	+		
		3	9 years	3 months	+		
		26	1½ years	2 weeks	+		
Tape Worm			years	months		+	
CS —	stress		4 months	2 months	+		
			1 year	3 months	+		
			8 months	2 months	+		
H.V.		14	2 years	6 weeks		+	
Entmba + +		19	15 years	1 month	+		
			years	1 month	+		
			25 years	2 months	+		
			2 years	1–2 months		+	
Entmba +		46	4 years	4 days	+		
	stress	18	2–3 years	N/A		+	

Copies of both of these studies are available from the Haworth Document Delivery Service (800–342–9678) or can be downloaded from *www.endfatigue.com*.

Discussion

We found that most patients [all but seven] had a combination of at least two underlying problems and forty-six patients had more than two problems. Previous trials have often shown disappointing results when only one underlying cause was sought or treated.

We found that patients—even those with fatigue of over ten years duration—experienced (usually rapid) resolution of their symptoms 57 percent of the time and significant improvement another 39 percent of the time if the multiple underlying problems were identified and treated. Frankly, we were surprised at the degree of improvement shown by our patients.

Why did these patients show such an assortment of problems? The patterns we observed suggested that the primary process might have been hypothalamic dysfunction (caused by viral or other infections) with secondary multiple endocrine (and possibly immune) abnormalities. As Dr. Sternberg notes in her excellent editorial on hypoimmune fatigue states,[8] and Dr. Behan and others note in their studies, hypothalamic-pituitary-adrenal (HPA) axis dysfunction appears to be common in chronic fatigue states.[9,10,11,12,13] This can manifest as borderline or overt adrenal insufficiency and borderline or overt hypothyroidism. In their study on fibromyalgia, Neeck et al.[9] examined baseline and TRH stimulated thyroid function. Although most fibromyalgia patients had normal baseline thyroid functions, their response to TRH stimulation was significantly blunted. The increase of TSH and T_4 after TRH stimulation was approximately 90 percent greater for TSH ($P < 0.05$) and over 800 percent greater for FT_4 ($P < 0.05$) in controls than in fibromyalgia patients. This, combined with a clinical picture suggestive of hypothyroidism, suggests that our current testing misses subtle, but clinically significant, hypothyroidism in these patients. This problem is often accentuated by a low normal TSH [secondary to hypothalamic dysfunction]. The low TSH can further mislead the clinician into thinking thyroid function is adequate. Impairment of receptors for thyroid and adrenal hormones may also impact here. In light of this, an empiric trial of 25 to 50 micrograms of Synthroid a day often resulted in marked improvement. It is suggested that the adrenal insufficiency be treated first. Otherwise, the administration of Synthroid may accelerate the metabolic breakdown of the patient's cortisol, exacerbating the patient's symptoms. Interestingly, many of our patients exhibited marked polydipsia with normal blood sugars. This raised the possibility of a mild diabetes insipidus component, although that possibility was not formally tested. Bakheit and Behan also noted upregulation of hypothalamic serotonin receptors in postviral fatigue syndrome.[11]

Patients with severe chronic fatigue states are sometimes found to exhibit immune dysfunction with associated recurrent and persistent infections. Infections like persistent bowel cryptosporidium or fungal overgrowth also suggest an immune suppressed state. We suspect that the immunologic abnormalities may be secondary to adrenal dysfunction. Chronic severe fatigue, myalgias, arthralgias and neuropsychiatric changes are often associated with persistently elevated interferon levels.[14,15] Cortisol also lowers interferon levels.[16] Interestingly, metoclopramide and naloxone have been reported to improve interferon induced fatigue,[14,15] although we've not tried these medications. It would be interesting to test interferon levels before and after treatment with cortisol and see if levels correlate with symptomatic improvement, as elevated interferon can mimic or cause many of the symptoms and signs (for example, achiness, muscle mitochondrial changes, and fatigue) seen in chronic fatigue patients.[14,15] This could offer another mechanism for cortisol's effectiveness. Other adrenal androgens (for example, testosterone, dehydroepiandrosterone [DHEA] and DHEA-S) also have significant effects on lymphokine production[16] and lower levels in females could explain their increased susceptibility. We recently tested DHEA-S levels in three patients with abnormal cortrosyn tests and found DHEA-S levels to be very low. ACTH is widely accepted as a regulating factor for adrenal androgen secretion under certain conditions.[16] Further studies of interleukin (IL) 2, 4, and 5 function in these patients would help define the immune dysfunction further. DHEA, for example, increases IL-2 and gamma-interferon (gamma-IFN). Testosterone decreases IL-4, IL-5 and gamma-IFN. Glucocorticoids inhibit gamma-IFN and IL-2.[16] Although the cause of the immune dysfunction is not clear, the above suggest possible mechanisms by which hypothalamic suppression could be involved.

Jefferies[4,5] noted several decades ago that severe fatigue and recurrent URIs following a severe viral infection were often caused by adrenal insufficiency and resolved with cortisol treatment. He theorized that the fatigue was caused by a transient, and at times permanent, inhibition of ACTH production by the viral infection. This theory was recently supported by the work of Demitrack and Dale.[10] In several thousand patient years of experience, Jefferies found these patients improved dramatically on low-dose cortisol. There was no toxicity (except mild gastritis) as long as the dosage was physiologic [for example, 5 milligrams of cortisol tid to qid] and not pharmacologic.[4,5] Our findings support Jefferies' experience. Patients with low adrenal reserve (for example, no doubling in one hour) usually did well with 5 milligrams of cortisol qam and, if needed, 2.5 milligrams at lunch. Patients with low baselines were more likely to need 5 to 7.5 milligrams of cortisol tid to qid (up to 30 milligrams a day, with morning doses being higher). Dr. Jefferies recommends that any patient who does not respond to bid dosing be given a trial of 2.5 to 5 milligrams of cortisol po qid. Patients with reactive hypoglycemia were likely to be hypoadrenal, as cortisol helps to maintain blood glucose levels.

Although at times they are secondary to the immune or other dysfunctions, the fibromyalgia and the parasitic, bacterial, and fungal infections need to be treated as well or the patient's fatigue will persist. Fibromyalgia appears to be a common endpoint of many physical, physiologic, and/or psychological stress states. We view it as predominately a sleep disorder. These patients have multiple tender points and occasionally muscle trigger points which could interfere with deep sleep. These patients tend to toss and turn a lot at night and remain in light sleep stages. The quality of the deep sleep stages that "recharge their batteries" appears to be disordered. Thus, despite many hours of sleep, these patients can be considered to have not (effectively) slept for many years. The stress of sleeping ineffectively leaves the patient functioning poorly and may alter the HPA axis.[13] This stress can aggravate the tender points and thus, the cycle continues. Treatment needs to be geared toward restoring the duration, and/or quality, of deep-stage sleep and resolving the patient's trigger and tender points.

Dr. Janet Travell, the personal physician to Presidents Kennedy and Johnson, is also one of the world's foremost experts on myofascial pain. In the *Trigger Point Manual,* Dr. Travell's and Dr. David Simon's book on myofascial pain,[17] there is an excellent chapter on perpetuating factors that must be treated. Our experience suggests that the perpetuating factors in myofascial pain syndrome and fibromyalgia are similar. We have found the a mix of therapies will usually cause fibromyalgia to improve or fully resolve. Our regimen consists of (a) Treatment with 10 to 50 milligrams of amitriptyline hs or 25 to 150 milligrams of trazodone hs or 5 to 10 milligrams of cyclobenzaprine hs. (b) Nutritional support, for example, Berocca Plus (or TwinLab Daily One Cap) vitamins one a day long term plus two tablets of magnesium chloride (Slow Mag) tid for six months. Correcting low Vitamin B_{12} and iron levels is important. (c) It is important to treat even borderline hypothyroidism and hypoadrenalisin (as discussed previously). (d) Exercise (when the patient starts to improve). (e) For our refractory patients, we've found a form of neuromuscular reeducation [Trager—per Milton Trager, M.D.] to be very beneficial. (f) Correcting structural perpetuating factors such as uneven leg lengths, small hemipelvis, short upper arms (adjust chair arms), et cetera, is important. (g) As noted below, it is also important to treat any occult underlying infections.

Chronic fatigue patients often have a mix of underlying infections caused by (and perhaps aggravating) their immune dysfunction. We found that treating these was critical. Most patients had a marked decrease in their recurrent viral infections on cortisol. Chronic sinusitis, UTI, and other bacterial infections are readily detectable. Bowel yeast overgrowth is harder to test for and, therefore, we considered treating the patient empirically if they had frequent antibiotic use or frequent vaginal or dermatologic fungal infections (that is, suggestive of increased risk of or a decreased resistance to fungal infections). We used 1 million units of nystatin po qid in this study. Our current experience suggests that adding 200 milligrams of itraconazole (Sporanox) po qd with food for three to four weeks, followed by 100 milligrams po qd (to the nystatin) may be more effective. Bowel parasites also needed to be treated and were surprisingly common (seven of nineteen patients tested). Samples should be obtained after a Phospho-Soda laxative[6] and tested for in a lab familiar with parasite detection (see methods). Otherwise, the low sensitivity will make this an unreliable test.

In many patients, the above problems appear to be associated with increased nutritional needs. Many patients with only mild to moderate fatigue (and therefore not included in this series) have their symptoms resolve fully, simply by taking a TwinLab Daily One Cap vitamin or Berocca Plus qd and two 67-milligram tablets of magnesium chloride (Slow-Mag) tid, and avoiding excess sugar, caffeine, and alcohol. This is an important part of the regimen for the severely fatigued patient in our current series as well.

Lindenbaum et al.[18] found that barely subnormal or occasionally even normal B_{12} levels can be associated with evidence of severe neuropsychiatric changes caused by cobalamin deficiency—even in the absence of anemia or macrocytosis. These included memory loss, fatigue, and personality changes. Similar findings were noted by Carmel.[19] Norman[20] also noted that as many as 40 percent of B_{12}-deficient individuals may have been missed by simply relying on serum B_{12} levels. These were found by checking urine methylmalonic acid. Lindenbaum et al.'s recent study confirms that B_{12} deficiency can occur even with vitamin B_{12} levels over 500 pg/ml.[21] Because the level at which neuropsychiatric changes cease to occur is not well defined, a trial of B_{12} 1 milligram IM a week for eight weeks was given in some patients with levels of up to 540 pg/ml to rule out subclinical B_{12} deficiency. Surprisingly, twenty-four of twenty-six patients had significant improvement. Some patients benefit from continuing with B_{12} injections 1 milligram IM every three to five weeks. Most others did not need this after the initial series of injections. A trial of iron treatment was also considered if ferritin levels were less than 40 ng/ml.

As in any other illness, psychological factors, including depression, anxiety, and psychological conflicts, are critical here and must be addressed. We found that lack of interests correlated well with depression being primary [found in only four of sixty-four patients]. If the patient had many interests, but was frustrated over not having the energy to fulfill them, the depression was usually considered to be secondary to the fatigue. This is corroborated by the common finding of high baseline cortisols in patients whose depression is primary. The frequency of low morning cortisol levels makes it unlikely that endogenous depression is common in chronic fatigue state patients.[12]

Patients may at times have intermittent exacerbations of their symptoms while physical and psychological issues are being worked through. Recurrence of previous problems (for example, low B_{12} or infections) occasionally occurs and requires retreatment. Continuing to guide and assist patients through this period is very important. Doing this, we have found that most patients maintained their improvement during the one to two year poststudy period.

Initially, we considered limiting the study to patients who met strict CFS (chronic fatigue syndrome) criteria. Recent reports, however, suggest that immunologic abnormalities seen in CFS patients [versus controls] are no different than those seen in other patients with severe fatigue.[22] Our experience also suggested that the underlying causes and the response to treatment were not affected by whether patients strictly met criteria for CFS. Because of these two reasons, we elected to study all patients who found their fatigue to be severe and persistent and whose constellation of symptoms was similar to CFS, even if they did not fulfill all of the criteria for CFS.

Ideally, we would have liked to have done a controlled crossover study for all variables and to test the effect of each treatment separately. Simultaneous treatment of the patient's underlying problems may be required, however, to cause the symptoms to resolve. We therefore chose, instead, to begin with an open clinical trial. At this point, we are planning a future controlled trial. Areas that would be good candidates for a controlled study within the above context would include: (1) Low-dose cortisol for patients with borderline low cortrosyn test baselines (cortisol of 6 to 13 mcg/dL) or borderline low adrenal reserve values; (2) A trial of itraconazole or fluconazole versus placebo in patients with recurrent fungal infections; (3) B_{12} injections as above versus placebo for patients with B_{12} levels of 208 to 540 pg/ml. The controlled trial may also decrease the problem of defining clearly which treatments are causing the improvement, as several treatments were often begun simultaneously.

Much of our experience confirms the old adage that "even a blind squirrel finds acorns." We are certain that there is much more to learn in this area. In the interim, it is hoped that the above report creates new avenues to explore in understanding the treatment of severe chronic fatigue.

Originally published in the *Journal of Musculoskeletal Pain* 3 (1995): 91–110. Used courtesy of Haworth Press. See references on page 414.

Yeast Questionnaire

SECTION A OF THIS QUESTIONNAIRE LISTS ASPECTS of your medical history that may promote growth of the common yeast *Candida albicans* and result in yeast-associated illness.

Sections B and C evaluate the presence of symptoms that are often found in individuals who suffer from yeast-connected illnesses.

For each "yes" answer in Section A, circle the point score. Total the points and record the score at the end of the section.

Next, go to Sections B and C and score as directed.

Section A: Your Medical History

POINT SCORE

1. Have you been treated for acne with tetracycline, erythromycin, or any other antibiotic for one month or longer?

2. Have you taken antibiotics for any type of infection for more than two consecutive months, or in shorter courses four or more times in any twelve-month period?

3. Have you ever taken an antibiotic—even for a single course?

4. Have you ever had prostatitis, vaginitis, or
    another infection or problem with your
    reproductive organs for more than one month?   (25)

5. Have you been pregnant:
    Two or more times?   5
    Once?   3

6. Have you taken birth control pills for:
    More than two years?   (15)
    Six months to two years?   (8)

7. Have you taken a corticosteroid such as
    prednisone, Cortef, or Medrol by mouth
    or inhaler for:
    More than two weeks?   15
    Two weeks or less?   (6)

8. When you are exposed to perfumes,
    insecticides, or other odors or chemicals,
    do you develop wheezing, burning eyes,
    or any other distress?
    Yes, and the symptoms keep me from
    continuing my activities.   20
    Yes, but the symptoms are mild and do not
    change my activities.   (5)

9. Are your symptoms worse on damp or humid
    days or in moldy places?   (20)

10. Have you ever had a fungal infection, such
    as jock itch, athlete's foot, or a nail or skin
    infection, that was difficult to treat and:
    Lasted more than two months?   20
    Lasted less than two months?   10

11. Do you crave:
    Sugar?   (10)
    Breads?   (10)
    Alcoholic beverages?   10

12. Does tobacco smoke cause you discomfort
    such as wheezing, burning eyes, or another problem?   10

TOTAL SCORE SECTION A   *147*

Section B: Major Symptoms

For each symptom that is present, enter the appropriate figure in the point score column:

If a symptom is occasional or mild   Score 3 points.
If a symptom is frequent and/or moderately severe   Score 6 points.
If a symptom is severe and/or disabling   Score 9 points.

Add the total score for this section and record it at the end of the section.

POINT SCORE

1. Fatigue or lethargy. — 6
2. Feeling of being "drained." — 6
3. Poor memory. — 3
4. Feeling "spacey" or "unreal." — 3
5. Inability to make decisions. — 6
6. Numbness, burning, or tingling. —
7. Insomnia. —
8. Muscle aches. — 6
9. Muscle weakness or paralysis. — 3
10. Pain and/or swelling in joints. — 6
11. Abdominal pain. — 6
12. Constipation. — 3
13. Diarrhea. —
14. Bloating, belching, or intestinal gas. — 6
15. Troublesome vaginal burning, itching, or discharge. — 6
16. Prostatitis. —
17. Impotence. —
18. Loss of sexual desire or feeling. — 3
19. Endometriosis or infertility. —
20. Cramps and/or other menstrual irregularities. —
21. Premenstrual tension. —
22. Attacks of anxiety or crying. — 6

23. Cold hands or feet and/or chilliness. $\underline{6}$

24. Shaking or irritable when hungry. $\underline{6}$

TOTAL SCORE SECTION B $\underline{81}$

Section C: Other Symptoms*

For each symptom that is present, enter the appropriate figure in the point score column:

If a symptom is occasional or mild	Score 1 point.
If a symptom is frequent and/or moderately severe	Score 2 points.
If a symptom is severe and/or persistent	Score 3 points.

Add the total score for this section and record it at the end of the section.

POINT SCORE

1. Drowsiness. $\underline{2}$

2. Irritability or jitteriness. $\underline{3}$

3. Incoordination. $\underline{2}$

4. Inability to concentrate. $\underline{3}$

5. Frequent mood swings. $\underline{3}$

6. Headache. $\underline{2}$

7. Dizziness, loss of balance. $\underline{2}$

8. Pressure above ears, feeling of head swelling. _____

9. Tendency to bruise easily. $\underline{2}$

10. Chronic rashes or itching. _____

11. Psoriasis or recurrent hives. _____

12. Indigestion or heartburn. _____

13. Food sensitivity or intolerance. $\underline{3}$

14. Mucus in stools. $\underline{2}$

15. Rectal itching. $\underline{2}$

*While the symptoms in this section occur commonly in patients with yeast-connected illness, they also occur commonly in patients who do not have Candida.

16. Dry mouth or throat.   _____

17. Rash or blisters in mouth.   _____

18. Bad breath.   2

19. Foot, hair, or body odor not relieved by washing.   _____

20. Nasal congestion or postnasal drip.   3

21. Nasal itching.   1

22. Sore throat.   3

23. Laryngitis, loss of voice.   _____

24. Cough or recurrent bronchitis.   2

25. Pain or tightness in chest.   3

26. Wheezing or shortness of breath.   3

27. Urinary frequency, urgency, or incontinence.   _____

28. Burning on urination.   3

29. Spots in front of eyes or erratic vision.   1

30. Burning or tearing of eyes.   1

31. Recurrent infections or fluid in ears.   1

32. Ear pain or deafness.   _____

TOTAL SCORE SECTION C   48

TOTAL SCORE SECTION B   81

TOTAL SCORE SECTION A   147

GRAND TOTAL SCORE (ADD UP TOTAL SCORES
FROM SECTIONS A, B, AND C)   276

The grand total score will help you and your physician decide if your health problems are yeast-connected. Scores in women will run higher, as seven items in the questionnaire apply exclusively to them, while only two apply exclusively to men.

Yeast-connected health problems are almost certainly present in women with scores *over 160* and in men with scores *over 140*.

Yeast-connected health problems are probably present in women with scores *over 120* and in men with scores *over 90*.

Yeast-connected health problems are possibly present in women with scores *over 60* and in men with scores *over 40*.

With scores of *less than 60* in women and *40* in men, yeast is less apt to be the cause of health problems.

Adapted from W. G. Crook, M.D., *The Yeast Connection and the Woman* (Jackson, TN: Professional Books, 1998) and *The Yeast Connection Handbook* (Jackson, TN: Professional Books, 1996). Used with permission.

Fibromyalgia Information Questionnaire

THIS QUESTIONNAIRE IS SIMILAR TO THE ONE ON our website (see Appendix J: Resources). The program will use this information to make a complete medical record for you and your doctor, and is a teaching program that will tailor treatment and recommendations specifically for *your* case.

Please describe briefly (in one sentence) what your main problem(s) are (you will be able to describe things at length later—toward the end of the questionnaire): _____

_____

_____

_____

_____

1A. How long have you been fatigued? _____

1B. What was the approximate date or time of onset? _____

2. How much has fatigue decreased your function? _____

3. Did symptoms begin ____ suddenly or ____ gradually?

4. What symptoms presented at onset? _____

5. What stresses were occurring in your life when the disease began?

_____

6. How many children do you have? _____ (list ages and names below)

NAME   AGE

_____ _____

_____ _____

_____ _____

_____ _____

7. Are you married, single, separated, divorced, widowed? (circle one)

8A. How many hours were you working (including commute but not including taking care of your family) weekly at the onset of your illness? _____

8B. How many hours were you spending weekly on your children's care at onset?_____

9A. How many hours per week are you working now? _____

9B. How many hours are you now spending weekly on your children's care?_____

10. What is your occupation? _____

11A. Do you have any family members with fibromyalgia/chronic fatigue syndrome? _____

11B. If so, who, and how old are they? _____

12. How old are you? _____ Date of birth: _____

13. Are you male or female? _____

14. How many doctors have you seen for your symptoms? _____

15. Check any of these that you have or have had:

Illness   *Year of Onset (approx.)*

_____ Stroke(s)   _____

_____ Multiple sclerosis   _____

_____ Neuropathies (if so, what type? _____)   _____

_____ Glaucoma   _____

_____ Cataracts   _____

_____ Lupus   _____

_____ Rheumatoid arthritis   _____

_____ Osteoarthritis ("wear & tear" arthritis)   _____

_____ Scleroderma   _____

_____ Other rheumatic diseases (please list below)

_____   _____

_____   _____

_____   _____

_____   _____

Phlebitis and/or Pulmonary Embolus

    If yes, did it go to your lungs?
    (i.e., pulmonary embolism) _____

_____ Angina or heart attack
(myocardial infarction)   _____

      _____ Angina; _____ Heart Attack; _____ Both

    1. Was this confirmed by- _____ EKG and/or

                            _____ exercise stress test and/or

                            _____ heart catheterization

    2. Did you have _____ angioplasty and/or _____ bypass

        If so, when? _____

_____ Mitral Valve Prolapse   _____

_____ Heart valve disease? (specify type below)   _____

    _____

_____ Are you on blood thinners?

If so, check which one and fill in dose

      _____ Coumadin/Warfarin _____ milligrams a day

      _____ Heparin _____ milligrams a day

      _____ Aspirin _____ milligrams a day

      _____ Other _____milligrams a day

_____ Abnormal heart rythym(s)? (specify type below)

_____

_____ Cancer? (check all that apply):

_____ breast

  1. Metastatic/Nonmetastatic _____

    If yes, to where? _____

  2. Did you have (check all that apply):

    _____ surgery; _____ radiation therapy;

    _____ chemotherapy;

    _____ other treatment? (please specify)

  3. Is the cancer _____ active or _____without recurrence?

_____ prostate (males only)

  1. Metastatic/nonmetastatic?_____

    If yes, to where? _____

  2. Did you have (check all that apply):

    _____ surgery; _____ radiation therapy; _____ chemotherapy

    _____ other treatment (please specify) _____

  3. Is the cancer _____ active or _____without recurrence?

_____ uterine (females only)

  1. Metastatic/nonmetastatic?_____

    If yes, to where? _____

  2. Did you have (check all that apply):

    _____ surgery; _____ radiation therapy; _____ chemotherapy

    _____ other treatment (please specify) _____

  3. Is the cancer _____ active or _____without recurrence?

_____ ovarian (females only)

  1. Metastatic/nonmetastatic?_____

    If yes, to where? _____

  2. Did you have (check all that apply):

    _____ surgery; _____ radiation therapy; _____ chemotherapy

    _____ other treatment (please specify) _____

3. Is the cancer _____ active or _____ without recurrence?

_____ other cancer (specify) _____

   1. Metastatic/nonmetastatic? _____

      If yes, to where? _____

   2. Did you have (check all that apply):

      _____ surgery; _____ radiation therapy; _____ chemotherapy

      _____ other treatment (specify type) _____

   3. Is the cancer _____ active or _____ without recurrence?

_____ Emphysema   _____

_____ Hypertension (high blood pressure)   _____

_____ Asthma   _____

_____ Stomach ulcers   _____

_____ Spastic colon or irritable bowel syndrome   _____

_____ Crohn's disease or ulcerative colitis (specify below)   _____

_____

_____ Depression   _____

_____ AIDS   _____

_____ Polio   _____

_____ Tuberculosis   _____

_____ Other chronic infection(s) (specify type)

_____

_____

_____ Reflex sympathetic dystrophy (RCPS)   _____
Which extremity? _____

_____ Recurrent prostatitis   _____
Has a bacterial culture ever been positive? _____

_____ Hepatitis (check all that apply)
      _____ Viral: _____ hepatitis A   _____

                           _____ hepatitis B   _____

                           _____ hepatitis C   _____

                           _____ with infectious mono   _____

_____ Any toxic chemical exposures? (list what and when)

_____   _____

_____   _____

_____   _____

_____ Lupus   _____

_____ Alcoholic   _____

_____ Other (specify type) _____ _____

_____ Unknown cause   _____

Are you using herbs? _____ (specify type)

_____

_____

Do you have cirrhosis? _____

Have you had a liver biopsy? _____

Have you had a blood test to check for high iron levels?

_____

_____Prostate enlargement   _____

_____Kidney stones   _____

_____Active disc disease (for example, sciatica)   _____

_____Kidney failure   _____

_____Other kidney problems? (describe below)

_____   _____

_____   _____

_____Diabetes

_____ juvenile onset   _____

_____ adult onset   _____

Are you taking tablets of niacin containing over 1,000

milligrams a day? _____

_____Pancreatitis (check all that apply):   _____

_____ from gallstones

_____ from alcohol

_____ other known cause (please specify) _____

_____

_____ unknown cause

16. Have you had any other operations? (please list below)

    Year (approx) _____ Type of surgery _____

    Year (approx) _____ Type of surgery _____

    Year (approx) _____ Type of surgery _____

17. Have you had any other hospitalizations? (please list below)

    Year (approx) _____ Reason _____

    Year (approx) _____ Reason _____

    Year (approx) _____ Reason _____

18. What other diagnoses do you have, if any? _____

19. Are you allergic to any medications ____ No ____ Yes (please list below)

    _____

20. Do you have any other allergies or sensitivities? (please list below)

    _____

    _____

21. Does your insurance pay for medications? _____ yes; _____ no

    If yes: _____% or $_____ copay; $_____ limit per year.

22. Please check where appropriate if you are taking or have taken any of the treatments listed below (Rx means by prescription only):

Treatment	Allergic or prohibitive side effects	Check if you are currently taking	Check if you took in the past and stopped	If discontinued the treatment give the single main reason (or add other)	Dose you are *currently* taking
Amitriptyline (Elavil) (Rx)	___ Yes ___ No	___ Helps ___ Doesn't help ___ Don't know if it helps	___ Yes	___ Side effects ___ Didn't work ___ Too expensive	___ mg; ___ times a day
Cyclobenzaprine (Flexeril) (Rx)	___ Yes ___ No	___ Helps ___ Doesn't help ___ Don't know if it helps	___ Yes	___ Side effects ___ Didn't work ___ Too expensive	___ mg; ___ times a day
Trazodone (Desyrel) (Rx)	___ Yes ___ No	___ Helps ___ Doesn't help ___ Don't know if it helps	___ Yes	___ Side effects ___ Didn't work ___ Too expensive	___ mg; ___ times a day
Zolpidem (Ambien) (Rx)	___ Yes ___ No	___ Helps ___ Doesn't help ___ Don't know if it helps	___ Yes	___ Side effects ___ Didn't work ___ Too expensive	___ mg; ___ times a day
Aprazolam (Xanax) (Rx)	___ Yes ___ No	___ Helps ___ Doesn't help ___ Don't know if it helps	___ Yes	___ Side effects ___ Didn't work ___ Too expensive	___ mg; ___ times a day
Clonazepam (Klonopin) (Rx)	___ Yes ___ No	___ Helps ___ Doesn't help ___ Don't know if it helps	___ Yes	___ Side effects ___ Didn't work ___ Too expensive	___ mg; ___ times a day
Carisprodol (Soma) (Rx)	___ Yes ___ No	___ Helps ___ Doesn't help ___ Don't know if it helps	___ Yes	___ Side effects ___ Didn't work ___ Too expensive	___ mg; ___ times a day
Armour Thyroid (Rx)	___ Yes ___ No	___ Helps ___ Doesn't help ___ Don't know if it helps	___ Yes	___ Side effects ___ Didn't work ___ Too expensive	___ mg; ___ times a day
Synthroid (Rx)	___ Yes ___ No	___ Helps ___ Doesn't help ___ Don't know if it helps	___ Yes	___ Side effects ___ Didn't work ___ Too expensive	___ mg; ___ times a day
Cortef (Rx)	___ Yes ___ No	___ Helps ___ Doesn't help ___ Don't know if it helps	___ Yes	___ Side effects ___ Didn't work ___ Too expensive	___ mg; ___ times a day
Fludrocortisone (Florinef) (Rx)	___ Yes ___ No	___ Helps ___ Doesn't help ___ Don't know if it helps	___ Yes	___ Side effects ___ Didn't work ___ Too expensive	___ mg; ___ times a day
Oxytocin (Rx) ___ Tablets ___ Injection ___ Other	___ Yes ___ No	___ Helps ___ Doesn't help ___ Don't know if it helps	___ Yes	___ Side effects ___ Didn't work ___ Too expensive	___ mg; ___ units a day
Natural Estrogen Brand Name	___ Yes ___ No	___ Helps ___ Doesn't help ___ Don't know if it helps	___ Yes	___ Side effects ___ Didn't work ___ Too expensive	___ mg; ___ times a day ___ every day ___ days per month

Treatment	Allergic or prohibitive side effects	Check if you are currently taking	Check if you took in the past and stopped	If discontinued the treatment give the single main reason (or add other)	Dose you are *currently* taking
Birth control pills Brand Name	_____ Yes _____ No	_____ Helps _____ Doesn't help _____ Don't know if it helps	_____ Yes	_____ Side effects _____ Didn't work _____ Too expensive	
_____ Natural progesterone or _____ Provera	_____ Yes _____ No	_____ Helps _____ Doesn't help _____ Don't know if it helps	_____ Yes	_____ Side effects _____ Didn't work _____ Too expensive	_____ mg; _____ times a day _____ every day _____ days per month
Testosterone (Rx) Brand Name	_____ Yes _____ No	_____ Helps _____ Doesn't help _____ Don't know if it helps	_____ Yes	_____ Side effects _____ Didn't work _____ Too expensive	_____ mg; _____ times a day _____ every day _____ days per month
Valacyclovir (Valtrex) (Rx)	_____ Yes _____ No	_____ Helps _____ Doesn't help _____ Don't know if it helps	_____ Yes	_____ Side effects _____ Didn't work _____ Too expensive	_____ mg; _____ times a day _____ every day _____ as needed
Famcyclovir (Famvir) (Rx)	_____ Yes _____ No	_____ Helps _____ Doesn't help _____ Don't know if it helps	_____ Yes	_____ Side effects _____ Didn't work _____ Too expensive	_____ mg; _____ times a day _____ every day _____ as needed
Acyclovir (Zovirax) (Rx)	_____ Yes _____ No	_____ Helps _____ Doesn't help _____ Don't know if it helps	_____ Yes	_____ Side effects _____ Didn't work _____ Too expensive	_____ mg; _____ times a day _____ every day _____ as needed
Nystatin (Rx)	_____ Yes _____ No	_____ Helps _____ Doesn't help _____ Don't know if it helps	_____ Yes	_____ Side effects _____ Didn't work _____ Too expensive	_____ mg; _____ times a day
Itraconazole (Sporanox) (Rx)	_____ Yes _____ No	_____ Helps _____ Doesn't help _____ Don't know if it helps	_____ Yes	_____ Side effects _____ Didn't work _____ Too expensive	_____ mg; _____ times a day
Metranidazole (Flagyl) (Rx)	_____ Yes _____ No	_____ Helps _____ Doesn't help _____ Don't know if it helps	_____ Yes	_____ Side effects _____ Didn't work _____ Too expensive	_____ mg; _____ times a day
Iodoquinol (Yodoxin) (Rx)	_____ Yes _____ No	_____ Helps _____ Doesn't help _____ Don't know if it helps	_____ Yes	_____ Side effects _____ Didn't work _____ Too expensive	_____ mg; _____ times a day
Doxycycline or tetracycline (Rx)	_____ Yes _____ No	_____ Helps _____ Doesn't help _____ Don't know if it helps	_____ Yes	_____ Side effects _____ Didn't work _____ Too expensive	_____ mg; _____ times a day
Nitroglycerin (Rx)	_____ Yes _____ No	_____ Helps _____ Doesn't help _____ Don't know if it helps	_____ Yes	_____ Side effects _____ Didn't work _____ Too expensive	_____ mg; _____ times a day
Ciprofloxacin (Cipro) (Rx)	_____ Yes _____ No	_____ Helps _____ Doesn't help _____ Don't know if it helps	_____ Yes	_____ Side effects _____ Didn't work _____ Too expensive	_____ mg; _____ times a day

Treatment	Allergic or prohibitive side effects	Check if you are currently taking	Check if you took in the past and stopped	If discontinued the treatment give the single main reason (or add other)	Dose you are *currently* taking
Sertraline (Zoloft) (Rx)	____ Yes ____ No	____ Helps ____ Doesn't help ____ Don't know if it helps	____ Yes	____ Side effects ____ Didn't work ____ Too expensive	____ mg; ____ times a day
Paroxetine (Paxil) (Rx)	____ Yes ____ No	____ Helps ____ Doesn't help ____ Don't know if it helps	____ Yes	____ Side effects ____ Didn't work ____ Too expensive	____ mg; ____ times a day
Fluoxetine (Prozac) (Rx)	____ Yes ____ No	____ Helps ____ Doesn't help ____ Don't know if it helps	____ Yes	____ Side effects ____ Didn't work ____ Too expensive	____ mg; ____ times a day
Venlafaxine (Effexor) (Rx)	____ Yes ____ No	____ Helps ____ Doesn't help ____ Don't know if it helps	____ Yes	____ Side effects ____ Didn't work ____ Too expensive	____ mg; ____ times a day
Nefazodone (Serzone) (Rx)	____ Yes ____ No	____ Helps ____ Doesn't help ____ Don't know if it helps	____ Yes	____ Side effects ____ Didn't work ____ Too expensive	____ mg; ____ times a day
Bupropion (Wellbutrin) (Rx)	____ Yes ____ No	____ Helps ____ Doesn't help ____ Don't know if it helps	____ Yes	____ Side effects ____ Didn't work ____ Too expensive	____ mg; ____ times a day
Bromocriptine (Parlodel) (Rx)	____ Yes ____ No	____ Helps ____ Doesn't help ____ Don't know if it helps	____ Yes	____ Side effects ____ Didn't work ____ Too expensive	____ mg; ____ times a day
Baclofen (Rx)	____ Yes ____ No	____ Helps ____ Doesn't help ____ Don't know if it helps	____ Yes	____ Side effects ____ Didn't work ____ Too expensive	____ mg; ____ times a day
Gabapentin (Neurontin) (Rx)	____ Yes ____ No	____ Helps ____ Doesn't help ____ Don't know if it helps	____ Yes	____ Side effects ____ Didn't work ____ Too expensive	____ mg; ____ times a day
Calcium	____ Yes ____ No	____ Helps ____ Doesn't help ____ Don't know if it helps	____ Yes	____ Side effects ____ Didn't work ____ Too expensive	____ mg; ____ times a day
Chromagen (iron)	____ Yes ____ No	____ Helps ____ Doesn't help ____ Don't know if it helps	____ Yes	____ Side effects ____ Didn't work ____ Too expensive	____ mg; ____ times a day
DHEA	____ Yes ____ No	____ Helps ____ Doesn't help ____ Don't know if it helps	____ Yes	____ Side effects ____ Didn't work ____ Too expensive	____ mg; ____ times a day
Thiamine pyrophosphate	____ Yes ____ No	____ Helps ____ Doesn't help ____ Don't know if it helps	____ Yes	____ Side effects ____ Didn't work ____ Too expensive	____ mg; ____ times a day
Creatine monohydrate	____ Yes ____ No	____ Helps ____ Doesn't help ____ Don't know if it helps	____ Yes	____ Side effects ____ Didn't work ____ Too expensive	____ mg; ____ times a week

Treatment	Allergic or prohibitive side effects	Check if you are currently taking	Check if you took in the past and stopped	If discontinued the treatment give the single main reason (or add other)	Dose you are *currently* taking
B-Complex	____ Yes ____ No	____ Helps ____ Doesn't help ____ Don't know if it helps	____ Yes	____ Side effects ____ Didn't work ____ Too expensive	____ mg; ____ times a day
Magnesium and malic acid	____ Yes ____ No	____ Helps ____ Doesn't help ____ Don't know if it helps	____ Yes	____ Side effects ____ Didn't work ____ Too expensive	____ mg; ____ times a day
Echinacea	____ Yes ____ No	____ Helps ____ Doesn't help ____ Don't know if it helps	____ Yes	____ Side effects ____ Didn't work ____ Too expensive	____ mg; ____ times a day
Monolaurin	____ Yes ____ No	____ Helps ____ Doesn't help ____ Don't know if it helps	____ Yes	____ Side effects ____ Didn't work ____ Too expensive	____ mg; ____ times a day
Vitamin B$_{12}$ ____ injections ____ sublingual	____ Yes ____ No	____ Helps ____ Doesn't help ____ Don't know if it helps	____ Yes	____ Side effects ____ Didn't work ____ Too expensive	____ mcg; ____ times a day
Acetyl-L-carnitine	____ Yes ____ No	____ Helps ____ Doesn't help ____ Don't know if it helps	____ Yes	____ Side effects ____ Didn't work ____ Too expensive	____ mg; ____ times a day
Artemesia annua	____ Yes ____ No	____ Helps ____ Doesn't help ____ Don't know if it helps	____ Yes	____ Side effects ____ Didn't work ____ Too expensive	____ mg; ____ times a day
Tricycline	____ Yes ____ No	____ Helps ____ Doesn't help ____ Don't know if it helps	____ Yes	____ Side effects ____ Didn't work ____ Too expensive	____ tabs; ____ times a day
Colostrom	____ Yes ____ No	____ Helps ____ Doesn't help ____ Don't know if it helps	____ Yes	____ Side effects ____ Didn't work ____ Too expensive	____ mg; ____ times a day
Rhus Toxicodendron	____ Yes ____ No	____ Helps ____ Doesn't help ____ Don't know if it helps	____ Yes	____ Side effects ____ Didn't work ____ Too expensive	____ times a day
Coenzyme Q$_{10}$	____ Yes ____ No	____ Helps ____ Doesn't help ____ Don't know if it helps	____ Yes	____ Side effects ____ Didn't work ____ Too expensive	____ mg; ____ times a day
L-Lysine	____ Yes ____ No	____ Helps ____ Doesn't help ____ Don't know if it helps	____ Yes	____ Side effects ____ Didn't work ____ Too expensive	____ mg; ____ times a day
Magnesium-potassium aspartate	____ Yes ____ No	____ Helps ____ Doesn't help ____ Don't know if it helps	____ Yes	____ Side effects ____ Didn't work ____ Too expensive	____ mg; ____ times a day
NADH	____ Yes ____ No	____ Helps ____ Doesn't help ____ Don't know if it helps	____ Yes	____ Side effects ____ Didn't work ____ Too expensive	____ mg; ____ times a day

Treatment	Allergic or prohibitive side effects	Check if you are currently taking	Check if you took in the past and stopped	If discontinued the treatment give the single main reason (or add other)	Dose you are *currently* taking
MSM (sulfur)	___ Yes ___ No	___ Helps ___ Doesn't help ___ Don't know if it helps	___ Yes	___ Side effects ___ Didn't work ___ Too expensive	___ mg; ___ times a day
St. John's wort	___ Yes ___ No	___ Helps ___ Doesn't help ___ Don't know if it helps	___ Yes	___ Side effects ___ Didn't work ___ Too expensive	___ mg; ___ times a day
Ginkgo biloba	___ Yes ___ No	___ Helps ___ Doesn't help ___ Don't know if it helps	___ Yes	___ Side effects ___ Didn't work ___ Too expensive	___ mg; ___ times a day
Ginger	___ Yes ___ No	___ Helps ___ Doesn't help ___ Don't know if it helps	___ Yes	___ Side effects ___ Didn't work ___ Too expensive	___ mg; ___ times a day

23. What other treatment(s) are you on?

Prescription:

1. _____; Dose _____ milligrams _____ times a day
2. _____; Dose _____ milligrams _____ times a day
3. _____; Dose _____ milligrams _____ times a day
4. _____; Dose _____ milligrams _____ times a day
etc.

Nonprescription:

1. _____; Dose _____ milligrams _____ times a day
2. _____; Dose _____ milligrams _____ times a day
3. _____; Dose _____ milligrams _____ times a day
4. _____; Dose _____ milligrams _____ times a day
etc.

24. Are you on Seldane, Hismanyl, Propulsid or Mevacor-family cholesterol lowering medication? _____

Symptom Checklist

Circle One   I. CFIDS Criteria

25. Yes No Has your fatigue *not* been lifelong (that is, you weren't born severely tired); and not the result of ongoing exertion; and

not substantially alleviated by rest; and results in substantial reduction in previous levels of occupational, educational, social, or personal activities?

26. Yes No   Do you have four or more of the following eight symptoms (check all that apply)? All of which must have persisted or recurred during six or more consecutive months of illness and must not have significantly predated the fatigue.

_____ a. Impairment in short-term memory or concentration severe enough to cause substantial reduction in previous levels of personal activity.

_____ b. Sore throat.

_____ c. Tender neck or axillary (armpit) lymph nodes.

_____ d. Muscle pain.

_____ e. Multijoint pain without joint swelling or redness.

_____ f. Headaches of a new type, pattern, or severity.

_____ g. Unrefreshing sleep.

_____ h. Postexertional fatigue lasting more than twenty-four hours?

Circle One   II. Fibromyalgia Criteria

27. Yes No   Have you had chronic widespread pain for more than three months in all four quadrants of the body (that is, above and below the waist and on both sides of the body) and also axial pain (that is, headache or pain around the spine or chest)? (These don't all have to be at the same time.)

28.   Has an M.D. or D.O. diagnosed you in the past with:

_____ Fibromyalgia   Date _____

_____ Chronic fatigue syndrome   Date _____

_____ Both   Date _____

29.   Please rate the following on a scale of 1 (near dead) to 10 (excellent) (circle the number that applies):

a. How is your energy?

1   2   3   4   5   6   7   8   9   10
1= "near dead" and 10= excellent

b. How is your sleep?

1   2   3   4   5   6   7   8   9   10

1= no sleep and 10= 8 hours of sleep a night without waking

c. How is your mental clarity?

1   2   3   4   5   6   7   8   9   10

1= "brain dead" and 10= good clarity

d. How bad is your achiness?

1   2   3   4   5   6   7   8   9   10

1= very severe pain and 10 = pain free

e. How is your overall sense of well-being?

1   2   3   4   5   6   7   8   9   10

1= "near dead" and 10= excellent

30. Give a representative blood pressure: _____/_____

31. How much do you weigh? _____ lbs; _____ kg

32. How tall are you? _____ inches; _____ cm

33. What are your average temperatures (oral—11 A.M. to 7 P.M.)? ___°F; ___°C

34. Adrenal checklist (place a check mark next to the symptoms you have)

_____ Hypoglycemia

_____ Shakiness relieved with eating

_____ Moodiness

_____ Recurrent infections that take a long time to go away

_____ Life was very stressful before symptoms began

_____ Low blood pressure

_____ Dizziness on first standing

_____ Sugar cravings

_____ Food sensitivity (if yes, please list foods) _____

_____ Have you been on cortisone (prednisone)? (If yes answer the following)

For how long? _____

What dose and form of cortisone/prednisone did you take? ___

_____

Did you feel better when you took it? _____ If yes, did you take it:

____ after your illness began

____ before your illness began

____ both

35. Thyroid checklist (place a check mark next to the symptoms you have)

____ Weight gain? (_____ lbs or _____ kg; over _____ years)

____ Low body temperature (under 98 degrees)

____ Achiness

____ High cholesterol

____ Cold intolerance

____ Dry skin

____ Thin hair

____ Heavy periods (females only)

36. Other hormones checklist (place a check mark next to all items that apply to you)

____ Premenstrual symptoms (females only). Describe: _____

_____

____ Are you menopausal? (females only) If yes, when did your periods stop?_____ years ago

____ Pallor (pale face) and cold extremities

____ Irregular periods (females only)

____ Decreased arm and leg hair growth

____ Decreased vaginal lubrication (females only)

____ Delayed orgasm

____ Decreased erections (males only)

____ Day or night sweats or hot flashes

____ Nipple discharge

    ____ One breast

    ____ Both breasts

Females only: Have you had:

1. A hysterectomy? _____ If yes, how long ago? _____

2. Ovaries removed? _____ One, _____ Both; How long ago? _____

3. A tubal ligation? _____ How long ago? _____

_____ Symptoms are worse the week before your period (females only)

_____ Decreased libido

37. Vasodepressor syncope (NMH) checklist (check all that apply)

_____ Dysequilibrium

_____ Did you ever have a tilt table test?

If yes, was it _____ positive _____ normal

_____ Do you feel like you've been "hit by a truck" the day after exercise?

38. Lyme disease checklist (check all that apply)

_____ History of frequent tick bites. If so, how many? _____

_____ Rash after tick bite

_____ Rash that looked like a "bull's-eye."

_____ Have you been treated for Lyme disease?

_____ Numbness or tingling in your fingers or feet

_____ History of a positive Lyme test

39. Prostatitis checklist (males only; check all that apply)

_____ Burning on urination

_____ Groin aching

_____ Discharge from your penis (not with ejaculation)

_____ Urine urgency with a small volume

40. Sinusitis/nasal congestion and other infection checklist (check all that apply)

_____ Chronic nasal congestion or postnasal drip

_____ Chronic yellow or green nasal discharge

_____ Chronic bad taste in your mouth or bad breath

_____ Headaches under or over eyes

_____ Scratchy/watery eyes

_____ Do you get cold sores or other viral sores (for example, herpes)?

_____ Chronic or intermittent low-grade fevers (over 99°F/37.2°C)

    1. If yes, how high does the fever go? _____

    2. Did your illness begin with a fever? _____

    3. Do you have lung congestion? _____

    4. How often do you have the fever? _____

_____ Has any antibiotic you've been on in the past even temporarily improved your chronic fatigue/fibromyalgia symptoms? If yes, which one? _____ How long did you take it? _____

41. Disordered sleep checklist (check all that apply)

    _____ Trouble _____ falling and/or _____ staying asleep? If yes, is it a _____ mild, _____ moderate, or _____ severe problem?

    _____ How many hours of uninterrupted sleep do you get a night? _____

    _____ Do you wake up during the night? If so, how often? _____

    _____ Do you wake at night to urinate?

    _____ Do your legs jump a lot or do you kick your spouse or kick your blankets off at night?

    _____ Do you snore? If yes:

        1. Are you more than twenty pounds overweight? _____

        2. Do you have periods when you stop breathing (ask your bed partner)? _____

        3. Do you have high blood pressure? _____

42. Seasonal affective disorder checklist (check all that apply)

    _____ Are your symptoms worse October to April?

    _____ Do you have weight gain and carbohydrate craving during the winter?

    _____ Are your symptoms worse during cloudy periods and less when it is sunny (for over one to two weeks)?

43. Yeast overgrowth checklist (check all that apply)

_____ Recurrent vaginal yeast infections (females only). If so, how often? _____

_____ Toenail or fingernail fungal changes

_____ Skin fungal infections (athlete's foot, jock itch, rash under bra)

_____ Do you get sores *in* your mouth (not on the lips) frequently?

_____ Do you get cold sores or herpes attacks before or during symptom flare-ups that seem to worsen your symptoms?

_____ Have you been on birth control pills? (females only)

If yes, how did you feel on them? _____ better _____ worse _____ no change

_____ Do small amounts of alcohol aggravate symptoms?

44. Parasite checklist (check all that apply)

_____ Did your problems begin with a diarrhea attack?

_____ Do you sometimes have diarrhea? If so, is it severe? _____

_____ Do you sometimes have problematic constipation?

_____ Do you have well water?

45. Vision/dental checklist (check all that apply)

_____ Double vision

_____ Constantly changing eyeglass prescriptions

_____ Blurred vision or halos around lights at night

_____ Have you had temporary vision loss in one eye?

If yes, which eye? _____ How many times? _____

How long did it last? _____

Is your sedimentation (sed) rate blood test over 30? _____

_____ Dry eyes

_____ Dry mouth

_____ Any evidence of dental infections?

_____ Migraine headaches

_____ Food and/or chemical sensitivities

_____ Did your symptoms begin within two months of:

getting a vaccination _____

moving into a new home _____

46. Do you have ringing in the ears? _____

47. Do you have any hearing loss? _____

48. Do you drink non-diet sodas or other sweetened drinks? If so, how much? _____ ounces a day.

49. Do you drink coffee? If so, how many 8-ounce/240-mL cups a day? _____ regular _____ decaf

50. Do you drink alcohol? If so, how many drinks per day on average? _____

51. Do you smoke cigarettes? If yes, how many packs a day? _____

52. How much can you exercise? _____

53. Besides your illness, what other stresses are going on in your life? _____

54. Do you have frequent and persistent infections? If yes, what kind?

55. Do you have frequent bladder infections? _____

56. Do you have a rash? _____ If yes, what does it look like?_____

_____

How long have you had it? _____

57. Do you have chest pain? _____ If yes (check all that apply):

If yes, how long have you had it? _____

Has it been _____ getting better, _____ getting worse, _____ staying the same?

Does it _____ increase, _____ decrease, or _____ stay the same with exercise (for example, walking up steps)?

With exercise, do you have:

_____ shortness of breath?

_____ chest tightness?

_____ pain radiating to your left arm?

_____ sweating?

Can you worsen the same chest pain by pushing on your chest muscles? _____

Is the pain _____ sharp, _____ dull, _____ worse with position change or deep breathing?

Are your chest pains mostly when you're relaxing (not exercising)? _____

During the chest pains, do you have (check all that apply):

_____ A feeling of being unable to have a deep enough breath?

_____ Numbness and/or tingling in your hands and toes?

_____ Numbness and/or tingling around the mouth?

_____ Spacey feelings?

_____ Feelings of panic or impending death?

Do you smoke cigarettes? _____ How many packs a day? _____ How long have you smoked: _____

Did your father, mother, sister(s) or brother(s) have angina? _____ If yes, did

they have it before age 65? _____

Do you have high cholesterol? _____ Approximately how high? _____

Do you have diabetes? _____

Do you have high blood pressure? _____

Do you have recurrent heart palpitations? _____ If yes (check all that apply):

_____ palpitations lasting longer than 20 seconds

_____ pulse _____ regular or _____ irregular

_____ pulse over 120/minute

_____ dizziness with palpitations

_____ taking thyroid hormone

58. Do you have shortness of breath? _____ If yes (check all that apply):

_____ It comes and go suddenly (not with exercise)

_____ Wake up short of breath at night

_____ Shortness of breath occurs if you are lying down flat. If yes, how many pillows do you sleep on? _____

_____ Worse with exertion. If yes, how many flights of steps does it take? _____

59. Do you have transient weakness/paralysis in one arm and/or leg? _____ If yes (check all that apply):

_____ Always on the same side of your body. If yes, which side?

_____

_____ Occurs in your arm when you're sleeping on it and goes away within five minutes of waking. If it doesn't go away within 5 minutes of waking, how many times has it occurred? _____ How long has it lasted? _____

60. Do you have ankle swelling? _____

61. Have you had any unusual weight loss? _____ If yes, _____ lb/kg, over _____ years, _____ years ago. Describe what happened:

_____

62. Do you have numbness or tingling around your lips or mouth? _____

63. Do you have panic attacks? _____

64. Do you have sudden attacks of inability to take a deep enough breath or shortness of breath? _____

65. Do you have blood in your stool? _____

Is it only bright red blood on your toilet tissue or on stool (not mixed in)?   _____

If yes, do you have hemorrhoids? _____ If no, answer the following:

Do you have bloody mucus with stools? _____ If yes, how often?

_____

Do you have painful bowel movements? _____

Has your doctor done a:

colonoscopy _____ If yes, when? _____ Result: _____

sigmoidoscopy _____ If yes, when? _____ Result: _____

barium enema _____ If yes, when? _____ Result: _____

none of these tests _____

Have your bowel movements gotten thinner (pencil-like)? _____

Have you had a lot of (check all that apply):

____ constipation

____ diarrhea

____ both

____ neither

66. Do you have abdominal pains? _____ If yes, describe: _____
_____

67. Do you cough up blood? _____ If yes, how long has it been going
on? _____
Have you had a chest x-ray since this began? ____ If yes, when? ____
What did it show? _____

68. Do you frequently cough up yellow mucus? _____ If yes, have you
had a chest x-ray since this began? _____ If yes, when? _____
What did it show? _____

69. Do you have a chronic cough? _____ If yes, how long have you had
it? _____ Have you had a chest x-ray since this began? _____
If yes, when? _____
What did it show? _____

70. Do you have chronic burning when you urinate and urinary urgency
even with small volumes? _____ If yes, have you had urine cultures
checked?

     If no, check urine culture during symptoms.

     If yes, do they usually show infection? _____ If no, for males,
do you have discharge from your penis when you wake in the
morning? _____ For females, is this a severe problem?
_____ (If no, take no action.)

71. Do you have pain in your feet? If yes, check all that apply:

____ Pain by heel that is worse with walking

____ Pain over most of the sole(s) of your feet when walking

____ Shooting/burning pain between two toes that is worse when
you squeeze that area

____ Horrible pain in one foot (the whole foot, not only one joint)
that has been occurring for more than six weeks and makes you
want to be sure no one touches it

_____ One foot that often feels cooler or warmer to the touch than the other and looks either pale or red

_____ Injury or surgery to this foot or the hip on the same side before the pain began

72. Do you have pain in your hands? If yes, check all that apply:

_____ Horrible pain in one hand (the whole hand, not only one joint) that's been occurring for more than six weeks and makes you want to be sure no one touches it

_____ One hand that often feels cooler or warmer to the touch than the other and looks either pale or red

_____ Injury or surgery to this hand or the shoulder on the same side before the pain began

73. Do you have chronic anal/rectal pain? _____

74. Do you have redness and swelling in one or more joints in hands or feet? _____ If yes, check all that apply:

_____ Redness and swelling in one hand

_____ Redness and swelling in one foot

_____ Redness and swelling in both hands

_____ Redness and swelling in both feet

_____ A history of gout

_____ A history of rheumatoid arthritis

_____ A history of other arthritis (specify type) _____

75. Do you have a breast lump that you have had for more than six weeks? _____ If yes:

Which breast? _____

Is there any nipple discharge? _____ If yes:

Are you breastfeeding? _____

Is it: _____ milky, _____ pus, _____ bloody, _____ clear?

Is it in the _____ right breast, _____ left breast, _____ both breasts?

How long have you had it? _____

76. Do you have any other lumps or bumps that are new or growing? _____ If yes, please describe: _____

_____

_____

77. Have you had problems with infertility? _____ If yes, do you still want to have a (or another) child? _____

78. If female, when was your last period?

_____ Over three months ago

_____ Days ago

79. Does food often stick in your foodpipe? _____ If yes:

How long has it been going on? _____

Is it worse for _____ solids, _____liquids, _____ the same for both?

Do you have a history of drinking over two alcoholic drinks/day, on average? _____

Have you used tobacco for over twelve years? _____

80. Does your tongue burn? _____ If yes:

Has your tongue become smooth, with cracks/fissures? _____

Do you have a white coating throughout your mouth? _____

Do you have a white coating on your tongue? _____

Do small tastebuds sometimes become inflamed and painful?

_____

81. Do you have any history of psychiatric illness? _____ If yes, describe: _____

_____

_____

82. Do you have any other symptom(s) or problem(s)? (Please don't be bashful, list them all.)

_____

_____

83. Are you married? _____ If yes:

    How long have you been married? _____

    Is your spouse supportive? _____

    What is your spouse's name? _____

    What is his or her occupation? _____

84. Did you have/need to change jobs or decrease how much you work because of your illness? If so, please describe: _____

    _____

85. Did your symptoms begin soon or immediately after ____ pregnancy or ____ an accident? If yes, how soon after? _____ If after an accident, give details:

    _____

    _____

86. Besides those already discussed:

    A. What things or treatments have you found helpful in the past?

    _____

    B. What things or treatments have you tried without benefit? _____

    _____

    C. What things or treatments have made you feel worse in the past?

    _____

87. What medical problems do or did your parents or siblings have? If they have died, note cause of death and approximate age at death.

    Mother: _____

    Father: _____

    Brothers: _____

    Sisters: _____

88. Do you feel depressed (as opposed to frustrated) over not being able to function)? _____

89. Do you have suicidal thoughts? _____

90. Please complete the Beck Depression Inventory, below.

Beck Depression Inventory

On this questionnaire are groups of statements. Please read each group of statements carefully. Then pick out the one statement in each group which best describes the way you have been feeling the past week, including today! Check the number beside the statement you picked. If several statements in each group seem to apply equally as well, circle the one that seems closest. Be sure to read all the statements in each group before making your choice.

A. _____ 0   I do not feel sad.
   _____ 1   I feel sad
   _____ 2   I am sad all the time and can't snap out of it.
   _____ 3   I am so sad or unhappy that I can't stand it.

B. _____ 0   I am not particularly discouraged about the future.
   _____ 1   I feel discouraged about the future.
   _____ 2   I feel I have nothing to look forward to.
   _____ 3   I feel that the future is hopeless and that things cannot improve.

C. _____ 0   I do not feel like a failure.
   _____ 1   I feel I have failed more than the average person.
   _____ 2   As I look back on my life, all I can see is a lot of failures.
   _____ 3   I feel I am a complete failure as a person.

D. _____ 0   I get as much satisfaction out of things as I used to.
   _____ 1   I don't enjoy things the way I used to.
   _____ 2   I don't get real satisfaction out of anything anymore.
   _____ 3   I am dissatisfied or bored with everything.

E. _____ 0   I don't feel particularly guilty.
   _____ 1   I feel guilty a good part of the time.
   _____ 2   I feel quite guilty most of the time.
   _____ 3   I feel guilty all of the time.

F. _____ 0   I don't feel I am being punished.
   _____ 1   I feel I may be punished.
   _____ 2   I expect to be punished.
   _____ 3   I feel I am being punished.

G. _____ 0 I don't feel disappointed in myself.

_____ 1 I am disappointed in myself.

_____ 2 I am disgusted with myself.

_____ 3 I hate myself.

H. _____ 0 I don't feel I am any worse than anybody else.

_____ 1 I am critical of myself for my weaknesses or mistakes.

_____ 2 I blame myself all the time for my faults.

_____ 3 I blame myself for everything bad that happens.

I. _____ 0 I don't have any thoughts of killing myself.

_____ 1 I have thoughts of killing myself, but would not carry them out.

_____ 2 I would like to kill myself.

_____ 3 I would kill myself if I had the chance.

J. _____ 0 I don't cry any more than usual.

_____ 1 I cry more now than I used to.

_____ 2 I cry all the time now.

_____ 3 I used to be able to cry, but now I can't cry even though I want to.

K. _____ 0 I am no more irritated now than I ever am.

_____ 1 I get annoyed or irritated more easily than I used to.

_____ 2 I feel irritated all the time now.

_____ 3 I don't get irritated at all by the things that used to irritate me.

L. _____ 0 I have not lost interest in other people.

_____ 1 I am less interested in other people than I used to be.

_____ 2 I have lost most of my interest in other people.

_____ 3 I have lost all of my interest in other people.

M. _____ 0 I make decisions about as well as I ever could.

_____ 1 I put off making decisions more than I used to.

_____ 2 I have greater difficulty in making decisions than before.

_____ 3 I can't make decisions at all anymore.

N.   _____ 0   I don't feel I look any worse than I used to.

_____ 1   I am worried that I am looking old or unattractive.

_____ 2   I feel that there are permanent changes in my appearance that make me look unattractive.

_____ 3   I believe that I look ugly.

O.   _____ 0   I can work about as well as before.

_____ 1   It takes an extra effort to get started at doing something.

_____ 2   I have to push myself very hard to do anything.

_____ 3   I can't do any work at all.

P.   _____ 0   I can sleep as well as usual.

_____ 1   I don't sleep as well as I used to.

_____ 2   I wake up one to two hours earlier than usual and find it hard to get back to sleep.

_____ 3   I wake up several hours earlier than I used to and I cannot get back to sleep.

Q.   _____ 0   I don't get more tired than usual.

_____ 1   I get tired more easily than I used to.

_____ 2   I get tired from doing almost anything.

_____ 3   I am too tired to do anything.

R.   _____ 0   My appetite is no worse than usual.

_____ 1   My appetite is not as good as it used to be.

_____ 2   My appetite is much worse now.

_____ 3   I have no appetite at all anymore.

S.   _____ 0   I haven't lost much weight, if any, lately.

_____ 1   I have lost more than five pounds.

_____ 2   I have lost more than ten pounds.

_____ 3   I have lost more than fifteen pounds.

T.   _____ 0   I am purposely trying to lose weight.

_____ 1   I am not purposely trying to lose weight.

U. _____ 0   I am no more worried about my health than usual.

_____ 1   I am worried about physical problems, such as aches and pains; or upset stomach; or constipation.

_____ 2   I am very worried about physical problems and it's hard to think of much else.

_____ 3   I am so worried about my physical problems that I cannot think about anything else.

V. _____ 0   I have not noticed any recent change in my interest in sex.

_____ 1   I am less interested in sex than I used to be.

_____ 2   I am much less interested in sex now.

_____ 3   I have lost interest in sex completely.

---

91. Had you traveled out of the country in the six weeks before your illness began? _____ If yes:

    Did you get diarrhea while traveling? _____

    Did you eat fish in the Caribbean area in the six weeks before your illness began? _____ If yes:

    Did you eat barracuda? _____

    Did you have unusual feelings in your teeth or a metallic taste in your mouth? _____

    Did you have a lot of numbness and tingling in your fingers and/or toes? _____

92. Are your energy and mental clarity, as well as your pain, improved when you take codeine (Darvon, Percocet, Vicoden, etc.)? _____

93. Do you have chronic vulvar or vaginal pain (females only)? _____ If yes, is it:

    _____ Only with intercourse

    _____ Even without intercourse

94. Please type your experience with the illness (up to two to three pages), including how it began, how it affects your life, what it feels like, significant factors, and anything else your doctor may find helpful.

95. Complete the Yeast Questionnaire (see Appendix C). Enter the total score here: _____.

96. Lab Values: Please put in the actual *number* result (not the letters or units that come after it) in the "result number" column and your lab's normal range for that test (often given in parentheses after, above, or below the result) in the normal range column. Pick the one(s) that most closely fit your lab's format: If a test is not available or has not been done, place a check mark in the box all the way to the left.

Not Done	Lab Test	Your Result	Normal Range
	ESR (Sed Rate: sedimentation rate)		Not needed
	Free T$_4$ (free thyroxine)		_____ to _____
	Total T$_3$ (triiodothyronine)		_____ to _____
	Free T$_4$ index (not T$_7$, T$_4$, or T$_7$ index)		_____ to _____
	TSH (thyroid stimulating hormone)		Not needed
	DHEA-S (DHEA-sulfate—not plain DHEA)		
	B$_{12}$ (Vitamin B$_{12}$)		Not needed
	Percent saturation (% sat; iron % saturation)		Not needed
	Ferritin		_____ to _____
	Free testosterone		_____ to _____
	Cortrosyn stimulation test 1. Cortisol (if drawn before 9:00 A.M., give first reading (or lowest reading if not clear which was first)		_____ to _____
	2. Cortisol (second reading)		Not needed
	3. Cortisol (third reading)		Not needed
	Do not give results of any cortisols drawn after 12:00 noon.		
	Hgb A1C (glycosylated hemoglobin) (not regular Hgb or hemoglobin)		Not needed
	Females only:		If confusing leave blank
	FSH (follicle-stimulating hormone)		_____ to _____
	LH (luteinizing hormone)		_____ to _____

Put down results for the tests below only if they are abnormal (high or low).

1. Blood count or CBC

Test Name	*Your Result (only if marked abnormal— high or low)*	Normal Values
WBC (white blood cells)	_____	(_____)
HCT (hematocrit)	_____	(_____)
MCV (mean cell or corpuscular volume)	_____	(_____)
Lymphs % (lymphocytes)	_____	(_____)
EOS % (eosinophils) (as %, not total)	_____	(_____)
Monocytes %	_____	(_____)
Atypical lymphocytes %	_____	(_____)
Platelet count	_____	(_____)
Bands	_____	(_____)

Does it list any of the cells below? _____ If yes, check all that apply:

_____ Promyelocytes

_____ Metamyelocytes

_____ Blast cells

_____ Target cells

2. Chemistry

Test Name	*Your Result (only if marked abnormal— high or low)*	Normal Values
Glucose (blood sugar)	_____	(_____)
BUN (blood urea nitrogen)	_____	(_____)
Creat (creatinine)	_____	(_____)
SGOT (ALT)	_____	(_____)
SGPT (AST)	_____	(_____)
Alk. phos (alkaline phosphatase)	_____	(_____)
Bilirubin	_____	(_____)

NA (sodium) _____ (_____)
K+ (potassium) _____ (_____)
Mg (magnesium) _____ (_____)
Ca (calcium) _____ (_____)
Cholesterol _____ (_____)
Uric acid _____ (_____)
Triglycerides _____ (_____)
HDL cholesterol _____ (_____)

3. Urine Analysis (U/A)

Test Name	*Your Result (only if marked abnormal— high or low)*	*Normal Values*
S.G. (specific gravity)	_____	(_____)
RBC (red blood cells)	_____	(_____)
WBC (leukocytes)	_____	(_____)

4. Estradiol (for females) _____ N/A

5. Somatomedin C (IGF-1) _____ (_____)

6. Lyme Test
_____ Positive
_____ Negative
_____ Not sure/indeterminate

7. Stool for *Clostridium difficile* (*C. diff* or toxin)
_____ Positive
_____ Negative

Test Name	*Your Result (only if marked abnormal— high or low)*	*Normal Values*
8. IgE	_____	(_____)

9. Antimicrosomal antibodies
   ____ Negative
   ____ Positive (above normal range) (> or = to _____)
   ____ Less than (<) 1: _____)
   ____ Greater than (>) 1: _____)

10. Antithyroglobulin antibody
    ____ Negative
    ____ Positive (above normal range) (> or = to _____)
    ____ Less than (<) 1: _____)
    ____ Greater than (>) 1: _____)

	Your Values	*Normal Values*
11. Antinuclear antibodies (FANA or ANA)	____ negative or	(negative or 1:80 or ____ 1:_____ less)
12. Rheumatoid factor (latex fixation)	____ negative or	(negative or 1:80 or ____ 1:_____ less)
13. Prolactin	_____	_____

If you have any abnormal blood tests results (whether or not they were listed above) please overline them or mark them in red on your lab results sheet and be sure your physician sees them!

E

Treatment Protocol Checklist for Chronic Fatigue Syndrome and Fibromyalgia

THIS SECTION CONTAINS THE LIST OF THE MOST commonly used treatments for CFIDS/FMS and instructions for how to use them. I have grouped them by category. As each patient is different, everyone needs a different mix of treatments. The educational program on our website (www.endfatigue.com, go to "How to get well now") will let you know which treatments you need for your specific case.

Dear Patient,
Below is a listing of the more common treatments used in treating CFIDS/FMS. I would use this list as a record of your treatments and have it with you for follow-up/phone visits. Put an "x" through the number in front of any treatment you stop and note the reason stopped and date. Put the date started in front of the other treatments. Although it can take six weeks to see a treatment's benefits, most of the medication's side effects will usually occur within the first few days of starting a treatment. Except for treatments 1 through 21, which can all be started in the first one to three days, add in one new treatment each one to three days. If a side effect occurs, stop the last two or three treatments for a few days and see if it goes away. If the side effect is worrisome, call your family doctor (or go to the emergency room) immediately. If needed, all treatments (except if you've been on numbers 27, 35, 41, 92 through 99 or 122, and 126 for over two

months—then taper these off) can be stopped until the situation is clarified. Do not get pregnant or drive on treatment if sedated. It is normal for a woman's periods to be irregular during the first three to four months of treatment. You can begin to slowly taper off most treatments when you feel well for six months. On average, it takes three months to start feeling better. Stop things one at a time (for example, one treatment every one to three weeks) so you can see if you still need it. If needed, any or all of these can be used forever (usually *not* necessary). For sources of the products and services listed here, see Appendix J: Resources.

Nutritional Treatments

_____ 1. From Fatigued to Fantastic powdered formula. Take ¾ to 1½ tablespoons a day blended with milk, water, or yogurt. Add stevia to taste (approximately 8 drops). If diarrhea occurs, start with a lower dose and work your way up or divide the daily dose into smaller doses and take several times of the day. Because this contains calcium, do not take it within two hours of taking thyroid hormone. You can substitute treatment numbers 3, 4, 5, 7, 12B, 13, 105, and 107, below.

_____ 2. CFS/FM Multi. Take one a day.

_____ 3. Natrol's My Favorite Multiple—Take One. Take one a day.

   Note: Read labels carefully. Do not confuse this formula with Natrol's My Favorite Multiple. That is a different product.

_____ 4. Fibrocare or Magnesium/Malic Acid Plus. Take two tablets three times a day for eight months, then two tablets a day (less if diarrhea is a problem). Start with one to two a day and slowly work up as you are able without getting uncomfortable diarrhea. You can take up to ten a day for constipation. Taking it with food may lessen diarrhea. If pain or fatigue recur on lowering the dose, increase it. Taken at bedtime, it helps sleep.

_____ 5. Calcium. Take 500 to 1,000 milligrams daily, with 400 international units of vitamin D (a chewable calcium, calcium citrate, or calcium chelate is recommended). If you get a nonchewable tablet, test it to see if it dissolves in two to three inches of vinegar over a period of one hour (swirl it around in the vinegar a few times). If it doesn't, it won't dissolve in your stomach, and you need to get a different brand. (Do not drink the vinegar). You can also avoid this problem by using capsules or liquid filled gelcaps. Taken at bedtime, calcium supplements may help sleep.

____ 6. Lipoic acid. Take 200 milligrams a day for six to nine months. This supplement protects the liver. It is especially important to take it if you are you're on Sporanox or Diflucan. If you have active hepatitis or cirrhosis, consider taking 300 to 2,000 milligrams a day, depending on the severity of your condition.

____ 7. Vitamin B_{12}. Take 1,000 to 5,000 micrograms sublingually (under your tongue) daily.

____ 8. Vitamin B_{12} injections. Get one 1-cc (3,000-microgram) intramuscular injection three to five times weekly for a total of fifteen doses, then as needed (for example, one to twelve times a month). This needs to be made by a holistic compounding pharmacy.

____ 9. N-Acetyl-L-cysteine (NAC). Take 500 milligrams a day for nine months, then take as needed. Makes glutathione.

____ 10. Chromagen FA (iron). Take one tablet a day. Do not take within six hours of thyroid hormone preparations or Cipro, as these can prevent their absorption. Take on an empty stomach (for example, take between 2:00 and 6:00 P.M., on an empty stomach). It is all right to miss up to three doses a week. Stop in four to six months, or when your ferritin blood test is over 40. Taking iron can turn your stools black. Taking 500 to 1,000 milligrams of vitamin C with each tablet may improve absorption.

____ 11. Flaxseed/borage oil. Take three 1,050-milligram capsules twice a day for nine months. Use flaxseed oil *without* borage oil if you have bipolar (manic-depressive) disorder. Dry eyes, mouth, and hair suggest a need for this. Use only Barlean's flaxseed oils.

____ 12. SAM-e. Take 200 milligrams one to four times a day. Use Nature's Made brand.

____ 12B. Vitamin C. Take 500 to 1,000 milligrams twice a day.

____ 13. Vitamin E. Take 400 international units of natural vitamin E a day.

____ 13B. Imuplus. Take one packet twice a day. This helps to the body to make glutathione.

____ 13C. Zinc sulfate. Take 25 milligrams twice a day for six weeks, then stop.

Mitochondrial Energy Treatments

Use these for nine months. Then drop the dose to the lowest dose that maintains the effect (or stop it if there has been no benefit).

____ 14. CFS/FM Energy Formula. Take three capsules a day

____ 15. Acetyl-L-carnitine. Take two 500-milligram capsules twice a day for three months. Then take 250 to 500 milligrams a day or stop it. Although important in CFS/FMS, it is even more important to take this if you also have mitral valve prolapse and/or elevated blood triglycerides. If the cost is prohibitive, you can take less or substitute L-carnitine.

____ 16. Coenzyme Q_{10}. Take 100 to 200 milligrams once a day. This is especially important if you are taking a cholesterol-lowering drug such as Mevacor. Take it with a meal that has fat, with oil supplements, or in an oil-based form to improve absorption.

____ 17. L-Lysine. Take 1,000 milligrams three times a day for three months, then take 1,000 milligrams a day. Also take this supplement if you have oral cold sores or genital herpes to suppress them.

____ 18. L-Arginine. Take 2,000 milligrams two to three times a day.

Note: Do not take this supplement if it causes flare-ups of herpes. Or take lysine with it.

____ 19. Magnesium/potassium aspartate. Take two 500-milligram capsules twice a day for three to four months. Be sure to use a "fully reacted" brand.

___ 20. Vitamin B complex. Take one or two 50-milligram tablets at night.

___ 21 NADH. Take two 5-milligram tablets each morning. Use the Enada brand. Take it on an empty stomach first thing in the morning (leave it by your bedside in the bottle or foil wrap with a glass of water) at least one-half hour before eating, drinking coffee or juice, or taking any medication or supplements (except thyroid, which you can take with the NADH). It takes two months to see if it works. Fifteen to 20 milligrams a day may be more effective and is safe. *Do not take vitamin C, malic acid, lipoic acid, or other acids within two to three hours of NADH, as acid destroys NADH.*

Sleep Aids for Fibromyalgia

You can try these in the order listed or as you prefer, based on your history. Adjust dose as needed to get seven to eight hours of solid sleep without waking or hangover. No going to the bathroom if you wake up unless you still have to go five to ten minutes later. Mixing low doses of several treatments is more likely to help you sleep without a hangover than a high dose of one medication. You can take up to the maximum dose of all checked-off treatments simultaneously. Do not drive if you have next day sedation. If you're not sleeping seven to eight hours a night without waking on the checked-off treatments, *do not* wait until your next appointment to let us know or contact your physician! Ambien, Klonopin, Xanax, and Soma are considered potentially addictive—I've never seen this happen, though, with the recommended dosing below. If you have next day sedation, try taking the medications (except the Ambien) a few hours before bedtime. The antidepressants (for example, Prozac or Paxil) can improve sleep a lot after six weeks. Taking your magnesium and/or calcium at night can also help sleep.

___ 22. Zolpidem (Ambien). Take one-half to one 10-milligram tablet at bedtime. If you tend to wake during the night, leave an extra one-half to one tablet at bedside and you can take it as needed to help you sleep through the night.

____ 23.   Trazodone (Desyrel). Take one-half to six 50-milligram tablets at bedtime. Although sedating, it can be used during the day (50 to 250 milligrams at a time) for anxiety. Do not take over 450 milligrams a day (or 150 milligrams a day if on other antidepressants).

____ 24.   Herbal Sleep Formula, containing 160 milligrams of valerian, 125 milligrams of kava kava, 100 milligrams of passionflower, 80 milligrams of lemon balm, 25 milligrams of 5-HTP, and 100 micrograms of melatonin. Take two to four tablets each night, or use up to four a day for anxiety.

____ 25.   Passionflower (*Passiflora*). Take 100 to 200 milligrams at night. This is also good for anxiety during the day.

____ 26.   Delta-wave sleep-inducing CDs or tapes. These help, with no side effects. Play to fall asleep and if you wake during the night. They can be played throughout the night if desired. You can use either of the two tapes or CDs.

____ 27.   Clonazepam (Klonopin). Begin slowly and work your way up as sedation allows. Take one-half of a ½-milligram tablet at bedtime, increasing up to six tablets at bedtime as needed. This can be very effective for sleep, pain, and restless leg syndrome.

____ 28.   Melatonin. Take one 300-microgram tablet (available at health food stores) at bedtime. Do not use a higher dose unless you find it to be more effective (³⁄₁₀ milligram is usually as effective as 5 milligrams—and may be safer).

____ 29.   Doxylamine (Unisom For Sleep). Take 25 milligrams at night. This is an antihistamine.

____ 30.   Carisprodol (Soma). Take one-half to one tablet at bedtime. This is very good if pain is severe.

____ 31.   Cyclobenzaprine (Flexeril). Take one-half to two 10-milligram tablets at bedtime. This is a muscle relaxant. It can cause dry mouth.

____ 32.   Kava kava. Take one to three 250-milligram capsules of 30 percent extract—at night. If a rash develops, add a 50-milligram B-complex at night—and stop taking the kava or decrease the dose or frequency of use. If the rash persists, see your family doctor.

____ 33. 5-Hydroxytryptophan (5-HTP). Take 100 to 400 milligrams at night. This supplement naturally stimulates serotonin. Don't take over 250 milligrams a day if you are on Prozac, Paxil, Zoloft, Desyrel, or Celexa.

____ 34A. Mirtazapine (Remeron). Take one to three 15-milligram tablets at bedtime. This is especially helpful if you feel like you're "hibernating" during the day.

____ 34B. Amitriptyline (Elavil). Take one-half to five 10-milligram tablets at bedtime. This is good for nerve pain and vulvadynia. It may cause weight gain or dry mouth.

____ 35. Alprazolam (Xanax). Take one-half to four ½-milligram tablets at bedtime. This is short-acting and gives a good three to five hours sleep with less hangover in the morning.

____ 36A. Brain wave unit.

____ 36B. Sinemet 10/100. Take one between 6:00 and 9:00 P.M. each evening for restless leg syndrome.

Hormonal Treatments

Several studies show that thyroid therapies can be very helpful in CFIDS/ FMS, even if your blood tests are normal. This treatment is, however, very controversial, even though it's usually very safe. All treatments (even aspirin) can cause problems in some people however. The main risks of thyroid treatment are:

1. Triggering caffeine-like anxiety or palpitations. If this happens, cut back the dose and increase by one-half to one tablet each six to eight weeks (as is comfortable) or slower. Sometimes taking 100 to 200 milligrams of vitamin B_1 (thiamine) a day will also help. If you have severe, persistent racing heart, call your family doctor and/or go to the emergency room.
2. Exercise (such as climbing steps). If you are on the edge of having a heart attack, thyroid hormone can trigger it.

In the long run, though, I suspect thyroid may decrease the risk of heart disease. If you have chest pain, go to the emergency room and/or call your family doctor. It will likely be chest muscle pain (not dangerous), but better safe than sorry. To put it in perspective, I've *never* seen this happen despite treating many hundreds of patients with thyroid. Increasing your thyroid dose to levels *above* the *upper* limit of the normal range may accelerate osteoporosis (which is already common in CFIDS/FMS). Because of this, you need to check your thyroid (total T_3 and free T_4—*not* TSH) levels after four to eight weeks on your optimum dose of thyroid hormone. All this having been said, we find treatments with thyroid hormone to be *safer* than aspirin and ibuprofen. If you have risk factors for angina, do an exercise stress test to make sure your heart is healthy before beginning thyroid treatment. Risk factors for angina include:

- Diabetes.
- Elevated cholesterol.
- Hypertension.
- Smoking.
- A personal or family history of angina.
- Gout.
- Age over fifty years old.

There are several forms of thyroid hormone, and one kind will often work when the other does not. Do not take thyroid hormone within six hours of iron supplements or two hours of calcium or you won't absorb the thyroid (take your multivitamin with iron and calcium at bedtime). I usually use Armour Thyroid.

___ 37. L-Thyroxine (Synthroid) 50 micrograms (100 micrograms equals 0.1 milligram).

___ 38. Armour Thyroid (natural thyroid glandular) ½ grain (equals 30 milligrams).

___ 39. Thyrolar ½ (this equals 25 micrograms of T_4 plus 6.25 micrograms of T_3). It needs to be refrigerated.

For each of these three forms, take one-half tablet each *morning* on an empty stomach for one week, and then one tablet each morning. Increase the dosage by one-half to one tablet each two to six weeks, until you are taking two tablets daily. Check a repeat total T_3 and free T_4 blood level when you have been on two tablets a day for four weeks. If okay, you can continue to raise the dose by one-half to one tablet each morning each six to nine weeks, up to a maximum of four tablets a day, and then recheck the total T_3 and free T_4 four weeks later. Adjust it to the dose that feels the best (lower the dose if you are shaky or if your pulse is regularly over 88 beats a minute). Do not go over four tablets a day without discussing it with your doctor. When you find your optimum dose, you can often get a single tablet at that strength.

___ 40. Sustained-release T_3 (T_3 SR, or activated thyroid). Get 7½- to 15-microgram capsules. When you are up to 60 micrograms a day, order 60-microgram capsules as well. It is much cheaper to get one large dose capsule than many smaller ones. In fibromyalgia, resistance to normal thyroid doses may occur and patients often need very high levels of activated T_3 SR thyroid to improve. One research group feels that the average dose needed in FMS is 125 micrograms each morning—*much* higher than your body's normal production. Because we are often going above normal levels with T_3 SR, the risks and potential side effects noted above increase. Because of this, if you have risk factors, it is more important to consider an exercise stress test to make sure your heart is healthy (no underlying angina) before beginning this protocol. Also, if your total T_3 blood test goes above normal (the free T_4 is normally low on this treatment), consider a Dexa scan to check for osteoporosis each six to eighteen months while on treatment. This having been said, in our experience this treatment has been quite safe and, for some FMS patients, dramatically effective. Begin with 7½ micrograms each *morning* and continue to increase by 7½ micrograms each three days until you're at 60 micrograms a day, and then increase by 15 micrograms a day each four to six weeks until one of the following happens (whichever comes first):

1. You reach 120 micrograms each morning (or 60 micrograms if you're over fifty years old, unless approved by your physician).
2. You feel healthy.

3. Your oral temperature is routinely at least 98.4°F during midday.

4. You get shakiness, worsening *significant* palpitations (occasional "flip-flops" are common) or other side effects.

Check a total T_3 level every two months and discuss with your doctor if it is above normal, which it may need to be. If you feel no better even on the maximum dose, taper off. Decrease by 7½ micrograms every three days until you're at 15 micrograms a day. Take 15 micrograms a day for three weeks. Then take 7½ micrograms a day for three weeks, and then stop.

After being on treatment for three to four months, many patients can lower the T_3 dose or stop it. Feel free to try dropping the dose. If you feel better initially and then worse (beginning more than four weeks after starting a new dose), you probably need to lower the dose.

Adrenal hormones help your body deal with stress and maintain blood pressure.

___ 41. Cortef. Take one-half to two and a half 5-milligram tablets at breakfast, one-half to one and a half tablets at lunch, and zero to one-half tablets at 4:00 P.M. Use the lowest dose that feels the best. Most patients find that one to one and a half tablets in the morning and one-half to one tablet at noon is optimal. Take it with food if it causes an acid stomach. Do not take over four tablets a day without discussing the risks with your physician. Take calcium (see item 1 or 5, above) if you are on Cortef. If taken too late in the day, Cortef can keep you up at night. You can double the dose for up to one to three weeks (to a maximum of seven tablets a day), during periods of severe stress (for example, infections—see or call your doctor for the infection and let him or her know you're raising the dose). If routinely taking over four tablets a day, wear a Medic Alert bracelet that says "on chronic cortisol treatment." Take 500 milligrams of vitamin C twice a day for adrenal support. Taking 100 milligrams of Asian (*Panax*) ginseng twice a day (taken in "six-weeks-on, two-weeks-off" cycles) can also help your adrenals to heal. After nine months, you can try to wean off the Cortef (decrease the dosage by one-half tablet a day every two weeks) if you feel all right (or no worse) without it.

___ 42.   Dehydroepiandrosterone (DHEA). Take this each morning or twice daily (lower the dose if acne or darkening of facial hair occurs). GNC has a good brand of timed-release DHEA tablets. Keep your DHEA-*sulfate* levels between 140 and 180 mcg/dL for females and 300 to 400 mcg/dL for males. If you have breast cancer, do not use without your physician's okay. See page 250 for dosing).

___ 43A.   Fludrocortisone (Florinef). Begin by taking one-quarter or a 0.1-milligram tablet each morning. Then increase the dosage by one-quarter tablet each three to seven days. Increase more slowly if headache occurs. Increase your water, salt, and potassium intake (for example, drink 12 ounces of V-8 juice and eat one banana a day). Check potassium level and blood pressure every six weeks for four months, and then each three to four months.

___ 43B.   Increase your salt intake to about 5 to 10 grams a day and water intake to approximately 1 gallon a day. If your mouth and lips are dry (and you're not on Elavil), you're dehydrated—drink more water or herbal tea or lemonade sweetened with stevia (see item 54b on page 328), *not* sodas or coffee.

Other hormones to consider include the following.

___ 44.   Oxytocin—10 units each morning by mouth or by intramuscular injection—as is helpful. The injections may sting. If so, you can add $\frac{2}{10}$ to $\frac{5}{10}$ cc lidocaine (*without* epinephrine) to the oxytocin.

___ 45.   Natural estrogen. Take 1 milligram of Estrace (estradiol) once or twice daily, *or* put a 0.05 to 0.1 milligram Climara patch on each Sunday, *or* take 2½ milligrams of biestrogen once or twice a day. If you have not had a hysterectomy, you *must* be on progesterone with the estrogen to prevent uterine cancer. If you are on the patch and it seems to stop working the last one to two days of the week, you can change the patch every five days. Use the estrogen _____ every day; _____ day one through twenty-five of your cycle (day one of your period is day one of your cycle). It is normal for your periods to be irregular for three to four months. If your symptoms (including migraines and anxiety) worsen for the week you are off the estrogen, we can add a 0.025-milligram Climara patch for that week. If they worsen a few hours before you take the estrogen by mouth, divide the dose up through the day (for example, one-half tablet four times a day versus two tablets each morning). If you order your estrogen/progesterone capsules from Professional Arts Pharmacy or Cape Apothecary, the pharmacist will work with you in adjusting the dose.

___ 46. Ortho-Novum 1/35. Start taking this the Sunday after this period. Its effectiveness as birth control begins after you've been on it the first week. If you miss a pill, add alternate contraception that cycle. Its effectiveness as birth control is decreased while on doxycycline or amoxicillin (Amoxil, Augmentin, Polymox, Trimox, Wymox) family antibiotics.

___ 47A. Natural progesterone (Prometrium—available in most pharmacies). Take 100 milligrams daily if you are over forty-eight years old. If you are under forty-eight years old, take 200 milligrams a day for the sixteenth through twenty-fifty day of your cycle. Take it at night.

___ 47B. Relaxin (Vitalaxin 20). Take one to two 20-microgram tablets one to two times a day. It often takes three months to see the benefit. You may have morning sickness and/or breast tenderness during the first month of use. Start with one tablet at night. If okay, take one tablet twice a day for five days.

___ 48A. Testosterone. Males should get a ½-cc (100 milligrams) shot every seven to ten days or apply 25 to 100 milligrams (order 100-milligram-per-gram cream) one or two times a day (less if acne occurs). Rub the cream into an area of thin skin on the abdomen, or inner arms.

___ 48B. Testosterone—Females should take 2 milligrams in tablets or cream (make 4-milligrams-per-gram cream) from one to two times a day (less if acne or darkening of facial hair occurs).

___ 49. Somatomed. Take two tablets *on an empty stomach* (*at least* two hours after eating), one hour before bedtime on weeknights (don't take it on Saturday and Sunday night). After three months, stay off it for two to four weeks. This helps the body to make growth hormone.

Antiviral Agents

___ 50. Famciclovir (Famvir). Take 750 milligrams three times a day. If you are feeling better in one month, continue Famvir until you feel well for two more months. If you're not feeling better in six weeks, stop it. Continue it as long as needed to feel well. Take echinacea (see item 62, below), lysine (see item 17, above) and thymic protein (see item 63, below) while on Famvir to make it more effective.

___ 50A. Valacyclovir (Valtrex) and cimetidine (Tagamet). Take one 1,000-milligram tablet of Valtrex and one 300-milligram tablet of Tagamet four times a day for six months. It takes four months to see the effect. Take echinacea (see item 62, below), lysine (see item 17, above) and thymic protein (see item 63, below) while on Valtrex to make it more effective.

___ 51. Lithium. Take 300 milligrams one to three times a day. If you have tremors, take two teaspoons of expeller-pressed safflower oil from a health food store (uncooked—for example, as salad dressing) daily or lower the dose. Check a lithium level one month after beginning medication. Then have a lithium and thyroid blood test (free T_4) every six to twelve months.

___ 52. Monolaurin. Take nine 300-milligram capsules once a day on an empty stomach for one week, followed by six capsules once a day for twenty days. Take 1,500 milligrams of lysine twice a day while on Monolaurin.

___ 53. Olive leaf extract. Take three to four 500-milligram capsules three times a day for ten to fourteen days for respiratory infections, or three to four capsules three times a day for six to twenty-four weeks for chronic infections (such as HHV-6, Epstein Barr, and so on).

Anti-Yeast Treatments

____ 54A. Avoid sweets—this includes sucrose, glucose, fructose, corn syrup, or any other sweets, until the doctor says that it is okay to include them in your diet again. Avoid fruit *juices,* which are naturally sweet. Having one or two pieces of fruit a day (the whole fruit as opposed to the juice) is okay. Stevia and Sweet Balance are great sugar substitutes.

____ 54B. Stevia. This herbal sweetener is wonderful. Use all you want. Sweet Balance is also excellent.

____ 55. Acidophilus or other milk bacteria (refrigerated is preferable). Take 3 to 6 billion units a day. Do *not* take within six hours of taking an antibiotic (for example, take it at midday if you take the antibiotic morning and night)

____ 56. Caprylic acid. Take one to three 500- to 650-milligram capsules three times a day with meals for three to four months and then 1,800 to 3,600 milligrams a day as needed.

____ 57. Garlic. Take one clove one to three times a day with meals. Crushed in olive oil with salt, it tastes great on bread.

____ 58. Mycelex oral lozenges (for thrush and/or "in the mouth" sores). Suck on a lozenge five times a day for one to four days, as needed. After sucking on it awhile (such as ten minutes), put pieces of the lozenge up against sore(s) until you are tired of it being there.

____ 59. Nystatin. Begin by taking one 500,000-unit tablet a day and increase by 1 tablet a day until you are up to two tablets two to three times a day. Your symptoms may initially flare as the yeast die off. If this occurs, decrease the dose and then increase the nystatin more slowly or stop for awhile until symptoms decrease. The nystatin is usually taken for five to eight months. If nausea occurs, take two twice a day and/or switch to the nystatin powder in capsules or mixed in water. Repeat nystatin for four to six weeks any time you take an antibiotic or have recurrent bowel symptoms.

____ 60. Fluconazole (Diflucan). Take 200 milligrams a day.

or

Itraconazole (Sporanox). Take two 100-milligram tablets each day (simultaneously) with food for six weeks.

Begin taking the Diflucan or Sporanox four weeks after beginning the nystatin. If the symptoms have improved and then worsen when you stop the antifungal, refill the prescription for another six weeks. (Note: A six-week supply costs over five hundred dollars!) If your symptoms flared when you began the nystatin, begin with one-quarter to one-half of the above dose for the first week. *Do not* take Seldane, Hismanyl, Propulsid, cholesterol-lowering agents related to Mevacor while on Sporanox or Diflucan! Two hundred milligrams of Diflucan a day may be substituted for Sporanox if you are on antacids. Take lipoic acid (see item 6, above) any time you take Sporanox or Diflucan. Also, taking betaine HCl to help digestion at the same time as the Sporanox can dramatically increase Sporanox's absorbtion and effectiveness. Lipoic acid may decrease the risk of liver inflammation from the Diflucan or Sporanox. If you need to stay on these medications more than three months, check liver blood tests (ALT, AST) every three months. If you feel well and symptoms (especially bowel symptoms) recur over time, consider re-treating yourself with nystatin and/or caprylic acid and oregano oil and/or Sporanox (or Diflucan) for one month as needed. If you have a low income and no prescription insurance, the company that makes Diflucan may supply it for free.

___ 61. Oregano oil (enteric coated). Take two capsules on an empty stomach three times a day for three to four months, then two a day as needed for yeast overgrowth.

Immune Stimulants

___ 62. Echinacea. Take 300 to 325 milligrams three times a day (also take while on Famvir). Stay off the echinacea for one week each month or it will stop working. It may also improve adrenal function.

_____ 63. Thymic protein, available as Proboost. Dissolve the contents of 1 packet *under your tongue*—any that is swallowed is destroyed!—three times a day for six weeks, then once a day for six weeks. Also take it three times a day at first sign of any infection until the infection resolves. It costs approximately two dollars a packet.

_____ 64. MgN3. Take two to four 250-milligram capsules four times a day for two weeks. Then take two twice a day. This natural product *triples* some important components (natural killer cells) of your immune system. It is expensive.

_____ 65. Selenium. Take 200 micrograms a day (in addition to the 200 micrograms of selenium in your multivitamin) for six months. You may get toxic if you take over 200 micrograms a day for over six months.

_____ 66. Cat's claw. Use the Saventaro form. Take one capsule three times a day for ten days, then once a day.

_____ 67. Inositol hexaphosphate (IP_6). Take 5 to 8 grams a day for one to two months, and then 1 gram twice a day.

For Brain Fog

_____ 68. Ginkgo biloba. Use a product standardized to 24 percent glycosides. Take one 60-milligram capsule twice a day for brain fog; two twice a day for depression or sexual dysfunction from antidepressants. It takes six weeks to work.

_____ 69. Vinpocetine plus ginkgo. Take one capsule supplying 10 milligrams of vinpocetine plus 60 milligrams of ginkgo two to three times a day.

_____ 70. Piracetam. Take 1,200 milligrams twice a day for two weeks, then take 2,400 milligrams twice a day for two weeks. Then adjust to optimum dose (up to 4,800 milligrams a day). It can be ordered from England. Take with Hydergine (see item 71, below).

_____ 71. Hydergine. Take 4 to 6 milligrams each morning.

_____ 72. Dimethylaminoethanol (DMAE). Take up to 400 milligrams a day.

For Migraines

Magnesium (see items 1 and 4, above) is also very important.

___ 73. Vitamin B$_2$ (riboflavin). Take 400 milligrams a day to prevent migraines.

___ 74. Feverfew. Take 250 milligrams one to three times a day to prevent migraines.

Treatment for Parasites

If your stool test shows parasites, recheck the stool test three to four weeks after finishing the treatment below.

___ 75. Metronidazole (Flagyl). Take 750 milligrams three times a day for ten days (or 750 milligrams of Flagyl ER twice a day), followed by Yodoxin (see below) for many parasites. For *Clostridium difficile* take 250 milligrams four times a day or 500 milligrams three times a day. It may cause nausea/vomiting (uncomfortable but usually not worrisome). Do not drink alcohol while on this medication as it will make you vomit. The extended-release form is easier on the stomach, as is the brand-name form. If you get numbness/tingling in your fingers, or it worsens if you usually have it, stop the Flagyl.

___ 76. Iodoquinol (Yodoxin). Take 650 milligrams three times a day for twenty days after Flagyl is completed.

___ 77. Tinidazole (Fasigyn). Take 2,000 milligrams once daily for three consecutive days with food (for *Entamoeba histolytica*) *or* three doses, each two weeks apart (for giardia or *Dientamoeba fragilis*).

___ 78. Paromomycin (Humatin). Take 500 milligrams three times a day for ten days (for *Cryptosporidium*). For blastocystis, add Yodoxin.

___ 79. Azithromycin (Zithromax). Take one 250-milligram tablet a day on an empty stomach for ten days, along with one Bactrim DS tablet twice a day for ten days (an alternate treatment for *Cryptosporidium*). Add *Artemisia* (see item 84, below).

____ 80. Bactrim DS. Take one tablet twice a day for 10 days, plus 650 milligrams of Yodoxin three times a day with food for ten days. Do not take folic acid supplements (for example, a B-complex or multivitamin) for these ten days (for blastocystis).

____ 81. Amphotericin-B. Take 100 milligrams twice a day by mouth plus 500 milligrams of tinidazole twice a day plus one tablet of furazolidone (Furoxone) twice a day. Take these three together with food for five to seven days.

____ 82. Lactoferrin. Take one to three 350-milligram capsules at bedtime.

____ 83. Multi-Pure water filter. Most other filters, except reverse osmosis, are ineffective.

____ 84. *Artemisia annua,* an herbal antiparasitic. Take two 500-milligram tablets three times a day for twenty days.

____ 85. Tricycline, an herbal antiparasitic. Take two tablets three times a day after meals for six to eight weeks (concentrated Artemisia).

____ 86. Colostrum (mother's milk). Take three capsules three times a day for eight to twelve weeks. Then stop or use the lowest dose needed for symptoms. If nausea or indigestion occurs, lower the dose to a comfortable level for one to two weeks till it passes. Take on an empty stomach.

____ 87. Quinacrine. Take 100 milligrams a day for five days. May be useful for empiric therapy of suspected, but not identified, parasites.

____ 88. Albendazole (Albenza). Take 400 milligrams a day for five days. May be useful for empiric therapy of suspected but not identified parasites.

Treatment for Bacterial, Mycoplasma, Chlamydial, Bladder Infections With E. Coli or Other Infections

These infections usually take months to years to eradicate. It is common for symptoms to flare up from the infection die-off during the first two to six weeks of treatment. Take the antibiotics for six months and, if better, then repeat six-week cycles till your symptoms stay gone. Antidepressants, Neurontin, and/or codeine may block the antibiotic's effectiveness. Be sure to take two tablets of nystatin twice a day and acidophilus while on the antibiotics. If you have occasional low-grade fever (that is, if your temperature is over 98.6°F), check your oral temperature occasionally to see if the antibiotic reduces or eliminates the fever. If so, stay on that antibiotic for at least six months.

___ 89A. Ciprofloxacin (Cipro). Take 750 milligrams twice a day for six months. Do not take magnesium products (for example, Fibrocare, some antacids, Pro Energy, From Fatigued To Fantastic powder formula) within six hours of Cipro or you won't absorb the Cipro).

or

___ 89B. Doxycycline (a tetracycline). Take 100 milligrams three times a day for six months. If symptoms *recur* when the doxycycline is completed, keep repeating six-week courses until the symptoms stay resolved. Take nystatin (at least two twice a day) while on the antibiotic. Birth control pills may not work while on doxycycline. *Do not* take any doxycycline tablets older than their expiration date (very dangerous).

or

___ 89C. Azithromycin (Zithromax). Take one 600-milligram tablet a day (take with food if it bothers your stomach). Don't take magnesium-containing products within six hours of the Zithromax.

___ 89D. Biaxin. Take 500 milligrams twice a day.

___ 89E. D-Mannose. Take ½ teaspoon (2.5 grams) stirred in water every two to three hours while awake for two to five days for acute bladder infections (may use long term for chronic infections) caused by *E. coli* (this causes approximately 90 percent of bladder infections). If not much better in twenty-four hours, get a urine culture and consider an antibiotic.

Nonspecific Treatments

Items 92 through 99 may help treat neurally mediated hypotension (NMH) and decrease pain, as well as helping energy.

____ 90A. Nambudripad allergy elimination technique (NAET).

____ 90B. Myers cocktail intravenous nutritional therapies. This can be very helpful.

____ 91. Antioxynol (grapeseed extract). Take one to two 50-mg capsules one to two times a day.

____ 92. Dextroamphetamine (Dexedrine). Take one to two 5-milligram tablets in the morning; plus one-half to one and a half tablets at noon; or up to one 200-milligram tablet of Provigil in the morning and one at noon, as needed for energy. Amphetamine family stimulants are similar to Ritalin and may be addictive. Take less if you have caffeine-like shakiness. Most patients use one tablet in the morning and one-half at noon.

____ 93. Sertraline (Zoloft). Take one to two 50-milligram tablet(s) each morning or evening.

____ 94. Paroxetine (Paxil). Take one to two 20-milligram tablet(s) each morning.

____ 95. Fluoxetine (Prozac). Take one to two 20-milligram capsule(s) each morning. Begin with 10 milligrams a day the first week if the full dose makes you hyper.

____ 96. Venlafaxine (Effexor). Take one to two 37½-milligram tablets one to two times a day.

____ 97. Nefazodone (Serzone). Take 100 milligrams twice a day for one week, then 150 milligrams twice times a day.

____ 98. Citaloprim (Celexa). Take one to two 20-milligram tablets a day.

___ 99. Bupropion (Wellbutrin). Take 100 milligrams two to three times a day.

___ 100. Selegiline (Deprenyl). Take 10 milligrams in the morning.

___ 101. Aspirin. Take 81 milligrams a day.

___ 102. Oxygen, 10 liters. Take this via a partial rebreather mask (set at FI02 of 35–40 percent) for one hour one to two times a day. The oxygen mask must expand and contract during breathing.

___ 103A. Heparin. This is a blood thinner. Take 4,000 to 6,000 units subcutaneously twice a day for one month. Avoid any traumatic injuries. If you have preloaded syringes, use one syringe twice a day. This is a blood thinner—call immediately if you have any bleeding problems. Check the platelet count and PTT blood tests (see item 147, below) every three days for nine days, then weekly while on heparin. Inject it into the fat (*not* muscle) in your abdomen. Use a different spot each time (you may get a bruise where the injection is given). Stop taking it immediately if your blood or platelet count drops.

___ 103B. Naltrexone (ReVia). Take 3 milligrams twice a day (stop in one month if not helping).

___ 104. Warfarin (Coumadin), another blood thinner. Take 2 to 3 milligrams each morning. Reacts with *many* medications. Be sure to check with your doctor before adding or deleting any medicines (even aspirin) while on Coumadin. Check PT/INR blood tests as noted in item 148, below. Begin three days before stopping heparin.

___ 105. Methylsulfonylmethane (MSM), a form of sulfur. Take six 500-milligram tablets twice a day for two to three months, then as needed for allergies, wound healing, and arthritis. Take 500 milligrams of vitamin C with each dose to improve absorption. This is okay to take even if you are sulfa-allergic.

___ 106A. Guaifenesin (Humibid). Take ½ to 2 600-milligram tablets one to two times a day. No aspirin or herbals can be taken while on guaifenesin.

___ 106B. For pesticide detoxification (usually takes three to ten months to start working and symptoms may initially flare). Add 50 grams of choline and 25 grams of vitamin C to 500 cc (about 1 pint) of flavored water. Take 10 cc (2 teaspoons) three times a day for one month, then 5 cc (1 teaspoon) two times a day. Choline can cause a fishy smell at a higher dose. If this is a problem, lower the dose.

___ 107. L-Serine. Take two to six 250-milligram capsules a day.

___ 108A. Iberogast, a digestive system herbal. Take 20 drops three times a day in warm water with meals. Very helpful for indigestion (takes four to eight weeks to work).

___ 108B. Interferon. Take 50 units under your tongue each morning.

___ 109. St. John's wort (Hypericum). Take 300 to 625 milligrams three times a day. It takes six weeks to see the antidepressant effect. Use one standardized to at least 0.3 percent hypericum. Can take two-thirds of the total daily dose at night to help sleep. You can take up to 2,000 milligrams a day if you are not on other antidepressants. Otherwise, limit it to 1,000 milligrams a day.

___ 110. Bromocriptine (Parlodel). Take one-half of a 2½-milligram tablet at night for one week, then one tablet at night.

___ 111A. Peppermint oil. Use enteric/stomach coated 0.2 cc capsules. Take one to two capsules three times a day between meals (*not* with food) for spastic colon.

___ 111B. Simethicone (Mylicon). *Chew* one 40- to 80-milligram tablet three times a day as needed for abdominal gas pains.

___ 111C. Turkey rhubarb. For constipation, take two at bedtime. If this does not solve the constipation then also take two in the morning (not with food).

Pain Treatments

Antidepressants (see items 93 through 99, above) or lithium (see item 51, above) often help FMS pain.

___ 112A. *Rhus toxicodendron* (Rhus tox), a homeopathic treatment. Dissolve under the tongue as directed on the bottle as needed for muscle pain.

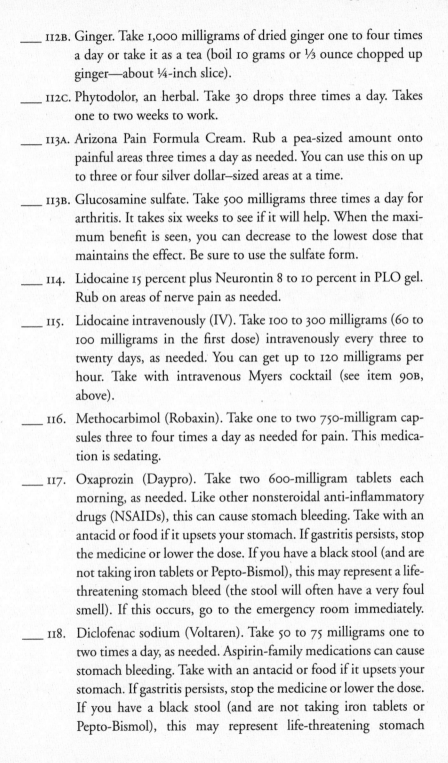

___ 112B. Ginger. Take 1,000 milligrams of dried ginger one to four times a day or take it as a tea (boil 10 grams or ⅓ ounce chopped up ginger—about ¼-inch slice).

___ 112C. Phytodolor, an herbal. Take 30 drops three times a day. Takes one to two weeks to work.

___ 113A. Arizona Pain Formula Cream. Rub a pea-sized amount onto painful areas three times a day as needed. You can use this on up to three or four silver dollar–sized areas at a time.

___ 113B. Glucosamine sulfate. Take 500 milligrams three times a day for arthritis. It takes six weeks to see if it will help. When the maximum benefit is seen, you can decrease to the lowest dose that maintains the effect. Be sure to use the sulfate form.

___ 114. Lidocaine 15 percent plus Neurontin 8 to 10 percent in PLO gel. Rub on areas of nerve pain as needed.

___ 115. Lidocaine intravenously (IV). Take 100 to 300 milligrams (60 to 100 milligrams in the first dose) intravenously every three to twenty days, as needed. You can get up to 120 milligrams per hour. Take with intravenous Myers cocktail (see item 90B, above).

___ 116. Methocarbimol (Robaxin). Take one to two 750-milligram capsules three to four times a day as needed for pain. This medication is sedating.

___ 117. Oxaprozin (Daypro). Take two 600-milligram tablets each morning, as needed. Like other nonsteroidal anti-inflammatory drugs (NSAIDs), this can cause stomach bleeding. Take with an antacid or food if it upsets your stomach. If gastritis persists, stop the medicine or lower the dose. If you have a black stool (and are not taking iron tablets or Pepto-Bismol), this may represent a life-threatening stomach bleed (the stool will often have a very foul smell). If this occurs, go to the emergency room immediately.

___ 118. Diclofenac sodium (Voltaren). Take 50 to 75 milligrams one to two times a day, as needed. Aspirin-family medications can cause stomach bleeding. Take with an antacid or food if it upsets your stomach. If gastritis persists, stop the medicine or lower the dose. If you have a black stool (and are not taking iron tablets or Pepto-Bismol), this may represent life-threatening stomach bleeding (the stool will often have a very foul smell). If this occurs, go to the emergency room immediately.

____ 119A. Tizanidine (Zanaflex). Take one to three 4-milligram tablets three times a day, with food, as needed for spasm and/or pain (sedating). Begin with 4 milligrams at night. If side effects occur raise dose more slowly. You can raise the dose by 2 milligrams every two to three days, to a maximum of 36 milligrams a day. May (rarely) cause hallucinations, delusions or liver inflammation and may lower blood pressure.

____ 119B. Clonidine patch (Catapres TTS 1). Wear one to three patches at a time and change them weekly. This is related to Zanaflex but cheaper and lowers blood pressure more.

____ 120. Dextromethorphan (DM). Take 50 milligrams four times a day with each dose of narcotic (for example, codeine or vicodin). This makes the narcotic more effective.

____ 121A. Copper/magnet bracelet.

____ 121B. Cetyl myristoleate. Take three 385-milligram capsules twice a day for ten days. You can raise the dose to a maximum of 17 grams a day. For arthritis and FMS pain—benefits often persist after the ten days of treatment.

____ 122A. Tramadol (Ultram). Take one to two 50-milligram tablets up to four times a day as needed for pain. *Caution:* This drug may rarely cause seizures or raise serotonin too high when combined with antidepressants. May cause nausea and vomiting.

____ 122B. Dantrolene (Dantrium). For muscle spasm, take one 25-milligram tablet a day for one week. Then take one tablet three times a day for one week, then two tablets three times a day for one week, then 100 milligrams three a day. Adjust to the lowest dose that feels the best. Stop or lower dose if severe diarrhea occurs. Check liver blood tests (see item 143, below) at six, twelve, and twenty-four weeks, and then each one to six months, to make sure there is no liver inflammation.

____ 123. Metaxalone (Skelaxin). Take one to two 400-milligram tablets four times a day as needed for pain. This is usually nonsedating.

____ 124. Orphenadrine (Norflex). Take one tablet twice a day.

____ 125A. Celecoxib (Celebrex). Take 100 to 200 milligrams one to two times a day for pain. Do not take if you're allergic to sulfa or aspirin (for example, hives). Do not use over 200 milligrams a day while on Sporanox or Diflucan.

____ 125B. Refecoxib (Vioxx). Take one-half to one 25-milligram tablet daily. Do not use if you are aspirin allergic (for example, hives).

____ 126. Gabapentin (Neurontin) Take 100 to 1,200 milligrams one to five times a day (to a maximum of 3,600 milligrams a day). Cut back if it causes any uncomfortable or unusual neurologic symptoms or excessive sedation. Begin with 300 milligrams at night, slowly increase to 300 milligrams three times a day as is comfortable.

____ 127. Baclofen (Lioresal). Take 10 to 20 milligrams one to three times a day. This medication is sedating.

____ 128A. Magnets. Start with spot magnets, insoles and seat. If they help in two months, consider a mattress pad.

____ 128B. Cod liver oil. Take ½ tablespoon (5,000 milligrams) a day. Do not use it if you are about to get pregnant—it has too much vitamin A.

Goldstein Protocol Treatments

____ 129. Nimodipine (Nimotop). Take 30 milligrams one to four times a day as is beneficial for symptoms.

____ 130. Nitroglycerin. Dissolve one-quarter to one tablet under the tongue as needed for muscle pain. May cause marked headache and/or dizziness the first three days it is used.

____ 131. Naphzoline 0.1-percent eye drops. Place 1 drop in each eye three to four times a day as needed for symptoms.

____ 132. TRH eyedrops (500 units in 9cc artificial tears). Place 1 drop in each eye three to four times a day as is helpful.

____ 133. Talcopone (Tasmar). Take 100 milligrams twice a day. Use this if it helps mental clarity and energy.

Follow Up Testing

____ 134. Stool for ova and parasites (O&P) at a laboratory specializing in parasite testing.

____ 135. Stool culture and sensitivity. Must be sent to Parasitology Center or Great Smokies Diagnostic Laboratories (see Appendix J: Resources).

____ 136. Sleep apnea study. Get insurance preauthorization—this can cost two thousand dollars.

____ 137. IGE food allergy blood test. *Ignore* the IgG Section—it is meaningless and will only make you nuts—look *only* at the IgE section.

____ 138. Dehydroepiandrosterone sulfate (DHEA-sulfate)—*not* DHEA—level.

____ 139. Free T_4 and total T_3 levels.

____ 140. Potassium level.

____ 141. Lithium level.

____ 141. Free testosterone level.

____ 142. Prolactin level.

____ 143. ALT, AST (liver tests). If taking Sporanox or Diflucan for more than three months, check every six to twelve weeks.

____ 144. HHV-6 (viral culture).

____ 145a. ISAC coagulation blood profile. Must send to Hemex Labs (see Appendix J: Resources).

____ 145b. Hereditary thrombotic panel. Send to Hemex Labs.

____ 146. Blood test for mycoplasma and chlamydia (general screens). Must be sent to The Institute For Molecular Medicine (see Appendix J: Resources).

____ 147. Platelet count and PTT blood test—each three days for nine days and then each one to two weeks while on heparin.

____ 148. PT/INR blood test—each two days for the first eight days on Coumadin, then every two weeks for six weeks, then each six to eight weeks while on Coumadin. Check two days after making *any* change to your medication and/or supplement regimen and consult your physician before making these changes. Keep the INR at the lowest level that leaves the patient feeling well, but not over 3.

____ 149. Dexa scan for osteoporosis.

____ 150. MRI of head and neck.

Stone Agers in the Fast Lane: An Evolutionary Approach to Fibromyalgia

by Jeffrey Maitland, Ph.D.

Why Did This Happen to Me?

As Nietzsche so astutely observed, when it comes to our own suffering, any explanation is better than none. If our suffering is the result of something simple like a cold we willingly accept the explanation that a virus is the cause. A cold or flu normally does not propel us into questions about the meaning of life because we know that we will be feeling better in a few days. But when our suffering continues unabated over longer and longer periods of time, we are less and less satisfied with the explanations that appeal to immediate causes, even when they are accurate. Ultimately we want to know why we suffer. As legend has it, when the Buddha allowed himself to be struck with the full significance of suffering, he set out on a course of spiritual illumination that ultimately changed the world. Every kind of suffering we might imagine, no matter how we try to explain it, is always a bodily event. The story of Christ's suffering on the cross and his resurrection is profound testimony to the universal struggle we all face as embodied beings.

It is easy to be content with explanations of intense suffering that appeal to immediate causes as long as the suffering is not ours. Anyone who has suffered the devastating effects of fibromyalgia knows the truth of this statement. As the reality of fibromyalgia begins to dawn on the sufferer, it is the rare person who is not tempted to wonder, "Why did this have to happen to me?" Haven't we all had moments in our life when we have asked similar questions? Even the hard-nosed scientist will be tempted to ask, "Why?" when his research grants are cut just as his wife dies of cancer and his house burns to the ground after being struck by lightning. After such a tragic series of events, it would be hard to imagine how he could be satisfied with a mere description of how cancer causes death or a detailed analysis of combustion.

Science, of course, is not meant to answer the ultimate questions about the meaning of life; and we should not blame it for not giving us such answers. But in between the kind of explanation that appeals to immediate or proximate causes and the kind that attempts to understand the meaning of life, there is another kind of scientific explanation that not only can give us a more satisfying answer to our "Why?" questions, but can also suggest new treatment strategies. This newly emerging science is the field of Darwinian Medicine. It promises an understanding of suffering and disease that goes beyond, but does not reject, the traditional medical answers that appeal to immediate causes. Unlike the physicists of his day, Darwin did not reject "Why?" questions. Rather he gave us a new and scientifically respectable way to ask and answer questions about purpose in biology and medicine.

In this article, I offer an evolutionary explanation of fibromyalgia as a means of adding to our understanding of this devastating condition. As with all evolutionary explanations of disease and suffering, the theory of fibromyalgia that I propose here is not intended as an alternate explanation to the proximate medical explanations that already exist. Evolutionary and proximate explanations of disease and suffering work together in expanding our understanding and treatment strategies. At this point in our understanding of fibromyalgia, an evolutionary explanation promises a broader understanding of the nature of this disorder. By understanding fibromyalgia in its broader evolutionary context, we may be better able to understand the peculiar nature of this disorder, predict who is likely to succumb to it, and hopefully devise even better treatment strategies. It will also help us to understand why the most important and yet most difficult treatment strategy for fibromyalgia sufferers to embrace is the need to change their way of living. In terms of the impact of such a theory on the sufferers themselves, perhaps they will see in it a more satisfying answer to their question, "Why did this happen to me?"

One of the more striking conclusions of this evolutionary approach is that fibromyalgia is, in part, a result of a useful adaptation to an environment that no longer exists. Fibromyalgia, then, should not be considered so much a disease in the usual sense, but rather as a fear disorder that is too sensitive for the chaos of the modern world. Like all evolutionary explanations, if this theory of fibromyalgia is properly constructed it should be capable of being tested and have certain predictive value. And if it, or some variation of it, is correct, it will not only support many of the observations and recommendations for treatment that have already arisen from the proximate theories, but it will also suggest new diagnostic and treatment strategies.

Once we understand that many of our evolved adaptations are better suited to a time when our ancestors were stone age hunters and gatherers (probably the Pleistocene savannah from 10,000 to 1,700,000 years ago), we will better appreciate the importance of critically examining how we are living our lives, especially in America, where fibromyalgia exists in alarming proportions—presently 12 to 15 million people in the United States are estimated to have fibromyalgia. People presently suffering from fibromyalgia are demonstrating to the rest of us certain warning signs that we would do well to heed. At this point in time they are more like the canaries that were taken into the mines as early detectors of poisonous gas than people who have fallen prey to some new disease. Their plight and ever increasing numbers, especially in America, are early warning signs that there is something terribly wrong in the way we are living our lives.

More so than with so many other causes of suffering, fibromyalgia is a condition that demands we change our lives. In many ways, it is one more among many signs of our spiritual crisis: a profound demonstration of our loss of connection to ourselves and our world. Even though a broader evolutionary approach can give us a deeper and more satisfying understanding of fibromyalgia, ultimately its significance lies in the spiritual crisis of our times.

We no longer need a prophet to tell us that we are out of touch with the wellsprings of life and living too fast. Not only have we lost touch with the rhythms of our bodies, but our fast-paced modern urban environments are chronically at odds with our biological inheritance. Under such conditions we must finally come to understand that no inoculation, drug, herb, diet, or manual therapy by itself or in combination can solve the problems that result from a world gone awry—unless, of course, we heed the all too obvious signs and change our ways.

Evolutionary Explanations

An evolutionary explanation of a disease or suffering of any kind is not, as I stated above, an alternative to or in competition with a proximate explanation. Both are necessary for understanding and treatment. "Proximate explanations answer 'What?' and 'How?' questions about structure and mechanism: evolutionary explanations answer 'Why?' questions about origins and functions . . . an evolutionary approach to disease studies not the evolution of the disease but the design characteristics that make us susceptible to the disease. . . . Evolutionary explanations thus predict what to expect in proximate mechanisms."[1]

An evolutionary or functional explanation can take one or a combination of four different forms. They are: (1) explanations that demonstrate how what appear to be disorders or diseases are actually defenses that have evolved to protect the organism, (2) explanations that demonstrate how an adaptation is the result of a genetic quirk, (3) explanations that show how certain genetic adaptations impose costs that are worth their benefit to the organism, and (4) explanations that point to true, but rare genetic defects.

As an example of the first kind of explanation, let us consider Margie Profet's functional understanding of morning sickness. A proximate explanation of morning sickness would tell us about the immediate causes and workings of nausea and vomiting, but it gives us little understanding as to why it happens. Profet argues that the nausea, vomiting, and food aversions that accompany early pregnancy evolved as a way to protect the developing fetus from toxins ingested by the mother. If her hypothesis is correct, one would expect morning sickness to begin when fetal-tissue differentiation begins and decrease as the fetus becomes less vulnerable. This prediction as it turns out is true, and Profet's theory is supported by substantial evidence.[2]

This evolutionary account of morning sickness has obvious and important consequences for the treatment and care of pregnant women. Once we realize that morning sickness is an adaptation that evolved as a way to protect the developing fetus, we immediately see that understanding it as a disease or abnormality could be a grave mistake. Any attempt, for example, to block the symptoms of morning sickness by drugs or other means could have dire consequences for the unborn child.

Some adaptations work quite well for the stone age environment in which they evolved and cause great difficulties for us in our present environment. These disorders are what Williams and Nesse call a "genetic quirk." Our modern couch potato is a good example. In the correct amounts, fat and sugar are an important source of nutrients. In the hunter gatherer phase of our distant ancestors, fat and sugar were not easily procured. Our ancestors adapted to a fat and sugar scarce environment by evolving a great and unbridled desire for these nutrients. So whenever fat or sugar became available, they would eat as much of it as they could in order to store it for leaner times. They would "pig out" as we would say today and lie around minimizing activity as a way to perhaps conserve their stores. Over consumption of these nutrients was not a problem for our ancestors for a number of related reasons: fat and sugar were not readily and always available, it took a considerable expenditure of energy (what we in the modern world consciously try to accomplish by exercise) just to survive and find food, and our ancestors did not live much past forty years when the damage of overconsumption usually appears. Since we have not yet evolved a "governor" for these unbridled tastes, in our present environment where we can find as much fat and sugar as we want, it is hardly surprising that we have developed a culture of couch potatoes.

Contrary to the wisdom of the day, we do not have to feel guilty for these desires. An evolutionary explanation shows that it is probably a mistake to think that some of us have addictive personalities and others don't just on the basis of our overwhelming desire to consume large quantities of fat and sugar. Certainly, such desires could very well become part of a psychologically driven eating disorder. The fact that psychologically driven eating disorders are rooted in adaptive biostrategies helps explain why these disorders are so difficult to treat. Ultimately however, the patient and therapist must come to terms with the fact that these desires will never go away and realize that a cure of an eating disorder cannot be predicated on the assumption that the desires must one day disappear. So it is not always necessary to go casting about for some childhood trauma or unconscious loss of mother love to explain why many of us eat too much fat and sugar. For many of us these desires are not due to an addictive personality rooted in childhood trauma. Clearly they are also not due to a genetic defect. Rather, they are due to a genetic "quirk": an adaptation that was selected for and worked well in the stone age environment, but doesn't work well in our modern enviroment.

Certain genetic adaptations can be understood by means of a cost/ benefit analysis. Their disadvantages to us are outweighed by their advantages. Sickle-cell anemia is a good example of a disease that has a genetic cause but which also provides a great advantage by protecting its bearers from malaria. As one would expect, since African Americans live in an environment in which malaria is rare, natural selection has been decreasing the frequency of the sickle-cell gene just as evolutionary theory predicts.

"Finally, there are 'outlaw' genes that facilitate their own transmission at the expense of the individual and thus bluntly demonstrate that selection acts ultimately to benefit genes, not individuals of species."[3] Genetic defects that cause disease and suffering are rare, however, because they are maladaptive. They are constantly being eliminated by environmental pressures and natural selection.

Before we look at the proximate and evolutionary theories of fibromyalgia, it is important to clear up a possible misunderstanding surrounding teleological explanations. Earlier I pointed out that evolutionary explanations provide respectable scientific answers to "Why?" questions. It is important to understand what this claim means. It does not mean that evolutionary theory rests on the view that natural selection involves any sort of consciousness that foresees or predicts a future that it then plans for in its design of organisms. Natural selection is not a form of planning or goal directedness. Rather natural selection operates blindly by means of a slow accretion of minute changes that make an organism a more fit reproducer for an environment or changing environments. Darwinian evolution should not be understood according to Spencer's misleading slogan "survival of the fittest" but more properly as the perpetuation of the best replicators. "Functional explanations in biology imply not future influences on the present but a prolonged cycling of reproduction and selection. A bird embryo develops wing rudiments in the egg because earlier individuals that failed to do so left no descendants. Adult birds lay eggs in which embryos develop wing rudiments for the same reason. In this sense, a bird's wing rudiments are preparation for its future but are caused by its past history."[4]

A Proximate Explanation of Fibromyalgia

One of the best and most easily accessible books on fibromyalgia and chronic fatigue was written by Dr. Jacob Teitelbaum, a physician who also suffered the devastating effects of chronic fatigue.[5] It is also an excellent example of a proximate explanation of fibromyalgia and a manual for its treatment. Since my purpose is to give an example of a proximate explanation in preparation for an evolution explanation, what follows is a rather brief over-simplification of Dr. Teitelbaum's theory.

Dr. Teitelbaum suggests that we view fibromyalgia as one among a number of related patterns of severe chronic fatigue states. Three patterns among many patterns of severe chronic fatigue that Dr. Teitelbaum elucidates are drop-dead flu, fibromyalgia, and the autoimmune triad. In the drop-dead flu pattern, the patient comes down with a "brutal flulike illness" that never goes away. A virus is suspected, of course, but even long after one would expect the virus to have been vanquished, symptoms persist. The functioning of the hypothalamus is suppressed by the disease. Since the hypothalamus coordinates and directs how the other glands function and work together, its dysfunction adversely affects other important glands like the adrenal and thyroid gland that also control our energy levels. The resulting hormonal dysfunctions also disrupt the immune system leaving the patient susceptible to chronic infections.

For most people, fibromyalgia and chronic fatigue are the same disorder. Fibromyalgia is accompanied by a sleep disorder and shortened achy muscles that have many trigger or tender points. Dr. Teitelbaum says that fibromyalgia patients rarely get a good night's sleep because they are unable to fall into a deep restorative slumber. Sleeping on achy muscles, he says, is like trying to spend the night sleeping on marbles. As in the case of the drop-dead flu, the hypothalamus, thyroid, adrenals, and the immune system are all adversely affected which in turn help perpetuate the disorder.

In the autoimmune triad the immune system attacks parts of the body as if they were invading organisms. This autoimmune reaction also creates fatigue by suppressing the hypothalamus, thyroid, adrenals, and the cells that aid in the absorption of B_{12}.

Fibromyalgia and chronic fatigue are peculiar in that any one of the problems mentioned in the three patterns or any other pattern can trigger the other problems thereby resulting in and perpetuating chronic fatigue.

Dr. Teitelbaum lists the following most common complaints of chronic fatigue and fibromyalgia: overwhelming fatigue and poor sleep, frequent infections, brain fog, achiness, increased thirst, allergies, anxiety, and depression. He also recognizes that most chronic fatigue patients are type-A personalities and that their perfectionism, their need to control, and their drivenness to succeed are ultimately rooted in the development of low self-esteem in childhood coupled with the feeling of not being able to defend their emotional boundaries. Given the peculiar nature of severe chronic fatigue, that problems in any pattern can trigger and perpetuate the disorder, Dr. Teitelbaum recommends a holistic approach that treats all the problems at once. He recommends a treatment program that includes various drugs, hormonal supplements, herbs, vitamins and mineral supplements, Rolfing, Trager, chiropractic, physical therapy, properly modulated exercise, and psychotherapy. If only one or two problems are treated, the existence of the other untreated problems will simply cause the chronic fatigue to reassert itself.

Dr. Teitelbaum mentions that there has never been a stable society in the history of human culture that has experienced the rapidity of change that we have. He fully recognizes that our fast-paced way of life is an aberration. And even though some people seem to thrive on it, more and more people are burning out from this chaotic way of living. He says, "I suspect that the physical processes that make up CFS [chronic fatigue syndrome] and fibromyalgia are manifestations of this [abnormal lifestyle]—and that we are just beginning to see the tip of the iceberg."[6] I couldn't agree more with Dr. Teitelbaum's assessment, and although he does not offer an evolutionary theory for fibromyalgia, his suspicions definitely point us in that direction.

The evolutionary approach will broaden and confirm why Dr. Teitelbaum's suspicions are correct. It will give us a way to articulate what fibromyalgia is, why it manifests as the complex of symptoms uncovered by the proximate explanation, and why certain people succumb to it. An evolutionary explanation will also allow us to understand why fibromyalgia is not a disease in the ordinary sense, but a fear disorder that involves the whole person and his world.

An Evolutionary Explanation of Fibromyalgia

One rather straightforward way to understand the nature of a genetic adaptation is to remove it or interfere with its effects and observe how the organism malfunctions. Take something simple like the experience of pain. We might be tempted to believe that a life free of all pain would be a great blessing, but clearly it is not. Those rare people who are born without the ability to feel pain usually die by the age of thirty. Since their bodies do not register pain, they often unknowingly damage parts of themselves. Since they never feel uncomfortable, they often sit too long in one position, develop pressure sores, and eventually ruin their joints. Pain is obviously an important adaptation that serves to protect the organism and without it our life would become a precarious affair.

The same considerations apply to the nature of fatigue. What would a life look like without the ability to feel fatigue? The answer is quite simple: remove our ability to feel fatigue and we would eventually destroy ourselves. But if fatigue functions this way, how is it that chronic fatigue sufferers have managed to override this adaptation and so thoroughly and profoundly burn themselves out? Part of the answer to this puzzling question lies in understanding the nature of emotion, and especially the nature of fear.

In order to understand the adaptive function of emotion, let us consider what life would be like without emotion or when emotions have been blocked or suppressed. We only have to look to the field of psychology to find ample information about the effects of suppressing or interfering with the natural expression of emotion. Studies of child rearing practices in Northern Germany, for example, revealed the existence of many strict, cold, and unfeeling mothers who were unable to properly contact their infants. The child raised by a contact-avoidant mother is also contact-avoidant and "is not only to a degree 'depressed' but also angry and likely to express this socially in later life. The angry avoidant individual may be brilliantly successful as the world knows but potentially dangerous to himself and others. A society dominated by such individuals, as Reich in various ways has already suggested, can be a danger to the world."[7]

Or consider what happens when people are subjected to abuse of any kind. To those who know nothing about the psychology of abuse, the existence of battered women unable to leave their abusive partners seems impossible to understand. Although the response to abuse is much less complicated in animals, we see some of the same pattern at work in humans. When animals are subjected to aversive stimulation that they can neither control nor escape they too become "helpless victims." After being subjected to the abusive experiments, and then placed in experimental situations where they could easily learn to escape by jumping a barrier, these animals failed to extricate themselves from their situation. They had lost their ability to protect themselves. Other animals that had not been subjected to the aversive conditions first, managed to escape quite easily.[8]

Unlike the more complicated human emotions like embarrassment or the more tonic emotions like joy, fear evolved as part of an alarm system designed to protect us from danger. This conclusion was dramatically demonstrated in an experiment with guppies. On the basis of how they responded to one of their predators, a small mouth bass, the guppies were divided into three groups: timid, ordinary, and bold. Each group was then put into a tank with a bass. After sixty hours, forty percent of the timid guppies and fifteen percent of the ordinary guppies had survived. None of the bold guppies made it.[9]

We no longer live in the kind of environment in which the adaptation of fear originally developed, but obviously a life without the ability to feel fear, like a life without the ability to feel pain, would probably be very short indeed. Fear is clearly a very important and useful adaptation. In the stone age environment those humans who were born with little or no fear probably did not survive. As a result their genes did not become part of the gene pool. Those who did survive developed a highly sensitive and responsive alarm system, so sensitive in fact that our ancestors often found themselves responding to many false alarms. But this is just what one would expect. This sort of adaptation is based on what Nesse and Williams call the smoke-detector principle: it is better to have a very sensitive smoke-detector that gives many false alarms than a house burned to the ground. With respect to fear, "The cost of getting killed even once is enormously higher than the cost of responding to a hundred false alarms."[10]

As phenomenologists have pointed out, human emotions are disclosive forms of intentionality.[11] They cannot be reduced to mere neurophysiological processes or to the release of chemicals like adrenaline or noradrenaline, because they are also forms of understanding. Emotions not only warn us when we are about to make wrong choices, they also can propel us toward exciting new opportunities. Emotions inform us about the nature of our world and guide us in knowing what we truly want. Before we find the right words to explain our actions, we often know that a course of action is wrong simply because it feels wrong. The great intellectual virtuosity that we modern people display is a quite recent development in our evolutionary history and we often forget that our ancestors relied primarily on feeling to understand and manage their world. The suppression of feeling and bodily sensation is an aberration of the modern world, not an evolutionary advance. A healthy, modern person would be one in whom the cognitive and feeling functions are integrated. The intellect of a healthy person does not attempt to understand the world at the expense of feelings and bodily sensations that have been suppressed. Nor is a healthy person an anti-intellectual or one who allows his conflicted emotional states to override appropriate cognitive functioning.

Without our emotions, we lose our sense of connectedness and our bearings. A situation that brings us great sadness also teaches us to avoid similar choices in the future. A low mood may prevent us from acting "precipitously to escape temporary difficulties, but as difficulties continue to grow and our life's energies are progressively wasted, this emotion helps to disengage us from a hopeless enterprise so that we can consider alternatives. Therapists have long known that many depressions go away only after a person finally gives up some long-sought goal and turns his or her energies in another direction."[12] Without the ability to mobilize our anger when attacked we would be unable to defend ourselves. Free flowing feeling and sensation connect us with nature and with others. Warm openhearted humans are not driven by perverse, unconscious desires to destroy their environment, abuse their children, or dominate others.

When we integrate the evolutionary perspective with the phenomenological and psychological, we see that our emotions evolved as a way to understand our world, and, in the case of fear and anger, as a forms of protection. Healthy emotion and feeling help to guide and direct our lives. In certain respects they are like the adaptations of pain and fatigue. When they are blocked or suppressed they can cause us and others great harm. But when they function properly, they are an integral part of how we come to understand, care about, manage, and find our place in the universe and our world.

By consolidating the above insights, we can understand the seemingly incomprehensible way that people with fibromyalgia override their bodies' defense against overexertion and end up exhausted. Fibromyalgia is not a disease in the usual sense, it is a fear disorder based on a genetic quirk. It is a maladaptive fear response that results when unrelenting stress and trauma, destructive parenting, and/or childhood trauma are coupled together in a highly sensitive individual who pursues the futile attempt to live in a chaotic world at odds with his or her bodily and psychic resources. Since fibromyalgia begins as a maladaptive fear response, it begins as a central nervous system disorder that then spreads to the entire body, but especially to the endocrine and immune systems.[13]

Ever since Hans Selye published his ground-breaking research on stress, there is hardly anyone who does not know how damaging stressors can be to our bodies and our immune systems. Recent evidence suggests, for example, that secretion of the stress hormone cortisol may actually be part of the way the body protects itself from the damage from other aspects of the stress response. A life free of stressors is impossible and probably not even desirable. In truth, only when stress becomes distress do problems result. Even though many fear responses are false alarms, in manageable numbers with enough time in between, such responses are still adaptive and not damaging to our bodies in the long run.

But consider what happens to people whose alarm systems are always being triggered. Their body would never have enough time to recuperate from the stress response. They would become hypervigilant and unable to experience the restorative nature of deep sleep or parasympathetic relaxation. They would always be getting ready to either defend themselves or flee, and their autonomic nervous system would be locked into a high state of sympathetic arousal. Their ability to experience deep restorative sleep would deteriorate further and over time they would become achy and exhausted. (Research demonstrates that when normal people are deprived of deep restorative sleep, they develop the symptoms of fibromyalgia within two weeks, including achy shortened muscles.) They would become cold and experience more thirst, and they would become susceptible to infections because their hypothalamus, thyroid, adrenals, and immune system would cease to function properly. This description is clearly the picture of fibromyalgia, but the question still remains, "How did these people get locked into this fear state, a state in which their alarms are constantly being triggered by their world?"

All animals and humans have an instinctive desire to discharge sympathetic arousal. If an animal or human is successful in dealing with a dangerous situation by fighting or fleeing, sympathetic arousal will be successfully discharged. The nervous system will shift from its state of high sympathetic arousal to the relaxed parasympathetic response. But if an animal is unable to successfully deal with an attack, it will "play possum." It will go into a high state of sympathetic arousal, a freezing immobilization response that mimics death. This immobilization response serves at least two functions: it anesthetizes the animal from pain, and it may deceive the predator long enough so that the animal can escape when the predator is not looking. If the trauma is unrelenting as in the study cited above where animals were put into abusive experimental conditions, the animal can remain stuck in fearful and helpless immobility unable any longer to defend itself.

In the face of threats or injuries that we can neither control nor escape, we humans also have the ability to immobilize ourselves. We do it by simultaneously freezing (becoming rigid) and falling into a disassociated state of collapse. Indeed, most traumatized people who have not received appropriate therapy show varying degrees of both the rigid freezing response and the collapsed dissociated response. Unrelenting or unresolved trauma leaves us fearful and helplessly immobilized in a state of high sympathetic arousal that we are unable to discharge. Not recognizing how their high sympathetic arousal and immobility are rooted in fear, many severely traumatized individuals become thrill seekers in an attempt to discharge their highly agitated state. Unfortunately, this unconscious strategy provides only a momentary illusion of discharge. In reality, it actually creates even more highly charged states of sympathetic arousal and immobility. Many also experience a kind of helpless immobility that leaves them unable to summon the volition and energy to defend themselves or leave their abusive situations. They become "victims." Since neither way of being allows for discharge, these people can never fully relax. Under such conditions exhaustion is the expected sequella.[14]

Fibromyalgia can be divided into two broad and sometimes overlapping types, posttraumatic and primary. Posttraumatic fibromyalgia seems to result from a series of traumatic events such as multiple car accidents or surgeries. Even though posttraumatic patients may not always exhibit the same psychological and emotional precursors that patients with primary fibromyalgia do, both types are clear examples of a chronic fear condition. For both types the world has become a fearful place.

As Dr. Teitelbaum points out, most primary fibromyalgia patients have low self-esteem; they are perfectionists who are driven to control their world and succeed in it. As he said in a lecture once, most of these patients, even if they were to receive four Nobel prizes, would still think they hadn't done enough. Due to their low self-esteem many have a fear of being seen as weak. As an unconscious strategy to get the approval they never received as children, they become driven overachievers and perfectionists. As a result, they burn out in the futile attempt to feel good about themselves by seeking external approval. Their low self-esteem is sometimes the result of having been abused or made to feel inadequate by destructive parents or significant care givers. As adults, many find themselves caught in seemly impossible no-way-out situations where their every action seems to make all the difference between imminent disaster and a momentary reprieve. Everything seems to depend on them and they seem incapable of ever extricating themselves from a life full of imminent disaster, stress, or danger. As a result they constantly sacrifice themselves and rarely do what makes them happy.

Like the abused experimental animals and many battered women, people with fibromyalgia have lost the ability to protect themselves and do what is best for their own well-being and happiness. Many unconsciously believe that they were the reason for the abuse that they suffered as children. As adults they often think that they are the cause of other people's outbursts. Like the abused experimental animals, they cannot jump the barrier and escape damaging and exhausting ways of living. Like most people with fear disorders, they suppress and deny their fear and, as a result, block their ability to trust. Unable to trust they often find themselves unable to open to the love we all want and expect. In place of defending themselves, many talk excessively about their situation, often complaining bitterly about how they have been mistreated and misunderstood. In the end, they are only looking for someone to give them the love, support, and sense of safety they never had. For only in a safe therapeutic environment is it possible for traumatized individuals to appropriately discharge their highly tuned states of sympathetic arousal.

Another very interesting characteristic of people with fibromyalgia is that they tend to be very sensitive people, hypervigilant and alert to what others are feeling around them, and often much better informed about their condition than most doctors. Some are even psychic. Their sensitivity may be the defensive result of the unresolved trauma suffered in childhood or the result of evolution—or both. It may be that our genetic susceptibility to fear can be placed on a continuum, and that fibromyalgia patients tend to be more sensitive than others. This kind of sensitivity was a great advantage in a stone age environment, and these kind of people were probably highly prized by their communities. But when this sensitivity is combined with destructive parenting, excessive unresolved trauma, and/or unrelenting stress, it produces fearful people. In the case of primary fibromyalgia, it produces driven people with perfectionist tendencies who have a need to prove themselves. When people with this kind of fear disorder, whether primary or posttraumatic, choose or are forced to compete in our chaotic modern environment with its high levels of stress and neverending onslaught of real and imagined dangers, they cannot help but find themselves in a constant state of fear as their alarm systems are continually being triggered. For such people, it is no wonder they become more and more exhausted and fall into severe chronic fatigue. When people with primary fibromyalgia meet our modern environment with their perfectionism, the consequences are deadly and the logic clear: driven to succeed, perfectionists can never reach their impossible goals, and exhaustion is the byproduct of all their efforts.

The extreme sensitivity of people with fibromyalgia brings them into conflict with the important people in their lives who often imply that their symptoms are "all in their head." They are often made to feel guilty about their suffering by their doctors, therapists, and significant others. This reaction is especially prevalent among those whose own feelings are deeply repressed, because such people find the sensitivity and pain of the fibromyalgia patient a threat to their tidy, overly intellectualized, and repressed world. It is no wonder that fibromyalgia sufferers become angry and depressed. Depression and anger are not the causes of fibromyalgia or necessarily part of the array of symptoms, but the secondary results of it. Anger is a natural response to a physical and/or verbal attack and not being understood. Abused people are understandably angry, but when anger is repressed, as it often is in fibromyalgia, it also leads to exhaustion and depression.

In studies of vervet monkeys, researchers discovered that the high ranking alpha males had twice the amount of serotonin levels than other males. "When these 'alpha males' lost their position, their serotonin levels immediately fell and they huddled and rocked and refused food, looking for all the world like depressed humans."[15] When Prozac was administered to these deposed alpha males, these behaviors did not appear. Even more surprisingly, when the alpha male was removed from a group and Prozac was administered to any randomly chosen male, he became the new alpha male every time. Prozac can raise serotonin levels, but when given to a person suffering from the fear driven nature of fibromyalgia, such a prescription may only be a temporary solution that masks a complicated disorder. If the driven nature of the fear disorder is ignored, Prozac may give the patient an illusory boost, but one that could propel him to take up his stress filled lifestyle once again. The eventual result would be to drive the patient into further exhaustion.

Loss of position and loving what we cannot have also leads to depression. Every fibromyalgia sufferer is either in the process of losing their position in the fast-paced modern world or has already lost it. Especially in the early days of treating their problem, many sufferers still dream of returning to the chaotic pace and competition of the world even though they no longer have the energy to compete and be successful in it. Many still want to return to this kind of chaos even when they know that this is the kind of existence that brought them to their present state of overwhelming exhaustion. If they get a momentary boost of energy from their treatment program, they often immediately jump back in to their fast-paced approach to life and work all the harder trying to make up for lost time. As a result, they create a terrible flare-up and are exhausted and nonfunctional for days. The hardest lesson the fibromyalgia patient has to learn, the most bitter pill they have to swallow, is that they cannot return to their old life. When they finally realize the truth of this life-giving recommendation and give up trying to achieve what they cannot have, their depression lifts and they can begin the process of overcoming their suffering.

Whether real or imagined, if our fear is constantly being triggered by the world in which we live, we will become frozen in the numbing immobility response that constitutes high sympathetic arousal. In such a state, if we persist in the futile effort of trying to keep up with a world that is at odds with our psychophysiological resources, the downward spiral of chronic fatigue is the likely outcome. When we are exhausted and no longer able to protect ourselves, the world becomes and is perceived as an even more dangerous place. A fear disorder begets more fear and, as a result, the sufferer's world becomes increasingly more alarming.

Under such conditions, it is easy to understand why people with chronic fatigue are subject to frequent infections. Since they are constantly responding to alarms that they can neither fight nor flee, their fear begets more fear; they are driven to higher and higher levels of sympathetic arousal that they are unable to discharge and, as a result, they become more and more exhausted. Their fear results in a state of constant neurological overdrive that eventually exhausts their entire organism, which then in turn depresses their immune system.

Through the pioneering research of Candice Pert, Ph.D., we now know that a group of molecules called peptides are both produced by and act as the communicating link between the nervous, endocrine, and immune systems. Every cell in the body has an abundance of specific receptor sites to which peptides can attach themselves. It is no longer possible to view the nervous, endocrine and immune systems as three separate systems serving different functions; rather they must be seen as one network in communication with the entire organism. "By interlinking immune cells, glands, and brain cells, peptides form a psychosomatic network extending throughout the entire organism. Peptides are the biochemical manifestation of emotions; they play a crucial role in the coordinating activities of the immune system; they interlink and integrate mental, emotional, and biological activities."[16] Peptides alter behavior and feeling states and some researchers suspect that each peptide may evoke unique emotional states. The entire intestine is filled with peptide receptors that allow us to experience our feelings at a "gut level." Recall the research summarized in footnote 13 that showed a connection between the central nervous system and increased sensitivity to visceral pain and it becomes very clear that a maladaptive fear response is a kind of neurological overdrive, which by virtue of the peptide communication system, must affect the entire organism. In the end, it cannot but exhaust and defeat the immune system's ability to ward off or resist disease.

By consolidating the broader evolutionary explanation within the phenomenological perspective, our examination of fibromyalgia as a maladaptive fear response reveals an even deeper, more far reaching understanding of immune system disorders than one might otherwise suspect. As I pointed out elsewhere,[17] a phenomenological approach to fear shows that it is an orientation toward the world in which the person does not want to be present. For most people, a loaded gun placed at their head accompanied by angry threats is enough to make them not want to be present. Fear mobilizes us for action. But as we have seen, if we are constantly subjected to the kind of pain, stress, or abuse that we can neither control nor escape, we will remain helplessly immobilized and unable to defend ourselves. In order not to be present to our suffering under such conditions, nature has given us a way to escape by providing us with a way to numb our experience. If we are unable to escape by running away or by fighting, we immobilize ourselves by going into high state of sympathetic arousal. If we remain stuck in this immobilization response, we, in effect, anesthetize the boundaries of self and body and cease being fully present in the present.

Living organisms are self-organizing. They persist because they are constantly in the process of forming boundaries in response to their ever-changing environments.[18] In a sense, an organism is like a water fountain whose constituent materials are being rapidly replaced while small but related variations of the form remain the same over time. But unlike a fountain where the form is maintained by outside forces, organisms have the inherent power to maintain and adapt their form to a changing environment. This is part of what it means to be alive. To be is to be a form. Every form has a boundary. Remove the boundaries of a form and it ceases to be. Since living forms are different from nonliving forms in that they are self-organizing, they must continually maintain and adjust their boundaries to ever-changing internal and external environments. Maintaining and evolving boundaries in the face of ever-changing environments is also part of what it means to be healthy and to have a self.

By numbing their boundaries through rigidity and collapse, people with fear disorders manage to escape their situation to some degree, but at a great cost. As we have already seen, they lose their ability to defend themselves. But the ability to defend oneself rests on the prior condition of having a clear sense of self and boundaries. In a very real sense, a fear disorder is a swoon into formlessness. People with fear disorders live a life in which their psychobiological form wants to become formless. Because identity and the on-going creation of boundaries go hand in hand, the swoon into formlessness is also a loss of the integrity of one's own identity. Without a clear sense of self-identity, defense of self is difficult.

With these considerations in mind let us turn our attention to the immune system. One obvious function of the immune system is to defend us against invading disease organisms. But more interesting than the question of the how the immune system accomplishes this amazing feat of defense is the logically prior question as to how the immune system distinguishes between self and not self in the first place. Defending oneself against an attacker and defending oneself from disease both require a sense of self identity. Although it may sound as though I am merely trading on metaphors to make this point about the self and the immune system, recent immunological theory and research is beginning to confirm Elie Metchnikoff's revolutionary and profoundly important insight that the immune system may be the biological ground of self-identity.

Metchnikoff (1845–1916), a Russian zoologist, was the first to recognize immunity as an active response of the host to infection. In marked contrast to genetic reductionism that claims that all biological properties of an organism, including morphology, are determined and can be explained by their genes, Metchnikoff pioneered a sophisticated holistic understanding of the whole organism that began with his investigations into the immune system. For Metchnikoff, "immunological processes are, above all, those activities that constitute organismic identity, and only as a consequence of secondary phenomena do they also *protect*. Correspondingly, these processes cannot be simply reduced to functions of recognition of other and/or protection of host. Rather, in Metchnikoff's more far-reaching view, self-identity arises from the dynamics of these immunological activities. The heuristic value of this information has yielded extraordinary insight."[19]

The inability of a person with a fear disorder to defend himself is the same as the immune system's inability to defend itself against infection. A person with a fear disorder has a problem in self-identity and hence, self-organization. Since the human organism is a unified being that includes an evolved consciousness, this problem of self-identity is not just a psychological problem: it exists all the way down from the psychological to the cellular level. The essential structure of biological organization is "shared at the cellular, individual, and ecological levels. . . . This reflects a highly dynamic, holistic vision of biology with the 'self' taking its rightful place as the unifying concept of actively developing, diverse selective systems."[20]

An organism that has lost some of its boundaries is an organism unable to protect itself at all levels. When human organisms cease to function without a clear sense of self and boundary, they can become "helpless victims" subject to infection and in danger of repeated insults from their world. They will also become subject to autoimmune diseases because they have trouble clearly distinguishing aspects of themselves from invading organisms. Likewise, they will become subject to self-destructive tendencies because they have trouble distinguishing themselves from their abusers. As I mentioned earlier, it is a well known fact that adults who were abused as children have the sense that they were somehow at fault and therefore brought the abuse upon themselves.

Our exploration of proximate and evolutionary explanations gives us the understanding that fibromyalgia is a fear disorder that begins in the nervous system and ultimately compromises the whole person. A phenomenological consolidation of these insights reveals that fibromyalgia cannot be fully understood unless we see it as an existential condition—a problem in the way in which the whole person lives his or her world. Since fibromyalgia is a disorder of the lived-reality of the whole person and his or her world, no one treatment, by itself, will turn the tide of chronic fatigue. A conventional corrective approach that only addresses the problem symptom by symptom cannot be successful. Fibromyalgia by its very nature requires a holistic approach.[21] Fortunately there is hope as Dr. Teitelbaum's research and holistic approach to treatment demonstrate. Gentle Rolfing, physical therapy, osteopathic manipulation, Trager, massage, hormone supplements, certain drugs, certain vitamins and minerals, diet, properly supervised exercise in the latter stages of treatment, herbs, acupuncture and the like are all helpful, but only when they are done together—and, most importantly, in the order that suits the unique requirements of each patient.

Since fibromyalgia is a fear response rooted in unresolved trauma and/or relentless stress that is constantly being triggered by the patient's world, it goes without saying that a form of psychotherapy that is capable of discharging chronic sympathetic arousal is an extremely important part of the treatment program. Since fibromyalgia is an existential condition that involves the whole person, its sufferers must first learn how to release themselves from the conflicts and fixations that stand in their way of protecting and caring for themselves. Then they must learn the more difficult task of how to live their lives differently in a chaotic world. By itself, psychotherapy is not enough, just as by itself, Rolfing or drug therapy is not enough. Unless all the therapies are employed in the correct sequence within a comprehensive holistic program, there is little hope for recovery. If the theory advanced in this article or some version of it is correct, then such a program of treatment must fully recognize that fibromyalgia is an existential condition, and address how this way of being is rooted in an immobilizing fear response that is constantly being triggered by the patient's world.

The Existential Crisis of Fibromyalgia

Our modern world is an aberration. It is filled with people who have lost touch with the wellsprings of life and being. Since we live in a world that has suppressed and does not value the kind of whole body feeling and sensation that connects us to our world and with one another, we live too fast and are in continual search of new thrills to stimulate our anesthetized bodies. Instead of using the wonderful discoveries of science and technology to care for our environment and others, we seek more ways to entertain ourselves while we destroy the very environment upon which our survival depends. We are the first species to systematically disassociate from our roots and soil our own nest.

The conceptual framework that supports the crisis of our modern world was first formulated 2,500 years ago by Plato and completed in the 1600s by Descartes. Plato asked the question, "What is being?" not by wondering how we experience it, but by asking the epistemological question, "How do we *know* being?" From the moment Plato asked the question this way he set the stage for how the Western world from then on would approach the nature of reality and self. Eventually this epistemological turn gave rise to science. Plato also argued that the mind is to the body as the pilot is to the ship. Everything that has to do with the ever changing earth plane, such as bodies, feelings, emotions, nature, and femininity are all imperfections to be eschewed for dwelling with the eternal masculine principles of mind and reason. Plato said that our true home is in a nonbodily, eternal, unchanging realm not of this earth.

Many centuries later Descartes attempted to lay the foundations of science by arguing that nature and living bodies are nothing but machines to be understood according to causal laws articulated in the language of mathematics. In Descartes' view, a human being is like a ghost that somehow mysteriously inhabits a body that is nothing more than a soft machine. By the nineteenth and twentieth centuries this mechanistic assumption had infected the way most people view their bodies and the nature of life in general. Like so many repressed people, both Plato and Descartes extol the virtues of reason and mind over the messiness of body and feeling. Both philosophies support an understanding of spirituality that stands in denial of our bodily being and connectedness to nature. Because these views are at the foundation of how conventional medicine approaches most disorders, and how many modern people think about themselves and their world, and because they support so many unhealthy ways of being, I prefer to call this kind of philosophy the metaphysics of disease.

The modern world and the rise of science are unthinkable without the philosophies of Plato and Descartes. We have both benefited and suffered enormously because of this conceptual framework. Because of it, many of us are now living in unbelievable and unprecedented material comfort while simultaneously experiencing a deep sense of disconnection from our bodies and environment. Meanwhile our cities are crumbling, many of our children have become drug addicts and hardened criminals, and people everywhere are complaining of stress and looking for the meaning of their life. We know that something is dreadfully wrong, but we have no idea what to do about it. It is as if we were on a fast train that we know is careening out of control, but that is so deliciously seductive and fascinating that we can't quite get off.

Fibromyalgia is but one manifestation of a world out of control. Like so many of our problems that require a whole system reorganization, it is often not recognized for what it is. Instead of recommending the much needed holistic treatment approach, ineffective piecemeal, mechanical solutions are typically all that are offered to patients. Chronic fatigue syndrome is a wake-up call for the rest of us and a profoundly important expression of the spiritual crises of our times. The word "crisis" means "turning point" and a true spiritual turning point is one that stops us dead in our tracks and demands one and only one solution—that we transform the way we live. The best hope for people with chronic fatigue is to see through the seductions of the modern world and get off the train. Anything short of transformation is nothing more than a mechanical stopgap measure, and simply the wrong solution.

A spiritual crisis arises when we reach the end of our belief in short term attempts to change the symptoms of our distress. At such moments we finally come to understand that the solution ultimately lies within ourselves. When we have reached the end of our rope, the solution is not to hang on for dear life, but to surrender. Surrender in this context does not mean to give up or submit unwillingly to outside demands, but to let go of our conflicted and fixated self in the profound sense embraced by all the world's great spiritual teachings. For it is in such moments of profound creative surrender that all healing happens.[22]

Creative surrender is not demanded when we know how to deal with a problem. When we have the flu or a flat tire, we are not tempted to ask about the meaning of life. But when we find ourselves caught in a true crisis, only creative surrender is capable of transforming our situation. The phenomenological consolidation of the proximate and evolutionary explanations is important because it helps us to understand how chronic fatigue is a fearful way of being-in-the-world that begins in the nervous system and ultimately compromises the entire person in relation to a world gone awry. But the ultimate solution to an existential condition is the one that reaches all the way to the spiritual crisis at the heart of the problem. The phenomenological consolidation of the proximate and evolutionary explanations is necessary and important, but the ultimate answer to the question, "Why did this happen to me?" is the transformation of the person who asks the question.

We have all the knowledge we need to change our world. What we are lacking is the kind of wisdom that is represented in traditional cultures and the great religions—the kind of wisdom which, because it transcends blind belief, dogma, and cultural bias, can transform a life and the world. "Wisdom is not out of reach. It requires a recalibration of the ego. The mental equipment is there but unused. Like chimpanzees who do not know how intelligent they are, we are only dimly beginning to perceive the possibilities of which our minds, operating in society, are capable."[23] Recalibration of the ego, or as I prefer to say, transformation of the whole person is indeed possible, but it also requires a transformation of the conceptual framework through which we view ourselves and nature. Since so much of our health care system rests on the assumption that the body is nothing but a soft machine, it is committed to treating their patients as if they were composed of symptomatic parts. The failure of fibromyalgia patients to respond to such an approach very clearly demonstrates the need for a holistic approach. Such an approach should be properly grounded in the holistic advances of the new biology, as well as sensitive to the unified nature of our whole being in relation to a world, and our inherent drive to understand our place in all of this of which of we are a part. A crisis is always at the heart of every turn toward transformation and the crisis of our times is no different. Its existence predicts a revolutionary shift toward a new kind of wisdom that embraces a science that is true to realization and fulfillment of our human being in relation to being itself.

The spiritual crisis at the heart of fibromyalgia is the same one at the heart of our modern world. On a small scale, any attempt to transform the life and world of a person with fibromyalgia is the same as the attempt to transform our shared world. All the signs are here, of course, but now is the time to resurrect our bodies, our deep biological feelings of connection, and to engage the whole of what we are in every attempt to understand and transform our world—not so that we can regress to a simpler stone age existence, but so that we may integrate our philosophy, science, technology, conventional, and complementary therapies to evolve a better world.

G

Myers Cocktail

FOR FURTHER INFORMATION ABOUT SOURCES OF the products and services mentioned in this section, see Appendix J: Resources.

1. The following are instructions for making up and administering the slow IV Myers Push (MP).

Supplies Needed	Amount
1. Bacteriostatic water	7 cc
2. Ascorbic acid (500 mg/ml), preservative-free	1–10 cc (*I often give 20–40 cc Vitamin C over* *30–40 minutes—see next page*)
3. Magnesium sulfate (MgSO₄), 50 percent (0.5 mg/ml)	2–4 cc
4. Pyridoxine (100 mg/ml), preservative-free	1 cc
5. Hydroxycobalamin (3,000 mcg/ml)	1 cc (give IM)
6. B-Complex 100	0.5–1 cc
7. Dexpanthenol (250 mg/ml)	0.5 cc
8. Glutathione, 200 mg per cc (optional)	2–5 cc (*Push in separately—do not mix in* *the same syringe with other nutrients*)
9. 20-cc or 25-cc syringes	

10.	18 gauge, 1 to 1½-inch needles
11.	25 gauge, ¾-inch butterfly sets
12.	Calcium gluconate, 10 percent, preservative-free (optional) 4–10 cc

Items 1 through 3 and 6 through 12 can be ordered (among other sources) from Harvard Drug Company. (800-783-7103). Item 4 can be obtained from compounding pharmacies, including Pathways and Wellness and Health Pharmaceuticals. Item 5 can be purchased from G.Y. and N. Most of the above items are also available from McGuff or Cape Apothecary.

To make the Myers Push (MP), draw up each ingredient using a separate syringe/needle and squirt it into the mouth of a 20-cc to 25-cc syringe. Attach the 25-gauge butterfly to the large syringe, pushing fluid through the butterfly tubing until the entire tubing and needle are filled. Now the mixture is ready for venipuncture and a slow IV push. The glutathione should be kept in the initial syringe (not mixed with other nutrients) and pushed in over one to ten minutes (1 cc every one to two minutes).

The dose of $MgSO_4$ typically begins at 2 cc. If the patient feels comfortable, without dizziness, nausea, or hypotension (warmth in the neck, face, chest, abdomen, groin, and/or extremities is normal, and is a sign of physiological action of the magnesium as a vasodilator), I usually increase the $MgSO_4$ to 4 cc and give it over ten to forty minutes. Alternately, all these nutrients can be added in an IV bag and allowed to drip in over thirty to sixty minutes.

The desired result is to inject at a rate at which the patient feels comfortable warmth without *excessive* flushing or feeling ill—that is, dizziness, nausea, and headache, symptoms that are rare.

Prior to the injection, it is important for the patient to be instructed to give frequent feedback about any developing warm feeling early on, so that the injection may be slowed down, or even temporarily stopped, before excessive, uncomfortable flushing occurs. Likewise, feedback by the patient needs to be given when the warm feeling has mostly subsided so that the injection may be resumed at a reduced rate. Eventually, the infusion will find the "happy medium" rate of injection, which maintains the "comfortable warmth" (see above).

Also, prior to the first few MP injections, explain that a taste of B vitamins usually appears during the infusion, often early in the push.

The physician needs to consider one major option, which has become routine in many quarters—the possible addition of calcium gluconate, 10 percent injectable. Some of the major reasons for deciding to include calcium are:

- If the patient feels consistently unwell for any reason after the MP (weakness, fatigue, sleepiness, palpitations—all rare and mild, if present).
- If the patient has a history, or laboratory evidence, of calcium deficit.
- If the physician's clinical judgement dictates it for any reason.

The dose of calcium gluconate 10 percent injectable varies from 4 cc to 10 cc, depending on the clinician's judgement. The key is to maintain balance without diluting the magnesium's positive effects.

A final caveat is that one needs to keep in mind the third of the troika—potassium. Over a period of time, IV magnesium may deplete potassium; the danger is that one may be tempted to increase the dose of magnesium, only to aggravate the low potassium picture. Always keep in mind that a potassium deficit may prevent magnesium repletion and vice-versa.

It is also, of course, possible to create calcium deficit by the MP. However, potassium depletion, in my experience, is clinically more frequent and more symptom-provoking, and at times alarming. (If needed, give the potassium by mouth—*not* I.V. *I.V. push potassium is FATAL.* I use Micro K Extendtabs, 10 MEQ, one to two times a day if potassium levels are under 4.0.)

2. Intravenous Vitamin C (I.V.C.)

The following are instructions for making up and administering the intravenous vitamin C (IVC.)

Supplies Needed	Amount
1. .45 percent NS infusion bag	150 cc
2. Ascorbic acid (500mg/ml), preservative-free	30 cc
3. Sodium bicarbonate, 8.4 percent	3 cc
4. 20-cc to 25-cc syringes	
5. 18-gauge, 1 to 1½-inch needles	
6. 3-cc syringes	
7. IV tubing	
8. 23-gauge, ¾-inch butterfly infusion sets	
9. Hypoallergenic tape	
10. Xylocaine, 1 to 2 percent (optional)	3 cc

All of the above supplies can be obtained from Harvard Drug Company.

To make up the IVC, add the ascorbic acid and the sodium bicarbonate to the IV bag. This infusion can be mixed one to two days before administration and stored in the refrigerator. It is best to bring the IV bag to room temperature before starting the infusion. This can be accomplished by taking the IV bag out of the refrigerator one to two hours ahead of time. Also, protect the IV bag from light.

The infusion is usually given over a period of forty-five to sixty minutes. It is best to select a large vein for the IV (that is, antecubital region) because the vitamin C can irritate the vessel wall. The 3 cc of sodium bicarbonate helps with the irritation problem. If the patient experiences pain or discomfort, slow down the infusion and apply a warm heating pad to the area. Also, squeezing and releasing the fist of the infused arm helps any discomfort.

It is rare for any patient not to tolerate the IVC. However, if discomfort continues and is unbearable, remove the needle and select a different vein. Another option is to add some IV-use procaine or lidocaine 2 percent to the infusion bag, starting with 3 cc (don't give more than 5 cc of 2 percent lidocaine per hour). Always make certain the patient is not sensitive to any of the "-caine" products, that it is for IV use, and that it does *not* contain epinephrine.

H

Qigong—A Chinese Energy Medicine Approach to CFIDS

by Kenneth S. Cohen, M.A.

Qigong is an ancient Chinese system of posture, gentle movement, respiratory technique and concentration used to improve health and prevent disease. It is the preventive and self-healing aspect of Chinese medicine.

Today, with an estimated 90 million practitioners in China and tens of thousands in the United States, Qigong is the most widely practiced form of alternative medicine in the world. Although Qigong can be used to combat specific illnesses, most practitioners consider Qigong a way to tap into hidden human potentials and enhance health and life beyond the "normal" or "average."

Chinese medicine is based on the belief that life energy, qi, flows through energy channels to reach all of the tissues of the body. When the flow is impeded, a person has too much energy on one side of the dam—creating a condition of congestion, inflammation, stagnation and/or pain and too little energy on the other side—leading to depletion, weakness and a feeling of disempowerment.

In the practice of acupuncture, fine needles are inserted into points that control qi flow. As obstructions dissolve, areas of excess are drained and places of insufficiency are filled. Thus homeostasis is restored.

Qigong has been called "acupuncture without needles." Instead of needles, the practitioner balances his or her own qi flow with meditative exercises and meditation. Qigong techniques appropriate for CFIDS require about as much energy as standing still for five to ten minutes and are thus non-taxing on energy reserves.

One of the greatest benefits of Qigong exercise is that most practitioners find that they have more energy after a session than before and the energy gain is cumulative with regular practice. The specific routine can be tailored to the needs and ability of the patient. If movement is impossible, qi can be mentally directed with Qigong healing imagery. Chinese Qigong literature is filled with thousands of visualizations. A typical one appropriate for CFIDS would be to imagine that as you inhale through the nose (allowing the abdomen to expand gently), deep, ocean-blue light suffuses the kidneys and adrenals with healing qi. While exhaling gently through the mouth, imagine that all of the stagnant, toxic or unneeded energy is leaving. By improving self-awareness and learning self-regulation skills, the practitioner learns to control aspects of the metabolism that are conventionally considered involuntary, such as hormonal levels, blood pressure, heart rate, oxygen delivery, etc.

Most importantly for CFIDS patients, Qigong emphasizes a systemic approach to healing: improving functioning in large areas of the body, rather than focusing exclusively on presenting symptoms of individual organs or body parts.

Qigong is complementary therapy and works well in conjunction with both allopathic medicine and other alternative modalities such as massage, orthomolecular medicine, biofeedback, and so on. Thousands of controlled scientific experiments have shown concrete evidence for Qigong's healing effects on conditions such as chronic pain, headaches, cancer, asthma, ulcers, bronchitis, hypertension and numerous other disorders.

A Qigong computerized data base is available in English that includes more than 1,000 complete research abstracts. Unfortunately, there has been no research to date on the effects of Qigong on CFIDS. Nevertheless, the experience of students and the clinical observations of Qigong therapists demonstrate that Qigong may be powerful therapy for CFIDS. Its multifaceted, systemic and holistic approach seems made-to-order for this complex condition. Qigong can lessen the intensity, duration and frequency of many CFIDS symptoms and improve overall vitality and quality of life. It has the strongest positive effects on:

1. *Fatigue*—Qigong reduces fatigue by energetically, yet gently stimulating the internal organs. Abdominal respiration (belly out on inhale,

belly in on exhale) massages the internal organs. When combined with deep relaxation and mental quietude, stress hormones and stress levels decrease.

According to Chinese medical theory, the body switches from an energy draining mode to one of energy conservation. Qi, life energy, is actually stored in the body, filling subtle energy reservoirs so that more is available for self-healing, self-repair and improved vitality.

In today's world, learning to conserve energy resources is important for everyone, besides CFIDS patients. Qigong teaches this essential stress-coping skill. The levels of positive hormones, such as DHEA increase (dehydroepiandrosterone, the body's most abundant hormone and precursor to the sexual hormones). DHEA levels are inversely linked with many CFIDS symptoms. Higher DHEA levels are correlated with improved immunity, memory, energy and decreased pain. According to C. Norm Shealy, M.D., Ph.D., founding president of the American Holistic Medical Association, "DHEA is the biological equivalent of qi."

Fatigue is also reduced by learning to tense only those muscles necessary for a task and eliminating unnecessary tension, such as that caused by poor posture, stress, pain or emotional reactions to pain. Qigong philosophy states, "If you need four ounces of force, do not use five." That extra ounce is unnecessary wear and tear on the body.

Recent research has shown that some biochemical processes occur as much as sixty times quicker in CFIDS patients compared to the general population. This may partially account for the tendency towards low adrenal function, decreased libido and an intolerance to stress, cold and prolonged exercise. Qigong's energy enhancing benefits may be due to a lowering of the metabolic rate in those areas that are on "overdrive" in CFIDS.

2. *Pain*—Musculoskeletal causes of pain can be significantly reduced by learning to use the body more intelligently. For instance, an important Qigong principle is *guan jie song kai,* "relax and open all the joints" (that is, do not lock the joints). Imagine them in a state of relaxed, open flexibility rather than tense contraction.

Let's look at a specific application of this principle: it is generally unwise to lock the knees. The knees are the body's shock absorbers. By keeping them slightly bent during Qigong practice and in such everyday activities as standing and walking, movement will not jar the spine. The lower back also remains more flexible and alive.

Qigong also reduces pain by improving relaxation skills. For instance, Qigong emphasizes sequential relaxation and sinking (*song chen*), imagining that each body part, starting at the head, is relaxing downwards; tension flows downhill like water and dissipates into the ground. Qigong promotes the release of endorphins, the body's good mood chemicals. Research shows that endorphins can reduce pain and stimulate the immune system.

3. *Brain Fog*—The brain, which comprises 2 percent of the body's weight, requires 20 percent of the body's available oxygen.

Brain fog is probably related to the 81 percent reduction in cerebral blood flow among CFIDS patients compared to controls. Numerous experiments have confirmed that Qigong can improve blood circulation in even the very small capillaries and areas most distant from the heart.

For instance, one way of testing peripheral blood flow is to use a medical device (the photoelectric sphygmograph) to shine a laser beam through the earlobe or finger tip. If there is more blood flow, the light beam is blocked and less light passes through the body part. Scientific experiments have demonstrated that Qigong practitioners, compared to controls, have significantly more blood flow. This means warmer hands and feet, less intolerance to cold and better brain blood supply.

Additionally, slow abdominal breathing, emphasized in Qigong, allows improved vasodilation and the most favorable conditions for oxygen delivery to cells. Qigong has the potential to improve concentration and optimize brain functioning.

Several studies have demonstrated the presence of a Qigong Electro-encephalogram (EEG), a unique brain-wave signature found among Qigong practitioners, consisting of an unusual quantity of alpha waves. Alpha waves indicate the ability to maintain a relaxed focus, as when one concentrates on a pleasant image. Qigong alpha waves have a strong electric charge (a high amplitude) indicating that the mind is less fragmented or disordered. Amplitude goes up when more of the brain cells are active.

4. *Empowerment*—CFIDS symptoms are augmented by a vicious cycle of disability and the emotional reaction to disability.

One of the most important benefits of Qigong is the sense of hope and self-efficacy: a feeling that you can make a difference in how you feel. This lessens anxiety, improves confidence and may increase the awareness of psychological options—perhaps reducing the hold of chemical depression.

The feeling of empowerment and inner strength engendered through Qigong make it essential training in the Chinese martial arts. For the CFIDS patient, Qigong may turn the odds more in their favor, giving them a better fighting chance against an enemy that seems to attack on all fronts.

Kenneth S. Cohen, M.A., health educator and China scholar, is the author of the internationally acclaimed book *The Way of Qigong: The Art and Science of Chinese Energy Healing* (Ballantine, 1997) and numerous healing visualization audiotapes (Sounds True Audio).

Recommended Reading

Books

Ali, M. *The Canary and Chronic Fatigue.* Denville, NJ: IPM Press, 1994. Focuses on the damage to enzyme systems by environmental stresses and nutritional-herbal-lifestyle therapeutics.

Crook, W. G. *The Yeast Connection and the Woman.* Jackson, TN: Professional Books, 1998. An excellent book. From *the* original teacher on yeast problems in CFIDS!

Forman, R. *How to Control Your Allergies.* Atlanta, GA: Larchmont Books, 1979. Diagnosis and treatment of food allergies.

Goldstein, J. *Betrayal by the Brain: The Neurologic Basis of Chronic Fatigue Syndrome, Fibromyalgia Syndrome and Related Neural Network Disorders.* Binghampton, NY: Haworth Press, 1996.

Goldstein, J. *Treatment Options in Chronic Fatigue Syndrome: A Guide for Physicians and Patients.* Binghamton, NY: Haworth Press, 1995.

Goldstein, J. *Tuning the Brain.* Binghamton NY: Haworth Press, 2001.

Ivker, R.S. *Sinus Survival.* New York, NY: Tarcher/Putnam. "Must reading" for patients with chronic sinusitis.

Jefferies, W.M. *Safe Uses of Cortisol,* 2nd ed. Springfield, IL: Charles C. Thomas, 1996. A landmark monograph on adrenal insufficiency. Written for physicians.

Rogers, S.A. *Tired or Toxic.* Syracuse, NY: Prestige Publishing, 1990. An extensive review of chemical sensitivity problems.

Rosenbaum, M., and M. Susser. *Solving the Puzzle of Chronic Fatigue Syndrome.* Tacoma, WA: Life Sciences Press, 1992. A good review of CFS treatments and also of infectious problems.

Travell, J.G., and D.G. Simons. *Myofascial Pain and Dysfunction: The Trigger Point Manual.* Baltimore, MD: Williams & Wilkins, 1983. A crucial text for anyone treating myofascial (muscle) pain. Chapter 4 discusses perpetuating factors, which are also important when treating fibromyalgia.

Journals and Newsletters

CFIDS Chronicle. A subscription comes with membership in the Chronic Fatigue and Immune Dysfunction Syndrome Association of America. Available from the Chronic Fatigue and Immune Dysfunction Syndrome Association of America, P.O. Box 220398, Charlotte, NC 28222-0398; 800–442–3437.

Fibromyalgia Network Newsletter. Available from the Fibromyalgia Network, P.O. Box 31750, Tucson, AZ 85751; 800–853–2929. From an excellent national FMS support group.

From Fatigued To Fantastic! Newsletter. $9/issue (2-4 issues per year). Helps you stay on the cutting edge of effective CFS/FMS therapy. Available from the office of Jacob Teitelbaum, 466 Forelands Road, Annapolis, MD 21401; 410–573–5389; http://www.endfatigue.com.

Journal of Chronic Fatigue Syndrome. For physicians. *Available from* Haworth Press, 10 Alice Street, Binghamton, NY 13904; 800–429–6784.

Journal of Musculoskeletal Pain. For physicians. Available from Haworth Press, 10 Alice Street, Binghamton, NY 13904; 800–429–6784.

Quarterly Review of Natural Medicine. Available from NPRC, 600 1st Avenue, No. 205, Seattle, WA 98104; telephone 206–623–2520.

Resources

Physicians Specializing in Chronic Fatigue Syndrome

PHYSICIAN ORGANIZATIONS

Holistic physicians are often familiar with effective CFIDS/FMS therapies. The following are organizations of physicians who take a holistic approach to medicine.

American College for Advancement of Medicine
P.O. Box 3427
Laguna Hills, CA 92654
http://www.apma.net

American Holistic Medical Association (AHMA)
4101 Lake Boone Trail, Suite 201
Raleigh, NC 27607
919–787–5146
Provides speakers through its Speakers Bureau.

INDIVIDUAL PRACTITIONERS

There are too many health practitioners who specialize in the treatment of CFIDS/FMS to list them all here. For a list of over 700 such practitioners worldwide, consult our website at http://www.endfatigue.com. If you are a practitioner and would like to add your name to our list, you can do so by visiting the website as well. The educational program at the website will also analyze your medical history (and laboratory test results, if available) to make a thorough medical record, a list of the most likely underlying problems in your case, and a treatment protocol tailored to your case. This will allow you to begin much of the protocol on your own and will assist and support your doctor in giving you the best possible care.

I see patients in consultation at my office, which is at the following address:

466 Forelands Road
Annapolis, MD 21401
410–573–5389
Fax: 410–266–6104

In addition, the following are doctors who specialize in treating certain specific aspects of CFIDS/FMS:

Joseph H. Brewer, M.D.
Plaza Internal Medicine Infectious Diseases, P.C.
4620 J.C. Nichols Parkway, Suite 415
Kansas City, MO
816–531–1550
Fax: 816–531–8277
www.plazamedicine.com
Dr. Brewer is possibly the foremost physician in the United States treating chronic active HHV-6 infection with ganciclovir.
Mike Rosner, M.D.

80 Doctors Drive, Suite 4
Hendersonville, NC 28792
828–684–1076
A neurosurgeon with extensive experience in treating CMI/CS in FMS/CFIDS. Dr. Rosner sees only patients who are referred to him by a physician.

Hotlines

CFIDS Association Hotline
800–442–3437

National Chronic Fatigue Syndrome and Fibromyalgia Association Hotline
816–313–2000

Products and Services

*Resources that are particularly noteworthy are marked with an asterisk.

Allergy Research Group–Nutricology Inc.
30806 Santana Street
P.O. Box 55907
Hayward, CA 94544
800–545–9960 800–782–4274 510–487–8526
Fax: 510–487–8530
E-mail: order@nutricology.com
www.nutricology.com
Sells Tricycline, an antiparasitic herbal preparation. A prescription is sometimes necessary. Also sells ImuPlus.

Amy Podd / A.P. Business Solutions
1109 Little Magothy View
Annapolis, MD 21401
410–757–7295
Sells therapeutic magnets.

Belmar Pharmacy
12860 West Cedar Drive
Lakewood, Colorado 80228
800–525–9473
www.belmarpharmacy.com

Carries oxytocin tablets. The physician phones in the prescription as well as the patient's credit card number, and Belmar mails the medication directly to the patient. They also carry colloidal gold for inflammatory diseases such as rheumatoid arthritis without a prescription.

Bernhard Industries
300 71st Street, Suite 435
Miami Beach, FL 33141
800–544–6425 305–861–2536
Sells a nasal steamer that is excellent for sinus problems.

Bio Brite
4340 East West Highway, Suite 401S
Bethesda, MD 20814
800–621–LITE (800–621–5483) 301–961–5940
Fax: 301–961–5943
www.biobrite.com
Sells light boxes and light visors for persons suffering from seasonal affective disorder.

Bio-Tech Pharmacal
P.O. Box 1992
Fayetteville, AR 72702
800–345–1199 501–443–9148
Fax: 501–443–5643
www.bio-tech-pharm.com
D-Mannose.

Body Ecology
1266 West Paces Ferry Road, Suite 505
Atlanta, GA 30327
800–4–STEVIA (800–478–3842)
Stevia; stevia cookbooks.

*Cape Apothecary
1384 Cape St. Claire Road
Annapolis, MD 21401
800–248–5978 410–757–3522 410–974–1788
Fax: 410–626–7226
www.rxstat.com/capedrug

Holistic compounding pharmacy that fulfills mail orders. Among other products, they can supply nystatin powder, low-dose naltrexone, interferon, pure dextromethorphan (DM), sustained-release T_3 (thyroid hormone), high-dose injectable vitamin B_{12}, natural biestrogen, and natural progesterone. Will work with you to adjust estrogen/progesterone formulations to provide the optimum dosage for you. Can also supply ingredients for Myers cocktails.

*CFIDS Buyers Club/Pro Health
800–366–6056
Variety of supplements and other products useful for the management of CFS/CFIDS, including CFS/MF Multi and CFS/FM Energy Formula. If you tell them that Dr. Teitelbaum referred you, they will make a charitable donation of a portion of your first purchase.

Clark's Pharmacy
15615 Bel-Red Road
Bellevue, WA 98008
800–480–3432 888–454–4941
Carries oral amphotericin B, tinidazole.

DiaSorin, Inc.
1990 Industrial Boulevard
Stillwater, MN 55082
800–328–1482 651–439–9710
Manufacturer of reagents used for Epstein-Barr IGM antibody testing.

Enzymatic Therapy
825 Challenger Drive
Green Bay, WI 54311
800–783–2286
www.enzy.com
Produces chewable deglycyrrhizinated licorice (DGL) tablets.

General Nutrition, Inc.
Customer Resources Department
300 Sixth Avenue
Pittsburgh, PA 15222
888–462–2548
www.gnc.com

Markets a good form of magnesium-potassium aspartate and timed-release DHEA. There are General Nutrition Centers (GNC) stores throughout North America. You can contact the company at the address above to find a store in your area.

*Great Smokies Diagnostic Laboratory
63 Zillicoa Street
Asheville, NC 28801
800–522–4762
Fax: 828–252–9303
www.gsdl.com
Stool culture and sensitivity tests; IgE food allergy blood test. Does an excellent job with stool testing for ova and parasites (O&P testing) and bacterial infections, as well as many other tests.

G.Y. and N.
877–864–5112
Carries ingredients for Myers cocktails.

Harvard Drug Company
800–783–7103
Carries ingredients for Myers cocktails.

*Hemex Labs
2505 West Beryl Avenue
Phoenix, AZ 85021-1461
800–999–CLOT (800–999–2568)
www.hemex.com
Blood testing, including CFIDS coagulation blood profile/immune system activation of coagulation (ISAC) panel test and hereditary thrombotic panel to see if heparin therapy may help.

Herb Finders
P.O. Box 3868
Salt Lake City, UT 84110-3868
800–780–6934
Carries turkey rhubarb.

*Immunosciences Lab, Inc.
8730 Wilshire Boulevard, Suite 305
Beverly Hills, CA 90211
800–950–4686 310–657–1077
Fax: 310–657–1053
www.immuno-sci-lab.com
Does CMV, HHV-6, and mycoplasma and chlamydia PCR testing.

*Institute For Molecular Medicine
15162 Triton Lane
Huntington Beach, CA 92649
714–903–2900
Fax: 714–379–2082
www.immed.com
For mycoplasma and chlamydia PCR testing, HHV-6 testing by Dr. Garth Nicolson.

Lab ISI
Napoli, Italy
39–583–719–935
Fax: 39–583–799–878
Supplier of CoCarboxylase (thiamine pyrophosphate, or TPP).

Lane Labs
110 Commerce Drive
Allendale, NJ 07401
800–526–3005 201–526–9090
Fax: 201–236–9091
www.lanelabs.com
A source for MgN3.

Medic Alert
2323 Colorado Avenue
Turlock, CA 95382
800–432–5378
Hotline: 209–634–4917 209–668–3333 (from Alaska or Hawaii)
Fax: 209–669–2495
www.medicalert.org
Provides bracelets that warn about serious chronic medical conditions.

*Meta Metrix
4855 Peachtree Ind. Boulevard
Norcross, GA 30092
800–221–4640
Fax: 770–441–2237
www.metametrix.com
For amino acid profile testing (#40 blood test).

Metagenics
100 Avenida La Pata
San Clemente, CA 92673
800–692–9400 949–366–0818
www.metagenics.com www.ultrabalance.com
Manufacturer of the UltraBalance Medical Foods line of products, including UltraClean, a hypoallergenic powdered food to use with bowel detoxification and elimination diets. This product, developed by nutritional biochemist Dr. Jeffrey Bland, is expensive, but it can help to determine food sensitivities.

Steven Nadell
4403 Vineland Road B-10
Orlando, FL 32811
800–647–6100
Distributor of Metagenics products, including UltraClear.

Nutricology. See Allergy Research Group-Nutricology Inc.

*Parasitology Center, Inc.
903 South Rural Road, Suite 101-318
Tempe, AZ 85281
480–777–1078 (call Urokeep at 602–545–9236 to get the stool test kit)
Fax: 480-777-1223
Does an excellent job with stool testing for ova and parasites (O&P test) and yeast.

*Pfizer Diflucan and Zithromax Patient Assistance Program
1101 King Street, Suite 600
Alexandria, VA 22314
800–869–9979 (Monday–Friday, 8:30 AM–5:30 PM Eastern time)

This is a program under which patients can apply for financial assistance to pay for Diflucan. Let them know you have immune suppression and fungal overgrowth. To qualify, single patients must have an income of less than $25,000; patients with dependents less than $40,000, with no Medicaid, private insurance, or AIDS programs benefits. The drugs must be for outpatient use. An application form is sent to the doctor's office; the doctor completes and signs the form, and attaches a prescription. The medicine is sent to the doctor's office. It generally takes four to five weeks to receive the medication. For more information about this and other programs to assist patients in obtaining medications they cannot otherwise afford, see the website www.needymeds.com.

PhytoPharmica
825 Challenger Drive
Green Bay, WI 54311
800–553–2370 920–469–9099
www.phytopharmica.com
Producer of Saventaro Cat's Claw, Iberogast, and Phytodolor.

Premier & Pacific Research Labs
800–325–7734
Olive leaf extract.

Professional Arts Pharmacy
1101 North Rolling Road
Baltimore, MD 21228
800–832–9285 410–747–6870
Fax: 410–788–5686
www.//voiceofwomen.com/VOW2_12150.proartpharm.html
Carries dexpanthenol (a form of pantothenic acid), natural biestrogen, and progesterone. Will work with you to adjust estrogen/progesterone formulations to provide the optimum dosage for you.

*Pure Water
Bren Jacobson
103 Second Street
Annapolis, MD 21401
888–801–8176 410–224–4877

Consultant on health and environmental concerns, especially water, and distributor of Multi-Pure water filters. Carries therapeutic magnets. Bren is also an excellent Rolfer, and does personal counseling in person or by phone.

*Ron's Wellness Store and Natural Pharmacy
701 North Highland Springs Avenue
Beaumont, CA 92223
800–400–7406 909–845–1101
Fax: 909–845–0971
An excellent source for pain and hormone creams, including Arizona Pain Formula Cream, 15-percent lidocaine in PLO gel, natural estrogen and progesterone, and testosterone cream.

*Serammune Physicians Laboratories
1890 Preston White Drive, Suite 201
Reston, VA 22091
800–553–5472
Performs ELISA-ACT blood test for food sensitivities, possibly the best blood test for food allergies.

*Jacob Teitelbaum, M.D.
466 Forelands Road
Annapolis, MD 21401
800–333–5287 410–573–5389
Fax: 410–266–6104
www.endfatigue.com
Many of the products recommended in this book available through my office and the Vitamin Shop section of my website. Among them are delta wave sleep-inducing CDs and tapes, D-mannose, olive leaf extract, Saventaro cat's claw extract, stevia, thymic protein (Pro-Boost), the From Fatigued To Fantastic Foundation powder multivitamin and mineral formula, and Dr. Teitelbaum's Sleep Formula. At our website, you can get the From Fatigued To Fantastic formulas, newsletters, and a program that will tailor a treatment protocol to your case, an extensive list of CFIDS/FMS support groups, a list of pratitioners who specialize in treating the disorder and who use a significant part of our protocol.

A word about products bearing my name: I developed these to meet the needs of my patients and others suffering from CFIDS/FMS. I know that when I see a "Dr. Smith's Formula," I worry that Dr. Smith "sold out." Because of this, I direct any company making my formulas to donate all of the money that I would have received for making them to charity. I also never accept any money from anyone whose products or services I recommend.

Thera Cane Company
P.O. Box 9220
Denver, CO 80209-0220
800–947–1470
Fax: 888–299–6577
http://www.theracane.com
Produces the Thera Cane self-massage device.

To Your Health
800–801–1406
Supplies Fibrocare (a source of magnesium glycinate), Valerian Rest, and other FMS products.

ViraCor
1210 NE Windsor Drive
Lee's Summit, MO 64086
800–305–5198
Fax: 816–347–0143
www/viracor.com
Performs rapid HHV-6 viral cultures.

*Women's International Pharmacy
5708 Monona Drive
Madison, WI 53716-3152
608–221–7800
Fax: 608–221–7819
    or
13925 West Meeker Boulevard, Suite #13
Sun City West, AZ 85375
623–214–7700
Fax: 623–214–7708
www.wipws.com
Supplies natural micronized estrogen, progesterone, and testosterone by mail order

Resource Organizations

Resources that are particularly noteworthy are marked with an asterisk.

American Association for Chronic Fatigue Syndrome
P.O. Box 895
Olney, MD 20830
An umbrella organization focusing on scientific research.

American Botanical Council*
P.O. Box 201660
Austin, TX 78720
800–373–7105 512–331–8868
Supplies information on specific herbs and publishes Herbalgram, *a magazine with information on helpful herbal remedies.*

Arthritis Foundation
P.O. Box 19000
Atlanta, GA 30326
(800) 283–7800

Association for Transpersonal Psychology
P.O. Box 3049
Stanford, CA 94309
415–561–3382
Fax: 415–561–3383
www.igc.org/atp/
For referrals to holistic counselors.

BioSET
P.O. Box 5356
Larkspur, CA 94977
877–927–0741 415–927–0741
www.BioSet-institute.com
Offers an allergy desensitization technique that also employs detoxification and enzyme therapy.

Brugh Joy, Inc.
P.O. Box 1059
Lucerne Valley, CA 92356
800–448–9187
For information on workshops that helping people to understand their deep psyches—to learn to accept and understand more fully who you really are.

*Chronic Fatigue and Immune Dysfunction Syndrome Association of America
P.O. Box 220398
Charlotte, NC 28222-0398
800–442–3437 704–365–2343
Fax: 704–365–9755
www.cfids.org
An excellent national patient support group and educational resource. One of the two organizations I would consult first.

Chronic Fatigue and Immune Dysfunction Syndrome Pathfinder
P.O. Box 2644
Kensington, MD 20891-2644

Chronic Fatigue Syndrome/Myalgic Encephalitis
Computer Networking Project
P.O. Box 11347
Washington, DC 20008
E-mail: cfs-me@sjuvin.stjohns.edu

Compuserve Chronic Fatigue and Immune
Dysfunction Syndrome Support Area
CFS/CFIDS/FMS Section (16)
Health and Fitness Forum (Good Health)
800–898–8199 (Compuserve information)

*Fibromyalgia Network
P.O. Box 31750
Tucson, AZ 85751
800–853–2929
www.fmnetnews.com

This is a "must join" group for fibromyalgia patients. One of the two organizations I would consult first.

Food Allergy and Anaphylaxis Network (FAAN)
10400 Eaton Place, Suite 107
Fairfax, VA 22030-2208
800–929–4040
www.foodallergy.org

Guild for Structural Integration
P.O. Box 1559
Boulder, Colorado 80306
800–447–0150
For practitioners of the Rolf method of structural integration.

*Myalgic Encephalitis Association of Canada
246 Queen Street, Suite 400
Ottawa, Ontario KIP 5E4
Canada
613–563–1565
An excellent source of general information for CFIDS and fibromyalgia patients, as well as a good source of important information for Canadian patients.

NAET
6714 Beach Boulevard
Buena Park, CA 90621
714–532–0800 714–523–8900
Fax: 714–523–3068
www.naet.com
Supplies information about the Nambudripad allergy elimination technique (NAET), including help with locating practitioners.

National CFIDS Fondation
The National CFIDS Foundation
103 Aletha Road
Needham, MA 02492
781–449–3535
Fax: 781–449–8606
www.ncf-net.org

National Chronic Fatigue Syndrome and Fibromyalgia Association
P.O. Box 18426
Kansas City, MO 64133

*National Fibromyalgia Research Association
P.O. Box 500
Salem, OR 97302
www.nfra.net
An excellent group currently focusing on Chiari malformation and cervical stenosis surgery for CFIDS/FMS.

National Myalgic Encephalitis/Fibromyalgia Action Network
3836 Carling Avenue Highway 17B
Nepean, Ontario K2H 7V2
Canada
613–829–6667

National Organization for Seasonal Affective Disorder
P.O. Box 40133
Washington, DC 20016

National Sanitation Foundation (NSF) International
P.O. Box 130140
789 North Dixboro Road
Ann Arbor, MI 48113-0140
800–NSF–MARK (800–673–6275) 734–769–8010
Fax: 734–769–0109
www.nsf.org
An independent, not-for-profit organization that tests and certifies drinking water treatment products.

Nightingale Research Foundation
383 Danforth Avenue
Ottawa, Ontario K2A OE3
Canada
www.nightingale.ca
An organization dedicated to the study of ME/CFS. Dr. Byron Hyde also offers expert legal counsel.

Qigong Research and Practice Center
P.O. Box 1727
Nederland, CO 80466
To receive information on Qigong, send them a self-addressed, stamped envelope.

Restless Leg Foundation
P.O. Box 314JH
514 Daniels Street
Raleigh, NC 27605
For information on restless leg syndrome.

Rolf Institute
205 Canyon Boulevard
Boulder, CO 80302
(303) 449–5903
(800) 530–8875
For information and referrals to a Rolfing practitioner in your area.

Trager Institute
21 Locust Avenue
Mill Valley, CA 94941
216–896–9383
Fax: 216–896–9385
www.trager.com
For referrals to Trager instructors, tutors, and practitioners.

Well Spouse Foundation
30 East 40th Street PH
New York, NY 10016
800–838–0879 212–685–8815
Fax: 212–685–8676
www.wellspouse.org
A resource organization for spousal caregivers.

Support Groups

There are too many local support groups for CFIDS/FMS patients to list them all here. For a list of such groups, consult our website at www.endfatigue.com. Please let us know if you would like to have your group added to our website list (go to the Q&A section).

Notes

Introduction

1. J. Teitelbaum and B. Bird, "Effective Treatment of Severe Chronic Fatigue: A Report of a Series of 64 Patients," *Journal of Musculoskeletal Pain* 3 (4) (1995): 91–110.

2. J.E. Teitelbaum, B. Bird, R.M. Greenfield, et al., "Effective Treatment of CFS and FMS: A Randomized, Double-Blind Placebo Controlled Study," *Journal of Chronic Fatigue Syndrome* 8 (2) (2001).

3. J. Teitelbaum and B. Bird, op cit.

4. Ibid.

Chapter 1: What Is Chronic Fatigue Syndrome?

1. G.P. Holmes, J.E. Kaplan, N.M. Gantz, et al., "Chronic Fatigue Syndrome: A Working Case Definition," *Annals of Internal Medicine* 108 (1988): 387–389.

R.K. Price, C.S. North, S. Wessely, et al., "Estimating the Presence of Chronic Fatigue Syndrome in the Community," *Public Health Reports* 107 (September-October 1992): 514–522.

R.B. Marchesani, "Critical Antiviral Pathway Deficient in Chronic Fatigue Syndrome Patients," *Infectious Disease News,* August 1993, p. 4.

2. L.A. Jason, J.A. Richman, A.W. Rademaker, et al., "A Community-Based Study of Chronic Fatigue Syndrome," *Archives of Internal Medicine* 159 (18) (11 October 1999): 2129-2137.

3. D.L. Goldenberg, "Fibromyalgia Syndrome: A Decade Later," *Journal of the American Medical Association* 159 (1999): 777–785.

4. S.E. Straus, S. Fritz, J.K. Dale, et al., "Lymphocyte Phenotype and Function in the Chronic Fatigue Syndrome," *Journal of Clinical Immunology* 13 (1) (January 1993): 30–40.

5. J. Teitelbaum and B. Bird, "Effective Treatment of Severe Chronic Fatigue: A Report of a Series of 64 Patients," *Journal of Musculoskeletal Pain* 3 (4) (1995): 91–110.

6. L.A. Jason, J.A. Richman, A.W. Rademaker, et al., op. cit.

7. J. Teitelbaum and B. Bird, op. cit.

8. D. Halpin and S. Wessely, "VP-1 Antigen in Chronic Postviral Fatigue Syndrome," *The Lancet* 1 (8645) (6 May 1989): 1028–1029.

G.E. Yousef, F J. Bell, G.F. Mann, et al., "Chronic Enterovirus Infection in Patients with Postviral Fatigue Syndrome," *The Lancet,* 1 (8578) (23 January 1988): 146–147.

L.E. Archard, N.E. Bowles, P.O. Behan, et al., "Postviral Fatigue Syndrome Persistence of Enterovirus RNA in Muscle and Elevated Creatine Kinase," *Journal of the Royal Society of Medicine* 81 (6) (June 1988): 326–329.

A. Martin Lerner, M. Zervos, and H.J. Dworkin, "New Cardiomyopathy: Pilot Study of Intravenous Ganciclovir in a Subset of the Chronic Fatigue Syndrome, *Infectious Diseases in Clinical Practice* 6 (1997): 110–117.

Nicolson, G.L, "Considerations When Undergoing Treatment for Chronic Infections Found in Chronic Fatigue Syndrome, Fibromyalgia, and Gulf War Illness," *Journal of Internal Medicine* 1 (1988): 115–117, 123–128.

Nicolson, G.L., M.Y. Nasralla, J. Haier, et al., "Mycoplasmal Infections in Chronic Illness: Fibromyalgia and Chronic Fatigue Syndrome, Gulf War Illness, Human Immunodeficiency Virus, and Rheumatoid Arthritis," *Medical Sentinel* 4 (1999): 172–176.

J. Brewer, K.K. Knox, and D.R. Carrigan, "Longitudinal Study of Chronic Active HHV-6 Viremia in Patients with CFS," paper presented at IDSA Conference, Philadelphia, PA, November 1999.

D. Wakefield, A. Lloyd, J. Dwyer, et al., "Human Herpesvirus 6 and Myalgic Encephalomyelitis," *The Lancet* 1 (8593) (7 May 1988): 1059.

Byron Hyde, Jay Goldstein, and Paul Levine, eds., *The Clinical and Scientific Basis of Myalgic Encephalitis and Chronic Fatigue Syndrome* (Ottawa, ON: Nightingale Research Foundation, 1992).

9. W. Jefferies, *Safe Uses of Cortisol,* monograph (Springfield, IL: Charles C. Thomas, 1981).

10. G. Neeck and W. Riedel, "Thyroid Function in Patients with Fibromyalgia Syndrome," *Journal of Rheumatology* 19 (7) (July 1992): 1120–1122.

M.A. Demitrack, K. Dale, S.E. Straus, et al., "Evidence for Impaired Activation of the Hypothalamic-Pituitary-Adrenal Axis in Patients with Chronic Fatigue Syndrome," *Journal of Clinical Endocrinology and Metabolism* 73 (6) (December 1991): 1223–1234.

G.A. McCain and K.S. Tilbe, "Diurnal Hormone Variation in Fibromyalgia Syndrome and a Comparison with Rheumatoid Arthritis," *Journal of Rheumatology* 25 (1993): 469–474.

A.M.O. Bakheit, P.O. Behan, T.G. Dinan, et al., "Possible Upregulation of Hypothalamic 5-HT Receptors in Patients with Postviral Fatigue Syndrome," *BMJ* 304 (6833) (18 April 1992): 1010–1012.

E.N. Griep, J.N. Boersma, and E.R. de Kloet, "Altered Reactivity of the Hypothalamic-Pituitary Axis in the Primary Fibromyalgia Syndrome," *Journal of Rheumatology* 20 (3) (March 1993): 469–474.

11. W. Jefferies, op. cit.

12. J. Teitelbaum and B. Bird, op. cit.

J.E. Teitelbaum, B. Bird, R.M. Greenfield, et al., "Effective Treatment of CFS and FMS: A Randomized, Double-Blind Placebo Controlled Study," *Journal of Chronic Fatigue Syndrome,* 8 (2) (2001).

13. W. Jefferies, op. cit.

J. Teitelbaum and B. Bird, op. cit.

J.E. Teitelbaum, B. Bird, R.M. Greenfield, et al., op. cit.

14. J. Teitelbaum and B. Bird, op. cit.

J.E. Teitelbaum, B. Bird, R.M. Greenfield, et al., op. cit.

15. C.A. Everson, "Sustained Sleep Deprivation Impairs Host Defense." *American Journal of Physiology* 265 (5 Part 2) (November 1993): R1148–1154.

S. Pillemer, L.A. Bradley, L.J. Crofford, et al., "The Neuroscience and Endocrinology of FMS—[An NIH] Conference Summary," *Arthritis and Rheumatism* 40 (11) (November 1997): 1928–1939.

Chapter 2: Going After the Easy Things First

1. R.M. Marston and B.B. Peterkin, "Nutrient Content of the National Food Supply," *National Food Review,* Winter 1980, pp. 21–25.

2. William G. Crook, *The Yeast Connection and the Woman* (Jackson, TN: Professional Books, 1995).

3. R.M. Marston and B.B. Peterkin, op. cit.

   J.H. Nelson, "Wheat: Its Processing and Utilization," *American Journal of Clinical Nutrition* 41, supplement (May 1985): 1070-1076.

4. H.A. Schroeder, "Losses of Vitamins and Trace Minerals Resulting from Processing and Preservation of Foods," *American Journal of Clinical Nutrition* 24 (5) (May 1971): 562–573.

5. S.B. Eaton and N. Konner, "Paleolithic Nutrition. A Consideration of Its Nature and Current Implications," *The New England Journal of Medicine* 312 (5) (31 January 1985): 283–289.

6. H.C. Trowell, ed., *Western Diseases: Their Emergence and Prevention* (Cambridge, MA: Harvard University Press, 1981).

7. W. Mertz, ed., "Beltsville 1 Year Dietary Intake Survey," *American Journal of Clinical Nutrition* 40, supplement (December 1984): 1323–1403.

8. J.G. Travell and D.G. Simons, *Myofascial Pain and Dysfunction: The Trigger Point Manual,* Vol. I (Baltimore, MD: Williams & Wilkins, 1983), pp. 103–164.

9. B. Kennes, I. Dumont, D. Brohee, et al., "Effect of Vitamin C Supplements on Cell-Mediated Immunity in Old People," *Gerontology* 29 (1983): 305–310.

   R.K. Chandra, "Effect of Macro and Micro Nutrient Deficiencies and Excess on Immune Response," *Food Technology,* February 1985, pp. 91–93.

   S. Chandra, et al., "Undernutrition Impairs Immunity," *Internal Medicine* 5 (December 1984): 85–99.

   R.K. Chandra, et al., "NIH Workshop on Trace Element Regulation of Immunity and Infection," *Nutrition Research* 2 (1982): 721–733.

   M.C. Talbott, L.T. Miller, and N.I. Kerkvliet, "Pyridoxine Supplementation: Effect on Lymphocyte Responses in Elderly Persons," *American Journal of Clinical Nutrition* 46 (4) (October 1987): 659–664.

S.N. Meydani, M.P. Barklund, S. Liu, et al., "Vitamin E Supplementation Enhances Cell-Mediated Immunity in Healthy Elderly Subjects," *American Journal of Clinical Nutrition* 52 (3) (September 1990): 557–563.

10. E. Braunwald, ed., *Harrisons Principles of Internal Medicine,* 11th ed. (New York: McGrawHill, 1987),(1), p. 1496.

S. Chandra, et al., "Undernutrition Impairs Immunity," op. cit.

R.K. Chandra, et al., "NIH Workshop on Trace Element Regulation of Immunity and Infection," op.cit.

T. Walter, S. Arredondo, M. Arevalo, et al., "Effect of Iron Therapy on Phagocytosis and Bactericidal Activity in Neutrophils of Iron-Deficient Infants," *American Journal of Clinical Nutrition* 44 (6) (December 1986): 877–882.

T.F. Kirn, "Do Low Levels of Iron Affect Body's Ability to Regulate Temperature, Experience Cold?" *Journal of the American Medical Association* 260 (5 August 1988): 607.

L.S. Darnell, "Abstract 21," *American Journal of Clinical Nutrition,* supplement.

11. D.C. Rushton, I.D. Ramsay, J.J. Gilkes, et al., "Ferritin and Fertility," letter to the editor," *The Lancet* 337 (8757) (22 June 1991): 1554.

12. J. Lindenbaum, E.B. Healton, D.G. Savage, et al., "Neuropsychiatric Disorders Caused by Cobalamin Deficiency in the Absence of Anemia or Macrocytoses," *The New England Journal of Medicine* 318 (26) (30 June 1988): 1720–1728.

13. W.S. Beck, "Cobalamin and the Nervous System," editorial, *The New England Journal of Medicine* 318 (1988): 1752–1754.

14. J. Lindenbaum, I.H. Rosenberg, P.W. Wilson, et al., "Prevalence of Cobalamin Deficiency in the Framingham Elderly Population," *American Journal of Clinical Nutrition* 60 (1) (July 1994): 2–11.

15. Karnaze, D.S., and R. Carmel, "Low Serum Cobalamin Levels in Primary Degenerative Dementia: Do Some Patients Harbor Atypical Cobalamin Deficiency States?" *Archives of Internal Medicine* 147 (3) (March 1987): 429–431.

16. B. Regland, M. Andersson, L. Abrahamsson, et al., "Increased Concentrations of Homocysteine in the Cerebrospinal Fluid in Patients with Fibromyalgia and Chronic Fatigue Syndrome," *Scandinavian Journal of Rheumatology* 26 (4) (1997): 301–307.

17. Ibid.

18. M.S. Seelig, "The Requirement of Magnesium by the Normal Adult," *American Journal of Clinical Nutrition* 14 (June 1964): 342–390.

F.L. Lakshmanad, et al., "Magnesium Intakes and Balances," *American Journal of Clinical Nutrition* 60 (6 Supplement) (December 1984): 1380–1389.

19. M.S. Seelig, op. cit.

20. M.J. Hoes, "Plasma Concentrations of Magnesium and Vitamin B_1 in Alcoholism and Delirium Tremens. Pathogenic and Prognostic Implications," *Acta Psychiatrica Belgica* 81 (1) (January-February 1981): 72–84.

Chapter 3: Hormones—The Body's Master Control System

1. J. Teitelbaum and B. Bird, "Effective Treatment of Severe Chronic Fatigue: A Report of a Series of 64 Patients," *Journal of Musculoskeletal Pain* 3 (4) (1995): 91–110.

2. J. Teitelbaum and B. Bird, "Effective Treatment of Severe Chronic Fatigue: A Report of a Series of 64 Patients," *Journal of Musculoskeletal Pain* 3 (4) (1995): 91–110.

   W.M. Jefferies, *Safe Uses of Cortisol*, 2nd edition, monograph (Springfield, IL: Charles C. Thomas, 1996).

3. W.M. Jefferies, *Safe Uses of Cortisol*, 2nd edition, monograph (Springfield, IL: Charles C. Thomas, 1996).

4. R.A. Anderson, et al., "Chromium and Hypoglycemia," abstract, *American Journal of Clinical Nutrition* 41 (4) (April 1985): 841.

5. Martine Le Gal, Pascal Cathebras, and Käthi Strüby, "Pharmaton Capsules in the Treatment of Functional Fatigue: A Double-Blind Study Versus Placebo Evaluated by a New Methodology," *Phytotherapy Research* 10 (1996): 49–53.

6. Christopher Hobbs, *The Echinacea Handbook* (Portland, OR: Eclectic Medical Publications, 1989).

7. F.E. Koen, "The Influence of Echinacea Purpurea On The Hypophyseal-Adrenal System," *Arzneimittel-Forschung* 3 (1953): 133–137.

8. *Medizinische Klinik* 4 (1969):1546–1547.

9. W.M. Jefferies, "Low-Dosage Glucocorticoid Therapy. An Appraisal of Its Safety and Mode of Action in Clinical Disorders, Including Rheumatoid Arthritis," *Archives of Internal Medicine* 119 (3) (March 1967): 265–278.

   J.E. Teitelbaum, B. Bird, R.M. Greenfield, et al., "Effective Treatment of CFS and FMS: A Randomized, Double-Blind Placebo Controlled Study," *Journal of Chronic Fatigue Syndrome* 8 (2) (2001).

10. W.M. Jefferies, *Safe Uses of Cortisol*, op. cit.

    W.M. Jefferies, "Low-Dosage Glucocorticoid Therapy. An Appraisal of Its Safety and Mode of Action in Clinical Disorders, Including Rheumatoid Arthritis," op. cit.

11. R. McKenzie, A. O'Fallon, J. Dale, et al., "Low-Dose Hydrocortisone for Treatment of Chronic Fatigue Syndrome: A Randomized Controlled Trial," *Journal of the American Medical Association* 280 (12) (23–30 September 1998): 1061–1066.

12. J.E. Teitelbaum, B. Bird, A. Weiss, et al., "Low Dose Hydrocortisone for Chronic Fatigue Syndrome," *Journal of the American Medical Association* 281 (1999): 1887–1888.

13. A.J. Cleare, E. Heap, G.S. Malhi, et al., "Low-Dose Hydrocortisone in CFS: A Randomized Crossover Trial," *The Lancet* 353 (9151) (6 February 1999): 455–458.

    J. Teitelbaum and B. Bird, "Effective Treatment of Severe Chronic Fatigue: A Report of a Series of 64 Patients," op. cit.

    J.E. Teitelbaum, B. Bird, R.M. Greenfield, et al., "Effective Treatment of CFS and FMS: A Randomized, Double-Blind Placebo Controlled Study," *Journal of Chronic Fatigue Syndrome* 8 (2) (2001).

14. P.M.J. Zelissen, R.J. Croughs, P.P. van Rijk, et al., "Effect of Glucocorticoid Replacement Therapy on Bone Mineral Density in Patients with Addison Disease," *Annals of Internal Medicine* 120 (3) (1 February 1994): 207–210.

15. J. Teitelbaum and B. Bird, "Effective Treatment of Severe Chronic Fatigue: A Report of a Series of 64 Patients," op. cit.

    J.E. Teitelbaum, B. Bird, R.M. Greenfield, et al., "Effective Treatment of CFS and FMS: A Randomized, Double-Blind Placebo Controlled Study," op. cit.

16. P.C. Rowe, I. Bou-Holaigah, J.S. Kan, et al., "Is Neurally Mediated Hypotension an Unrecognized Cause of Chronic Fatigue?" *The Lancet* 345 (8950) (11 March 1995): 623–624.

17. A. Susmano, A.S. Volgman, and T.A. Buckingham, "Beneficial Effects of Dextro-Amphetamine in the Treatment of Vasodepressor Syncope," *Pacing and Clinical Electrophysiology* 16 (1993): 1235–1239.

    B.P. Grubb, D.A. Wolfe, D. Samoil, et al., "Usefulness of Fluoxetine Hydrochloride for Prevention of Resistant Upright Tilt Induced Syncope," *Pacing and Clinical Electrophysiology* 16 (1993): 458–464.

    B.P. Grubb, D. Samoil, D. Kosinski, et al., "Use of Sertraline Hydrochloride in the Treatment of Refractory Neurocardiogenic Syncope in Children and Adolescents," *Journal of the American College of Cardiology* 24 (1994): 490–494.

18. I. Bou-Holaigah, P.C. Rowe, J. Kan, et al., "The Relationship Between Neurally Mediated Hypotension and the Chronic Fatigue Syndrome," *Journal of the American Medical Association* 274 (12) (27 September 1995): 961–967.

    P.C. Rowe, I. Bou-Holaigah, J.S. Kan, et al., op. cit.

    B.P. Grubb, D.A. Wolfe, D. Samoil, et al., op. cit.

    B.P. Grubb, D. Samoil, D. Kosinski, et al., op. cit.

19. P.C. Rowe, personal communication.

Johns Hopkins Hospital information sheet on neurally mediated hypotension.

20. A.W. Meikle, R.A. Daynes, B.A. Araneo, et al., "Adrenal Androgen Secretion and Biologic Effects," *Endocrine and Metabolic Clinics of North America* 20 (2) (June 1991): 381–421.

Parker, L.N., "Control of Adrenal Androgen Secretion," *Endocrine and Metabolic Clinics of North America* 20 (2) (June 1991): 401–421.

E. Barrett-Connor, R.T. Khaw, and S.C. Yen, "A Prospective Study of DHEA, Mortality and Cardiovascular Disease," *The New England Journal of Medicine* 315 (1986): 1519–1524.

21. G.R. Skinner, R. Thomas, M. Taylor, et al., "Thyroxine Should be Tried in Clinically Hypothyroid but Biochemically Euthyroid Patients," *British Medical Journal* 314 (7096) (14 June 1997): 1764.

22. G.R.B. Skinner, D. Holmes, A. Ahmad, et al., "Clinical Response to Thyroxine Sodium in Clinically Hypothyroid but Biochemically Euthyroid Patients." *Journal of Nutritional and Environmental Medicine* 10 (2) (June 2000): 115–125.

23. R.A. Nordyke, T.S. Reppun, L.D. Madanay, et al., "Alternative Sequences of Thyrotropin and Free Thyroxine Assays for Routine Thyroid Function Testing. Quality and Cost," *Archives of Internal Medicine* 158 (3) (9 February 1998): 266–272.

24. J. Teitelbaum and B. Bird, "Effective Treatment of Severe Chronic Fatigue: A Report of a Series of 64 Patients," op. cit.

25. J.G. Travell and D.G. Simons, *Myofascial Pain and Dysfunction: The Trigger Point Manual,* Vol. 1 (Baltimore, MD: Williams & Wilkins, 1983), pp. 103–164.

J. Travell, "Identification of Myofascial Trigger Point Syndromes: A Case of Atypical Facial Neuralgia," *Archives of Physical Medicine and Rehabilitation* 62 (1981): 100–106.

D.G. Simons, "Myofascial Pain Syndrome Due to Trigger Points," *International Rehabilitation Medicine Association Monograph Series* 1 (November 1987).

26. J.C. Lowe, R.L. Garrison, A.J. Reichman, et al., "Effectiveness and Safety of T_3 Therapy for Euthyroid Fibromyalgia: A Double-Blind, Placebo-Controlled Response Driven Crossover Study," *Clinical Bulletin of Myofascial Therapy* 2 (2/3) (1997): 31–58.

J.C. Lowe, A.J. Reichman, and J. Yellin, "The Process of Change During T_3 Treatment for Euthyroid Fibromyalgia: A Double-Blind, Placebo-Controlled, Crossover Study," *Clinical Bulletin of Myofascial Therapy* 2 (2/3) (1997): 91–124.

27. L. Hallberg, "Does Calcium Interfere with Iron Absorption?" editorial, *American Journal of Clinical Nutrition* 68 (1) (July 1998): 3–4.

28. M. Brock, *Acta Neurochirurgica* 47, supplement (1990): 127–128.

J.S. Jenkins, "The Role of Oxytocin: Present Concepts," *Clinical Endocrinology* 34 (1991): 515–525.

29. M.L. Vance, "Hypopituitarism," *The New England Journal of Medicine* 330 (23) (9 June 1994): 1651–1662.

30. S. Pillemer, L.A. Bradley, L.J. Crofford, et al., "The Neuroscience and Endocrinology of FMS—[An NIH] Conference Summary," *Arthritis and Rheumatism* 40 (11) (November 1997):1928–1939.

31. A.M.O. Bakheit, P.O. Behan, W.S. Watson, et al., "Abnormal Arginine-Vasopressin Secretion and Water Metabolism in Patients with Post-Viral Fatigue Syndrome," *Acta Neurologica Scandinavica* 87 (3) (March 1993): 234–238.

32. P.C. Rowe, H. Calkins, K. DeBusk, et al., "Fludrocortisone Acetate to Treat Neurally Mediated Hypotension in Chronic Fatigue Syndrome: A Randomized Controlled Trial," *Journal of the American Medical Association* 285 (1) (3 January 2001): 52–59.

33. A. Susmano, A.S. Volgman, and T.A. Buckingham, op. cit.

B.P. Grubb, D.A. Wolfe, D. Samoil, et al., op. cit.

B.P. Grubb, D. Samoil, D. Kosinski, et al., op. cit.

Chapter 4: When Your Defenses Are Down— Those Persistent Infections

1. J.R. Quesada, M. Talpaz, A. Rios, et al., "Clinical Toxicity of Interferon in Cancer Patients: A Review," *Journal of Clinical Oncology* 4 (February 1986): 234–243.

F. Adams, J.R. Quesada, and J.U. Gutterman, "Neuropsychiatric Manifestations of Human Leukocyte Interferon Therapy in Patients with Cancer," *Journal of the American Medical Association* 252 (7) (17 August 1984): 938–941.

2. A.W. Meikle, R.A. Daynes, B.A. Araneo, et al., "Adrenal Androgen Secretion and Biologic Effects," *Endocrine and Metabolic Clinics of North America* 20 (2) (June 1991): 381–421.

3. E. Barker, S.F. Fujimura, M.B. Fadem, et al., "Immunologic Abnormalities Associated with Chronic Fatigue Syndrome," *Clinical Infectious Diseases* 18, supplement 1 (1994): S136–S141.

T. Aoki, H. Miyakoshi, Y. Usuda, et al., "Low NK Syndrome and Its Relationship to Chronic Fatigue Syndrome," *Clinical Immunology and Immunopathology* 69 (December 1993): 253–265.

4. J. Savolainen, K. Lammintausta, K. Kalimo, et al., "Candida Albicans and Atopic Dermatitis," *Clinical Experimental Allergy* 23 (4) (April 1993): 332–339.

5. William G. Crook, *The Yeast Connection and the Woman* (Jackson, TN: Professional Books, 1995).

6. G. Reid, K. Millsap, and A.P. Bruce, "Implantation of *Lactobacillus casei* var. Rhamnosus into Vagina," *The Lancet* 344 (8931): 1229.

7. J. Edman, J.D. Sobel, and M.L. Taylor, "Zinc Status in Women with Recurrent Vulvovaginal Candidiasis," *American Journal of Obstetrics and Gynecology* 155 (1986): 1082–1088.

   R. Boyne, *Journal of Nutrition* 116 (1982): 816–822.

8. J. Avorn, M. Monane, J.H. Gurwitz, et al., "Reduction of Bacteriuria and Pyuria After Ingestion of Cranberry Juice." *Journal of the American Medical Association* 271 (10) (9 March 1994): 751–754.

9. Procter and Gamble Pharmaceuticals, in-house research data.

10. R.J. Deckelbaum, "ELISA More Accurate Than Microscopy for Giardia," *Infectious Diseases in Children,* October 1993, p. 30.

11. G.P. Holmes, J.E. Kaplan, N.M. Gantz, et al., "Chronic Fatigue Syndrome: A Working Case Definition," *Annals of Internal Medicine* 108 (1988): 387–389.

    L. Galland, M. Lee, H. Bueno, et al., "Giardia as a Cause of Chronic Fatigue," *Journal of Nutritional Medicine 1* (1990): 27–32.

    Ann Louise Gittleman, *Guess What Came to Dinner: Parasites and Your Health* (Garden City Park, NY: Avery Publishing Group, 1993).

    D.G. Simons, "Myofascial Pain Syndrome Due to Trigger Points," *International Rehabilitation Medicine Association Monograph Series I* (November 1987).

    J.G. Travell and D.G. Simons, *Myofascial Pain and Dysfunction: The Trigger Point Manual,* Vol. I (Baltimore, MD: Williams & Wilkins, 1983), pp. 103–164.

12. L. Galland, M. Lee, H. Bueno, et al., op. cit.

    Ann Louise Gittleman, op. cit.

    D.G. Simons, op. cit.

    J.G. Travell and D. G. Simons, op. cit.

13. W.C. Reeves, F.R. Stamey, J.B. Black, et al., "Human Herpesviruses 6 and 7 in Chronic Fatigue Syndrome: A Case-Control Study," *Clinical Infectious Diseases* 31 (1) (July 2000): 48–52.

14. A. Martin Lerner, Marcus Zervos, Howard J. Dworkin, et al., "New Cardiomyopathy: Pilot Study of Intravenous Ganciclovir in a Subset of the Chronic Fatigue Syndrome," *Infectious Disease in Clinical Practice* 6 (1997): 110–117.

15. S.E. Straus, J.K. Dale, M. Tobi, et al., "Acyclovir Treatment of the Chronic Fatigue Syndrome. Lack of Efficacy in a Placebo-Controlled Trial," *The New England Journal of Medicine* 319 (26) (29 December 1988): 1692–1698.

16. S. Naylor, "Role of Fungi in Allergic Fungal Sinusitis and Chronic Rhinosinusitis, *Mayo Clinic Proceedings* 75 (5) (May 2000): 540–541.

17. Ibid.

Chapter 5: Fibromyalgia—The Aching-All-Over Disease

1. J.G. Travell and D.G. Simons, *Myofascial Pain and Dysfunction: The Trigger Point Manual,* Vol. 1 (Baltimore, MD: Williams & Wilkins, 1983), pp. 103–164.

2. G.A. McCain and K.S. Tilbe, "Diurnal Hormone Variation in Fibromyalgia Syndrome and a Comparison with Rheumatoid Arthritis," *Journal of Rheumatology* 25 (1993): 469–474.

3. G. Neeck and W. Riedel, "Thyroid Function in Patients with Fibromyalgia Syndrome," *Journal of Rheumatology* 19 (7) (July 1992): 1120–1122.

   J. Teitelbaum and B. Bird, "Effective Treatment of Severe Chronic Fatigue: A Report of a Series of 64 Patients," *Journal of Musculoskeletal Pain* 3 (4) (1995): 91–110.

   J.E. Teitelbaum, B. Bird, R.M. Greenfield, et al., "Effective Treatment of CFS and FMS: A Randomized, Double-Blind Placebo Controlled Study," *Journal of Chronic Fatigue Syndrome* 8 (2) (2001).

4. H. Moldofsky, "Sleep and Chronic Fatigue Syndrome," in *Chronic Fatigue Syndrome,* ed. D. Dawson and S. Sabin (Boston, MA: Little, Brown and Company, 1993).

5. R.M. Bennett, R.A. Gatter, S.M. Campbell, et al., "Cyclobenzaprine Versus Placebo in Fibromyalgia," *Arthritis and Rheumatism* 31 (December 1988): 1535–1542.

   R.A. Gatter, "Pharmacotherapeutics in Fibromyalgia," *American Journal of Medicine* 81 (3A) (29 September 1986): 63–66.

6. H. Dressing and D. Riemann, "Insomnia: Are Valerian/ Melissa Combinations of Equal Value to Benzodiazepine?" *Therapiewoche* 42 (1992): 726–736.

Chapter 6: A Good Night's Sleep— The Foundation of Getting Well

1. C.A. Everson, "Sustained Sleep Deprivation Impairs Host Defense," *The American Journal of Physiology* 265 (5 Part 2) (November 1993): R1148–R1154.

2. S. Pillemer, L.A. Bradley, L.J. Crofford, et al., "The Neuroscience and Endocrinology of FMS–[An NIH] Conference Summary," *Arthritis and Rheumatism* 40 (11) (November 1997):1928–1939.

3. Ibid.

4. H. Moldofsky and P. Scarisbrick, "Induction of Neuresthenic Musculoskeletal Pain Syndrome by Selective Sleep Stage Deprivation," *Psychosomatic Medicine* 38 (1) (January-February 1976): 35–44.

A.M. Drewes, K.D. Nielson, S.J. Taagholt, et al., "Slow Wave Sleep in FMS," abstract, *Journal of Musculoskeletal Pain* 3 (Supplement 1) (1995): 29.

5. H. Dressing and D. Riemann, "Insomnia: Are Valerian/ Melissa Combinations of Equal Value to Benzodiazepine?" *Therapiewoche* 42 (1992): 726–736.

6. R. Cluydt, "Insomnia Treatment—A Postgraduate Medicine Special Report," 114–123.

7. B.P. Grubb, D.A. Wolfe, D. Samoil, et al., "Usefulness Of Fluoxetine HCL For Prevention of Resistant Upright Tilt Induced Syncope," *Pacing and Clinical Electrophysiology* 16 (1993): 458–464.

8. N.C. Netzer, R.A. Stoohs, C.M. Netzer, et al., "Using the Berlin Questionnaire to Identify Patients at Risk for Sleep Apnea Syndrome," *Annals of Internal Medicine* 131 (7) 5 October 1999): 485–491.

9. Millman, R.P, "Do You Ever Take A Sleep History?" *Annals of Internal Medicine* 131 (7) (October 1999): 535–536.

10. E.G. Lutz, "Restless Legs, Anxiety and Caffeinism," *Journal of Clinical Psychiatry* 39 (9) (September 1978): 693–698.

11. H.J. Roberts, "Spontaneous Leg Cramps and Restless Legs Due to Diabetogenic (Functional) Hyperinsulinism: A Basis For Natural Therapy," *Journal of the Florida Medical Association* 60 (5) (1973): 29–31.

12. K.A. Ekbom, "Restless Leg Syndrome," *Neurology* 10 (1960): 868–873.

13. S. Ayres and R. Michan, "Restless Leg Syndrome:Response to Vitamin E," *Journal of Applied Nutrition* 25 (1973): 8–15.

14. M.I. Boutez, et al., "Neuropsychological Correlates of Folic Acid Deficiency: Facts and Hypothesis," in *Folic Acid and Neurology, Psychiatry and Internal Medicine,* ed. M.I. Boutez and E.K. Reynolds (New York, NY: Raven Press, 1979).

Chapter 7: Pain, Pain, Go Away—
Natural and Prescription Pain Relief

1. K.C. Srivastava and T. Mustafa, "Ginger (Zingiber officinale) in Rheumatism and Musculoskeletal Disorders," *Medical Hypotheses* 39 (4) (December 1992): 342–348.

Chapter 8: Jump-Starting Your Body's Energy Furnaces

1. P.O. Behan, "Post-Viral Fatigue Syndrome Research," in *The Clinical and Scientific Basis of Myalgic Encephalitis and Chronic Fatigue Syndrome,* ed. Byron Hyde, Jay Goldstein, and Paul Levine (Ottawa, Ontario, Canada: Nightingale Research Foundation, 1992), p. 238.

2. J.T. Hicks, "Treatment of Fatigue: A Double Blind Study," *Clinical Medicine,* January 1964; pp. 85–90.

   D.L. Shaw, et al., "Management of Fatigue," *American Journal of Medical Science,* June 1962, pp. 758–769.

   C.A. Kruse, "Treatment of Fatigue with Aspartic Acid Salts," *Northwest Medicine,* June 1961, pp. 597–603.

   A. Gaby, "Potassium-Magnesium Aspartate," *Nutrition and Healing,* October 1995, pp. 3–11.

3. J.T. Hicks, op. cit.

4. D.L. Shaw, et al., op. cit.

   J.T. Hicks, op. cit.

5. A. Gaby, op. cit.

6. Byron Hyde, Jay Goldstein, and Paul Levine, eds., *The Clinical and Scientific Basis of Myalgic Encephalitis and Chronic Fatigue Syndrome* (Ottawa, ON: Nightingale Research Foundation, 1992).

7. J. Eisenger, *L.M.M. Medicine du-sud-est* 25 (7/8) (April 1989): 12371.

   J. Eisenger, "Transketolase Stimulation in Fibromyalgia," *Journal of the American College of Nutrition* 9 (1) (1990): 56–57.

8. J. Eisenger, "Transketolase Stimulation in Fibromyalgia," op. cit.

9. A.V. Plioplys and S. Plioplys, "Amantadine and L-Carnitine Treatment of Chronic Fatigue Syndrome," *Neuropsychobiology* 35 (1) (1997): 16–23.

H. Kuratsune, K. Yamaguti, M. Takahashi, et al., "Acylcarnitine Deficiency in Chronic Fatigue Syndrome," *Clinical Infectious Disease* 18 (3 Supplement 1) (January 1994): S62–S67.

10. V. Tanphaichitr and P. Leelahagul, "Carnitine Metabolism and Human Carnitine Deficiency," review article, *Nutrition* 9 (3) (May-June 1993): 246–252.

11. R.E. Keith, "Symptoms of Carnitine Like Deficiency in a Trained Runner Taking DL-Carnitine Supplements," letter, *Journal of the American Medical Association* 255 (9) (7 March 1986): 1137.

12. H.E.F. Davies, et al., "Ascorbic Acid and Carnitine in Man," *Nutrition Reports International* 36 (1987): 941.

13. J.G.D. Birkmayer, "NADH: The Energizing Coenzyme," pamphlet (New York, NY: Menuco Corporation, 1996).

    J.G.D. Birkmayer, interview, *Clinical Pearl News* 7 (1) (January 1997): 1–2.

    J.G.D. Birkmayer, "Coenzyme Nicotinamide Adenine Dinucleotide: New Therapeutic Approach for Improving Dementia of Alzheimer's Type." *Annals of Clinical and Laboratory Science* 26 (1) (January-February 1996): 1–9.

14. Daniel Malone, N. Wei, and P. Hitzig, "Treatment of 76 Patients with Primary FMS with Combined Dopaminergic and Serotonergic Drugs," abstract submitted to the Annual Scientific Meeting of the American College of Rheumatology, 1996.

15. J.G.D. Birkmayer, "The Coenzyme Nicotinamide Adenine Dinucleotide as a Biological Antidepressive Agent," *New Trends in Clinical Neuropharmacology*; 5 (1991): 19–25.

16. J.G.D. Birkmayer, C. Vreko, D. Volc, et al., "Nicotinamide Adenine Dinucleotide (NADH)—A New Therapeutic Approach to Parkinson's Disease. Comparison of Oral and Parenteral Application," *Acta Neurologica Scandinavica* 146 (Supplement) (1993): 32–35.

17. Wayne M. Becker, Jane B. Reece, Martin F. Poenie, et al., *The World of The Cell*, 3rd Edition (San Francisco, CA: Benjamin Cummings, 1996).

18. J.D. Loike, D.L. Zalutsky, E. Kaback, et al., "Extracellular Creatine Regulates Creatine Transport in Rat and Human Muscle Cells," *Proceeds of the National Academy of Sciences USA* 85 (3) (February 1988): 807–811.

19. P.L. Greenhaff, A. Casey, A.H. Short, et al., "Influence of Oral Creatine Supplementation on Muscle Torque During Repeated Bouts of Maximal Exercise in Man," *Clinical Science*; 84 (5) (May 1993): 565–571.

    Glenn Caldwell, personal communication, 8 March 1996.

20. P.L. Greenhaff, "Creatine and its Application as an Ergogenic Aid," *International Journal of Sports Nutrition* 5 (Supplement) (1995): 100–110.

21. M. Harris, et al., "Alterations in Leg Extension Power of Meat Eating and Non-Meat Eating (Vegetarian) Females with Creatine Supplementation," updated, poster presentation, Proceedings of Experimental Biology, Federation of American Societies for Experimental Biology, Anaheim, CA, 24–28 April 1994.

22. Laurie Gould, personal communication, 21 April 1997.

    Glenn Caldwell, personal communication, 8 March 1996.

    Ray Sahelian, *Creatine: Nature's Muscle Builder* (Garden City Park, NY: Avery Publishing Group, 1997), p. 104.

23. P.L. Greenhaff, "Creatine and its Application as an Ergogenic Aid," op. cit.

24. K. Folkers, S. Shizukuishi, K. Takemura, et al., "Increase in Levels of IgG in Serum of Patients Treated with Coenzyme Q_{10}," *Research Communications in Chemical Pathology and Pharmacology* 38 (2) (1982): 335–338.

    K. Folkers, P. Langsjoen, Y. Nara, et al., "Biochemical Deficiencies of Coenzyme Q_{10} in HIV Infection and Exploratory Treatment," *Biochemical and Biophysical Research Communications* 153 (2) (1988): 888–896.

    K. Lockwood, S. Moesgaadr, T. Hanoike, et al., "Apparent Partial Remission of Breast Cancer in "High Risk" Patients Supplemented with Nutritional Antioxidants, Essential Fatty Acids and Coenzyme Q_{10}," *Molecular Aspects of Medicine* 15 (Supplement) (1994): S231–S240.

    K. Lockwood, S. Moesgaard, T. Yamamoto, et al., "Progress on Therapy of Breast Cancer with Coenzyme Q_{10} and the Regression of Metastases," *Biochemical and Biophysical Research Communications* 212 (1) (6 July 1995): 172–177.

    P. Mayer, H. Hamberger, and J. Drew, "Differential Effects of Ubiquinone Q_7 and Ubiquinone Analogs on Macrophage Activation and Experimental Infections in Granulocytopenic Mice," *Infection* 8 (1980): 256–261.

    E. Bliznakov, A. Casey, and E. Premuzic, "Coenzymes Q: Stimulants of Phagocytic Activity in Rats and Immune Response in Mice," *Experientia* 26 (1970): 953–954.

25. L. Van Gaal, I.D. de Leeuw, S. Vadhanavikit, et al., "Exploratory Study of Coenzyme Q_{10} in Obesity," in K. Folkers and Y. Yamamura, eds., *Biomedical and Clinical Aspects of Coenzyme Q*, Vol. 4 (New York, NY: Elsevier Publishers, 1984), pp. 235–373.

26. A. Gaby, "The Role of Coenzyme Q_{10} in Clinical Medicine. Part I," *Alternative Medicine Review* 1 (1) (1996): 11–17.

27. Y. Ishihara, Y. Uchida, S. Kitamura, et al., "Effect of Coenzyme Q_{10}, a Quinone Derivative, on Guinea Pig Lung and Tracheal Tissue," *Arzneimittelforschung* 35 (1985): 929–933.

Chapter 9: More Natural Remedies

1. K.C. Srivastava and T. Mustafa, "Ginger (Zingiber officinale) in Rheumatism and Musculoskeletal Disorders," *Medical Hypotheses* 39 (4) (December 1992): 342–348.

2. A. Tamborini and R. Taurelle, "Value of Standardized Ginkgo Biloba Extract (EGb 761) in the Management of Congestive Symptoms of Premenstrual Syndrome," *Revue Francaise de gynecologie et d'Obstetrique* 88 (7-9) (July-September 1993): 447–457.

3. J.P. Haguenauer, F. Cantenot, H. Koskas, et al., "Treatment of Equilibrium Disturbances with Ginkgo Biloba—A Multicenter, Placebo Controlled Study," *Presse Medicale* 15 (31) (25 September 1986): 1569–1572.

   P.F. Smith and C.L. Darlington, "Can Vestibular Compensation Be Enhanced by Drug Treatment: A Review of Recent Evidence," review, *Journal of Vestibular Research* 4 (3) (May-June 1994): 169–179.

4. E. Grassel, "Effect of Ginkgo Biloba Extract on Mental Performance," *Fortschritte der Medizin* 110 (5) (February 1992): 73–76.

   W. Hopfenmuller, "Proof of the Therapeutic Effectiveness of a Ginkgo Biloba Extract—A Meta Analysis of 11 [Placebo Controlled] Trials in Aged Patients with Cerebral Insufficiency," *Arzneimittel-Forschung* 44 (9) (September 1994): 1005–1010.

   I. Hindmarch, "Activity of Ginkgo Biloba Extract on Short Term Memory," *Presse Medicale* 15 (31) (September 1986): 1592-1594.

5. Y.N. Singh and M. Blumenthal. "Kava: An Overview." *Herbalgram* 39 (Spring 1997): 33–55.

   Gary Piscopo, "Kava Kava: Gift of the Islands," *Alternative Medicine Review* 2 (5) (1997): 355–364.

6. Ibid.

7. Ibid.

8. Ibid.

9. Ibid.

10. D.F. Neri, D.Wiegmann, R.R. Stanny, et al., "The Effects of Tyrosine on Cognitive Performance During Extended Wakefulness," *Aviation, Space, and Environmental Medicine* 66 (4) (1995): 313–319.

11. R.H. Wolbling, et al., "Local Therapy of Herpes Simplex with Dried Extract From Melisa Officianalis," *Phyto Medicine* 1 (1994): 25–31.

12. W. Rees, B.K. Evans, and J. Rhodes, "Treating Irritable Bowel Syndrome with Peppermint Oil," *British Medical Journal* 2 (6194) (6 October 1979): 835–836.

Chapter 10: *Other Areas to Explore*

1. S.B. Miller, "IgG Food Allergy Testing by ELISA/EIA—What Do They Really Tell Us," *Townsend Letter for Doctors and Patients,* January 1998, pp. 62–66, 106.

2. R.M. Jaffe, "A Novel Treatment for Fibromyalgia Improves Clinical Outcomes in a Community Based Study," study presented before the American Association for the Advancement of Science, Baltimore, MD, 9 February 1996.

3. Sherry Rogers, *Tired or Toxic* (Syracuse, NY: Prestige Publishing, 1990).

   S. Rogers, "Chemical Sensitivity: Breaking the Paralyzing Paradigm. Part I.," *Internal Medicine World Report* 7 (3): 1.

   S. Rogers, op. cit.

4. A.C. Chester, "Chronic Fatigue of Nasal Origin: Possible Confusion with Chronic Fatigue Syndrome," in *The Clinical and Scientific Basis of Myalgic Encephalitis and Chronic Fatigue Syndrome,* ed. B.M. Hyde (Ottawa, Ontario, Canada: Nightingale Research Foundation, 1992), pp. 260–266.

5. J. Liebermann and D.S. Bell, "Serum Angiotensin-Converting Enzyme as a Marker for the Chronic Fatigue-Immune Dysfunction Syndrome: A Comparison to Serum Angiotensin-Converting Enzyme in Sarcordosis," *American Journal of Medicine* 95 (1993): 407–412.

6. Conference handout, Chronic Fatigue and Immune Dysfunction Syndrome Conference. Sponsored by the Chronic Fatigue and Immune Dysfunction Syndrome Association of America, Fort Lauderdale, FL, 7–9 October 1994.

   J. Goldstein, "Fibromyalgia Syndrome: A Pain Modulation Disorder Related to Altered Limbic Function?" *Bailliere's Clinical Rheumatology* 8 (November 1994): 777–800.

7. J. Goldstein, op. cit.

8. S. Ruhrmann and S. Kasper, "Seasonal Depression," *Medizinische Monatsschrift für Pharmazeuten* 15 (1992): 293–299.

Chapter 11: *Am I Crazy?*

1. H. Smythe, "Fibrositis Continues to Present Clinical Challenges," Rheumatology for the Practicing Physician, January 1989, pp. 13–14.

   E.N. Griep, J.N. Boersma, and E.R. de Kloet, "Altered Reactivity of the Hypothalamic-Pituitary Axis in the Primary Fibromyalgia Syndrome," *Journal of Rheumatology* 20 (3) (March 1993): 469–474.

Appendix A: For Physicians

1. F. Wolfe, K. Ross, J. Anderson, et al., "The Prevalence and Characteristics of Fibromyalgia in the General Population," *Arthritis and Rheumatism* 38 (1) (January 1995): 19–28.

2. J. Teitelbaum and B. Bird, "Effective Treatment of Severe Chronic Fatigue: A Report of a Series of 64 Patients," *Journal of Musculoskeletal Pain* 3 (4) (1995): 91–110.

   J.E. Teitelbaum, B. Bird, R.M. Greenfield, et al., "Effective Treatment of CFS and FMS: A Randomized, Double-Blind Placebo Controlled Study," *Journal of Chronic Fatigue Syndrome* 8 (2) (2001).

3. M.A. Demitrack, K. Dale, S.E. Straus, et al., "Evidence for Impaired Activation of the Hypothalamic-Pituitary-Adrenal Axis in Patients with Chronic Fatigue Syndrome," *Journal of Clinical Endocrinology and Metabolism* 73 (6) (December 1991): 1223–1234.

   J. Teitelbaum, "Estrogen and Testosterone in CFIDS/FMS," *The From Fatigued To Fantastic Newsletter,"* February 1997.

   P.O. Behan, "Post-Viral Fatigue Syndrome Research," in *The Clinical and Scientific Basis of Myalgic Encephalitis and Chronic Fatigue Syndrome,* ed. Byron Hyde, Jay Goldstein, and Paul Levine (Ottawa, Ontario, Canada: Nightingale Research Foundation, 1992), p. 238.

4. P.O. Behan, op. cit.

5. G. Faglia, L. Bitensky, A. Pinchera, et al., "Thyrotropin Secretion in Patients with Central Hypothyroidism: Evidence for Reduced Biological Activity of Immunoreactive Thyrotropin," *Journal of Clinical Endocrinology and Metabolism* 48 (6) (June 1979) 989–998.

6. G.R.B. Skinner, D. Holmes, A. Ahmad, et al., "Clinical Response to Thyroxine Sodium in Clinically Hypothyroid but Biochemically Euthyroid Patients,*" Journal of Nutritional and Environmental Medicine* 10 (2) (June 2000): 115–125.

   R.A. Nordyke, T.S. Reppun, L.D. Madanay, et al., "Alternative Sequences of Thyrotropin and Free Thyroxine Assays For Routine Thyroid Function Testing. Quality and Cost," *Archives of Internal Medicine* 158 (3) (9 February 1998): 266–272.

7. G.R.B. Skinner, D. Holmes, A. Ahmad, et al., op. cit.

8. M.A. Demitrack, K. Dale, S.E. Straus, et al., op. cit.

   E.N. Griep, J.N. Boersma, and E.R. de Kloet, "Altered Reactivity of the Hypothalamic-Pituitary Axis in the Primary Fibromyalgia Syndrome," *Journal of Rheumatology* 20 (3) (March 1993): 469–474.

G.A. McCain and K.S. Tilbe, "Diurnal Hormone Variation in Fibromyalgia Syndrome and a Comparison with Rheumatoid Arthritis," *Journal of Rheumatology* 25 (1993): 469–474.

9. W.M. Jefferies, *Safe Uses of Cortisol,* 2nd edition, monograph (Springfield, IL: Charles C. Thomas, 1996).

10. W.M. Jefferies, "Low-Dosage Glucocorticoid Therapy. An Appraisal of Its Safety and Mode of Action in Clinical Disorders, Including Rheumatoid Arthritis," *Archives of Internal Medicine* 119 (3) (March 1967): 265–278.

11. J. Teitelbaum and B. Bird, "Effective Treatment of Severe Chronic Fatigue: A Report of a Series of 64 Patients," op. cit.

W.M. Jefferies, *Safe Uses of Cortisol,* op. cit.

12. J.E. Teitelbaum, B. Bird, A. Weiss, et al., "Low Dose Hydrocortisone for Chronic Fatigue Syndrome," *Journal of the American Medical Association* 281 (1999): 1887–1888.

13. J.E. Teitelbaum, B. Bird, R.M. Greenfield, A. Weiss, L. Muenz, and L. Gould, "Effective Treatment of CFS and FMS: A Randomized, Double-Blind Placebo Controlled Study," op. cit.

14. W.M. Jefferies, *Safe Uses of Cortisol,* op. cit.

15. A.J. Morales, J.J. Nolan, J.C. Nelson, et al., "Effects of Replacement Dose of Dehydroepiandrosterone in Men and Women of Advancing Age, *Journal of Clinical Endocrinology and Metabolism* 78 (6) (June 1994): 1360–1367.

16. Elizabeth Lee Vliet, *Screaming To Be Heard: Hormone Connections Women Suspect . . . and Doctors Ignore* (New York, NY: M. Evans and Company, 1995).

17. Ibid.

18. Ibid.

19. Conference on the Neuroscience and Endocrinology of Fibromyalgia Syndrome, sponsored by the National Institutes of Health, 16–17 July 1996.

20. H. Dressing and D. Riemann, "Insomnia: Are Valerian/Melissa Combinations of Equal Value to Benzodiazepine?" *Therapiewoche* 42 (1992); 726–736.

21. M.B. Yunus and J.C. Aldag, "Restless Legs Syndrome and Leg Cramps in Fibromyalgia Syndrome: A Controlled Study," *British Medical Journal* 312 (7042) (25 May 1996): 1339.

22. P.C. Rowe, I. Bou-Holaigah, J.S. Kan, et al., "Is Neurally Mediated Hypotension an Unrecognized Cause of Chronic Fatigue?" *The Lancet* 345 (8950) (11 March 1995): 623–624.

23. Robert S. Ivker, *Sinus Survival* (New York, NY: Tarcher/Putnam, 2000).

24. J. Teitelbaum and B. Bird, "Effective Treatment of Severe Chronic Fatigue: A Report of a Series of 64 Patients," op. cit.

25. Wayne M. Becker, Jane B. Reece, Martin F. Poenie, et al., *The World of The Cell,* 3rd Edition (San Francisco, CA: Benjamin Cummings, 1996).

    J.Teitelbaum, "Mitochondrial Dysfunction [in CFS/FMS]," *From Fatigued to Fantastic Newsletter,* 1 (2) (1997).

26. B. Regland, M. Andersson, L. Abrahamsson, et al., "Increased Concentrations of Homocysteine in the Cerebrospinal Fluid in Patients with Fibromyalgia and Chronic Fatigue Syndrome," *Scandinavian Journal of Rheumatology* 26 (4) (1997) 301–307.

27. J. Lindenbaum, I.H. Rosenberg, P.W. Wilson, et al., "Prevalence of Cobalamin Deficiency in the Framingham Elderly Population," *American Journal of Clinical Nutrition* 60 (1) July 1994): 2–11.

28. J. Lindenbaum, E.B. Healton, D.G. Savage, et al., "Neuropsychiatric Disorders Caused by Cobalamin Deficiency in the Absence of Anemia or Macrocytoses," *The New England Journal of Medicine* 318 (26) (30 June 1988): 1720–1728.

29. W.S. Beck, "Cobalmin and the Nervous System," editorial, *The New England Journal of Medicine* 318 (26), (30 June 1988): 1752–1754.

30. J.Teitelbaum, "Mitochondrial Dysfunction [in CFS/FMS]," *From Fatigued to Fantastic Newsletter,* 1 (2) (1997).

31. W.S. Beck, op. cit.

32. J. Teitelbaum and B. Bird, op. cit.

    J.E. Teitelbaum, B. Bird, R.M. Greenfield, et al., "Effective Treatment of CFS and FMS: A Randomized, Double-Blind Placebo Controlled Study," op. cit.

Appendix B: Studies of Treatment Modalities for Chronic Fatigue and Fibromyalgia

STUDY #1. EFFECTIVE TREATMENT OF FIBROMYALGIA AND CHRONIC FATIGUE SYNDROME—A RANDOMIZED, DOUBLE-BLIND STUDY

References for this study can be found beginning on page 244.

STUDY #2. EFFECTIVE TREATMENT OF SEVERE CHRONIC FATIGUE: A REPORT OF A SERIES OF 64 PATIENTS

1. R.K. Price, C.S. North, S. Wessely, et al., "Estimating the Presence of Chronic Fatigue Syndrome in the Community," *Public Health Reports* 107 (September-October 1992): 514–522.

2. R.B. Marchesani, "Critical Antiviral Pathway Deficient in Chronic Fatigue Syndrome Patients," *Infectious Disease News,* August 1993, p. 4.

3. D.L. Goldenberg, "Fibromyalgia Syndrome: An Emerging but Controversial Condition," *Journal of the American Medical Association* 257 (1987): 2782–2787.

4. W. Jefferies, *Safe Uses of Cortisol,* monograph (Springfield, IL: Charles C. Thomas, 1981).

5. W.M. Jefferies, "Low-Dosage Glucocorticoid Therapy. An Appraisal of Its Safety and Mode of Action in Clinical Disorders, Including Rheumatoid Arthritis," *Archives of Internal Medicine* 119 (3) (March 1967): 265–278.

6. Michael Rosenbaum and Murry Susser, *Solving the Puzzle of Chronic Fatigue Syndrome* (Tacoma, WA: Life Sciences Press, 1992).

7. Medical Letter 34 (14 February 1992).

8. E.M. Sternberg, "Hyperimmune Fatigue Syndromes: Disease of the Stress Response?" editorial, *Journal of Rheumatology* 20 (3) (March 1993): 418–421.

9. G. Neeck and W. Riedel, "Thyroid Function in Patients with Fibromyalgia Syndrome," *Journal of Rheumatology* 19 (7) (July 1992): 1120–1122.

10. M.A. Demitrack, K. Dale, S.E. Straus, et al., "Evidence for Impaired Activation of the Hypothalamic-Pituitary-Adrenal Axis in Patients with Chronic Fatigue Syndrome," *Journal of Clinical Endocrinology and Metabolism* 73 (6) (December 1991): 1223–1234.

11. A.M.O. Bakheit, P.O. Behan, T.G. Dinan, et al., "Possible Upregulation of Hypothalamic 5-HT Receptors in Patients with Postviral Fatigue Syndrome," *BMJ* 304 (6833) (18 April 1992): 1010–1012.

12. E.N. Griep, J.N. Boersma, and E.R. de Kloet, "Altered Reactivity of the Hypothalamic-Pituitary Axis in the Primary Fibromyalgia Syndrome," *Journal of Rheumatology* 20 (3) (March 1993): 469–474.

13. G.A. McCain and K.S. Tilbe, "Diurnal Hormone Variation in Fibromyalgia Syndrome and a Comparison with Rheumatoid Arthritis," *Journal of Rheumatology* 25 (1993): 469–474.

14. J.R. Quesada, M. Talpaz, A. Rios, et al., "Clinical Toxicity of Interferon in Cancer Patients: A Review," *Journal of Clinical Oncology* 4 (February 1986): 234–243.

15. F. Adams, J.R. Quesada, and J.U. Gutterman, "Neuropsychiatric Manifestations of Human Leukocyte Interferon Therapy in Patients with Cancer," *Journal of the American Medical Association* 252 (7) (17 August 1984): 938–941.

16. A.W. Meikle, R.A. Daynes, B.A. Araneo, et al., "Adrenal Androgen Secretion and Biologic Effects," *Endocrine and Metabolic Clinics of North America* 20 (2) (June 1991): 381–421.

17. J.G. Travell and D.G. Simons, *Myofascial Pain and Dysfunction: The Trigger Point Manual,* Vol. I (Baltimore, MD: Williams & Wilkins, 1983), pp. 103–164.

18. J. Lindenbaum, E.B. Healton, D.G. Savage, et al., "Neuropsychiatric Disorders Caused by Cobalamin Deficiency in the Absence of Anemia or Macrocytoses," *The New England Journal of Medicine* 318 (26) (30 June 1988): 1720–1728.

19. R. Carmel, "Pernicious Anemia—The Expected Findings of Very Low Serum Cobalamin Levels, Anemia and Macrocytosis Are Often Lacking," *Archives of Internal Medicine* 148 (8) (August 1988): 1712–1714.

20. E.J. Norman and J.A. Morrison, " Screening Elderly Populations for Cobalamin (Vitamin B_{12}) Deficiency Using Urinary Methylmalonic Acid Assay by Gas Chromatography Mass Spectrometry," *American Journal of Medicine* 94 (6) (June 1993): 589–594.

21. J. Lindenbaum, I.H. Rosenberg, P.W. Wilson, et al., "Prevalence of Cobalamin Deficiency in the Framingham Elderly Population," *American Journal of Clinical Nutrition* 60 (1) (July 1994): 2–11.

22. S.E. Straus, S. Fritz, J.K. Dale, et al., "Lymphocyte Phenotype and Function in the Chronic Fatigue Syndrome," *Journal of Clinical Immunology* 13 (1) (January 1993): 30–40.

Appendix F: Stone Agers in the Fast Lane: An Evolutionary Approach to Fibromyalgia

1. Randolf M. Nesse and George C. Williams, *Why We Get Sick: The New Science of Darwinian Medicine,* (New York, NY: Vintage, 1994), p. 7. The title, "Stone Agers in the Fast Lane," as well as many of examples I use in this article come from this book. After a number of stimulating discussions with Bruno D'Udine (formerly senior researcher of the Italian National Research Council responsible for bilateral research projects with the Universities of Cambridge and Edinburgh, and presently at Parma University, Italy), I was encouraged to write this article on fibromyalgia. Along with many other important articles and books, he recommended that I read Nesse and William's work in evolutionary medicine. I am grateful for his support and untiring efforts at pointing me in all the right directions. I also especially want to thank Jacob Teitelbaum, M.D., and Thomas Romano, M.D., for reading an earlier version of this paper and offering their thoughtful criticisms and insights.

2. Ibid., pp. 88-90.

3. Ibid., p. 10.

4. Ibid., p. 243.

5. Jacob Teitelbaum, M.D., *From Fatigued to Fantastic*, (Garden City Park, NY: Avery Publishing Group, 1996).

6. Ibid., p. 74.

7. John H. Crook, *The Evolution of Human Consciousness*, (Oxford, 1980), pp. 285–292.

8. Ibid., p. 291.

9. Nesse and Williams, op. cit., p. 213.

10. Ibid., p. 213.

11. Jeffrey Maitland, *Spacious Body: Explorations in Somatic Ontology*, (Berkeley, CA: North Atlantic Books, 1995). See especially Chapters Two and Three for an explication of intentionality and a theory of emotion that includes an analysis of the important differences between fear and anxiety. Fear and anxiety are obviously related physiologically, but phenomenologically they are quite different. Fibromyalgia is not a panic or anxiety disorder, even though panic attacks and anxiety are often experienced in this disorder. My attempt in this article is to consolidate the proximate and broader evolutionary explanations within a phenomenological perspective in an effort to show how fibromyalgia is an existential condition rooted in a maladaptive fear response that is constantly being triggered by the sufferer's world. The proximate and evolutionary explanations show that fibromyalgia is a fear disorder that begins in the nervous system and ultimately compromises the entire person. The phenomenological perspective shows how fibromyalgia is a problematic way of being-in-the-world—an existential condition that involves the whole person in relation to his or her way of living a world gone awry.

   From the point of view of how to treat fibromyalgia, this broader evolutionary and phenomenological perspective is important for two related reasons: 1) it explains why any corrective treatment protocol that addresses this disorder symptom by symptom cannot be effective, and 2) it supports and explains why the holistic approach to fibromyalgia is so critically important to its proper treatment.

12. Nesse and Williams, op. cit., p. 217.

13. Some studies suggest an important link between the central nervous system and chronic fatigue. Researchers John LaManca, Ph.D., and Benjamin Natelson, M.D., compared the ability to concentrate of patients with chronic fatigue to normal controls after exercise. They found that the cognitive functioning of chronic fatigue patients was significantly impaired. One hour after exercise their ability to concentrate was significantly impaired and twenty-four hours later it had diminished even further.

Daniel Clauw, M.D., discovered that not only is pain sensitivity increased in the peripheral muscles of people with fibromyalgia but also in their smooth muscles of the viscera. Both of these discoveries point in the direction of CNS dysfunction in fibromyalgia. These results were reported in the *Fibromyalgia Network*, 36th edition, January, 1997, Tucson, Arizona, p. 7 and p. 10 respectively. I am grateful to my colleague and well-known expert in chronic fatigue and fibromyalgia syndrome Darice Putterman, P.T., who shared the above research with me. Her valuable insights and knowledge have been of great benefit to me in writing this article.

14. My understanding of the immobilization response to shock-trauma comes from the pioneering work of Dr. Peter Levine, a physiological psychologist, therapist, and Rolfer, and my fellow instructor at the Rolf Institute of Structural Integration who is also a gifted trauma specialist, William Smythe. For more information on this important work, see Peter Levine's *Waking the Tiger: Healing Trauma* (Berkeley, 1997). Also important to my understanding of the sympathetic and parasympathetic response is the work of researcher, Rolfer, and physical therapist, John Cottingham. Cottingham and his colleague Steven Porges, a physiological psychologist, were able to demonstrate that the application of the Rolfing holistic approach of manual therapy not only changed structure, but also significantly boosted the parasympathetic response. There are many important insights to be gleaned from their studies, but one of the more interesting is the comparison of the effects of a symptomatic or corrective approach to a holistic approach on the parasympathetic response. As it turns out, only the holistic approach to manual therapy produces a significant and long lasting parasympathetic response. See the following publications by John T. Cottingham: *Healing Through Touch: A History and Review of the Physiological Evidence*, (Boulder: Rolf Institute, 1985); "Effect of Soft Tissue Mobilization on Pelvic Inclination Angle, Lumbar Lordosis, and Parasympathetic Tone: Implications for Treatment of Disabilities Associated with Lumbar Degenerative Joint Disease," presented to the National Center of Medical Rehabilitation Research of the National Institute of Child Health and Human Development, March 19, 1992, Bethesda, Maryland and reprinted in *Rolf Lines*, Rolf Institute, (Spring, 1992), pp. 42–45; "Soft Tissue Mobilization (Rolfing pelvic lift) and Associated Changes in Parasympathetic Tone in Two Age Groups," co-authors Steven W. Porges and T. Lyon, *Physical Therapy*, Vol. 68, 1988, pp. 352–356; and "Shifts in Pelvic Inclination Angle and Parasympathetic Tone Produced By Rolfing Soft Tissue Manipulation," co-authors Steven W. Porges and K. Richmond, *Physical Therapy*, Vol. 68, 1988, pp. 1364–1370.

15. Nesse and Williams, op. cit., p. 219.

16. Fritjof Capra, *The Web of Life: A New Scientific Understanding of Living Systems*, (New York, 1996), pp. 282–283. See also *Molecules of Emotion: Why You Feel the Way Feel* by Candice Pert (New York, NY: Doubleday, 1997).

17. Jeffrey Maitland, op. cit.

18. Francisco J. Varela, *Principles of Biological Autonomy*, (New York, 1979).

19. Alfred I. Tauber, *The Immune Self: Theory or Metaphor*, (New York, NY: Cambridge University Press, 1994), p. 43.

20. Ibid., p. 96.

21. The holistic approach to many problems is often more successful than the corrective approach. For a case study that compares the holistic and corrective approach to the treatment of chronic low back pain, see "A Third Paradigm Treatment Model Using Soft Tissue Mobilization and Guided Movement-Awareness techniques For Patients with Chronic Low Back Pain: A Case Study" by John Cottingham, P.T., and Jeffrey Maitland, Ph.D., *The Journal of Orthopaedic and Sports Physical Therapy*, September, 1997, Vol. 26, No. 3, pp. 155–167.

22. For a more detailed examination of what it means to surrender in the contexts of healing, creativity, and transformation, see my book, *Spacious Body*, (Berkeley, 1995), especially Chapter Four. Also relevant are my articles, "Creativity" in *The Journal of Aesthetics and Art Criticism*, (Vol. XXXIV, No. 4, Summer, 1976), pp. 397–409; and "Creative Performance: The Art of Life" in *Research in Phenomenology*, (Vol. X, 1980), pp. 278–303.

23. John H. Crook, op. cit., p. 411.

Bibliography

Books

Ali, Majid. *The Canary and Chronic Fatigue.* Denville, NJ: IPM Press, 1994.

Becker, Wayne M., Jane B. Reece, Martin F. Poenie, and Wayne F. Poenie. *The World of The Cell,* 3rd Edition. San Francisco, CA: Benjamin Cummings, 1996.

Behan, P.O., "Post-Viral Fatigue Syndrome Research." In *The Clinical and Scientific Basis of Myalgic Encephalitis and Chronic Fatigue Syndrome,* ed. Boutez, M.I., and E.K. Reynolds, eds. *Folic Acid and Neurology, Psychiatry and Internal Medicine.* New York, NY: Raven Press, 1979.

Braunwald, E., ed. *Harrisons Principles of Internal Medicine,* 11th ed. New York: McGraw-Hill, 1987.

Crook, William G. *The Yeast Connection.* Jackson, TN: Professional Books, 1983.

Crook, William G. *The Yeast Connection and the Woman.* Jackson, TN: Professional Books, 1995.

Dawson, D., and S. Sabin, eds. *Chronic Fatigue Syndrome.* Boston, MA: Little, Brown and Company, 1993.

Folkers, K., and Y. Yamamura, eds. *Biomedical and Clinical Aspects of Coenzyme Q,* vol. 4. New York, NY: Elsevier Publishers, 1984.

Forman, R. *How to Control Your Allergies.* Atlanta, GA: Larchmont Books, 1979.

Gittleman, Ann Louise, *Guess What Came to Dinner: Parasites and Your Health.* Garden City Park, NY: Avery Publishing Group, 1993.

Goldstein, J. *Betrayal by the Brain: The Neurologic Basis of Chronic Fatigue Syndrome, Fibromyalgia Syndrome and Related Neural Network Disorders.* Binghamton, NY: Haworth Press, 1996.

Goldstein, J. *Treatment Options in Chronic Fatigue Syndrome: A Guide for Physicians and Patients.* Binghamton, NY: Haworth Press, 1995.

Goldstein, J. *Tuning The Brain.* Binghamton NY: Haworth Press, 2001.

Hobbs, Christopher, *The Echinacea Handbook.* Portland, OR: Eclectic Medical Publications, 1989.

Hyde, Byron, Jay Goldstein, and Paul Levine, eds. *The Clinical and Scientific Basis of Myalgic Encephalitis and Chronic Fatigue Syndrome.* Ottawa, Ontario, Canada: Nightingale Research Foundation, 1992.

Ivker, Robert S. *Sinus Survival.* New York, NY: Tarcher/Putnam, 2000.

Rogers, Sherry. *Tired or Toxic.* Syracuse, NY: Prestige Publishing, 1990.

Rosenbaum, Michael, and Murry Susser, *Solving the Puzzle of Chronic Fatigue Syndrome.* Tacoma, WA: Life Sciences Press, 1992.

Sahelian, Ray. *Creatine: Nature's Muscle Builder.* Garden City Park, NY: Avery Publishing Group, 1997.

Teitelbaum, Jacob. *From Fatigued To Fantastic!* Garden City Park, NY: Avery Publishing Group, 1996.

Travell, J.G., and D. G. Simons. *Myofascial Pain and Dysfunction: The Trigger Point Manual,* Vol. 1. Baltimore, MD: Williams & Wilkins, 1983.

Trowell, H.C., ed. *Western Diseases: Their Emergence and Prevention.* Cambridge, MA: Harvard University Press, 1981.

Vliet, Elizabeth Lee. *Screaming To Be Heard: Hormone Connections Women Suspect . . . and Doctors Ignore.* New York, NY: M. Evans and Company, 1995.

Articles

Abraham, G.E., and J. Fletchas. "Management of Fibromyalgia: Rationale for the Use of Magnesium and Malic Acid." *Journal of Nutritional Medicine* 3 (1992): 49–59.

Adams, F., J.R. Quesada, and J.U. Gutterman. "Neuropsychiatric Manifestations of Human Leukocyte Interferon Therapy in Patients with Cancer." *Journal of the American Medical Association* 252 (7) (17 August 1984): 938–941.

Alexander, W. *Internal Medicine World Report* (1–14 January 1995): 32.

Anderson, R.A., et al., "Chromium and Hypoglycemia." abstract, *American Journal of Clinical Nutrition* 41 (4) (April 1985): 841.

Aoki, T., H. Miyakoshi, Y. Usuda, and R.B. Herberman. "Low NK Syndrome and Its Relationship to Chronic Fatigue Syndrome." *Clinical Immunology and Immunopathology* 69 (3) (December 1993): 253–265.

Archard, L.E., N.E. Bowles, P.O. Behan, E.J. Bell, and D. Doyle. "Postviral Fatigue Syndrome Persistence of Enterovirus RNA in Muscle and Elevated Creatine Kinase." *Journal of the Royal Society of Medicine* 81 (6) (June 1988): 326–329.

Arenas, J., J.R. Ricoy, A.R. Encinas, P. Pola, S. D'Iddio, M. Zeviani, S. Didonato, and M. Corsi, "Carnitine in Muscle, Serum and Urine of Nonprofessional Athletes." *Muscle and Nerve* 14 (7) (July 1991): 598–604.

Avorn, J., M. Monane, J.H. Gurwitz, R.J. Glynn, I. Choodnovskiy, and L.A. Lipsitz, "Reduction of Bacteriuria and Pyuria After Ingestion of Cranberry Juice." *Journal of the American Medical Association* 271 (10) (9 March 1994): 751–754.

Ayres, S., and R. Michan. "Restless Leg Syndrome: Response to Vitamin E." *Journal of Applied Nutrition* 25 (1973): 8–15.

Bakheit, A.M.O., P.O. Behan, T.G. Dinan, C.E. Gray, and V. O'Keane. "Possible Upregulation of Hypothalamic 5-HT Receptors in Patients with Postviral Fatigue Syndrome." *BMJ* 304 (6833) (18 April 1992): 1010–1012.

Bakheit, A.M.O., P.O. Behan, W.S. Watson, and J.J. Morton. "Abnormal Arginine-Vasopressin Secretion and Water Metabolism in Patients with Post-Viral Fatigue Syndrome." *Acta Neurologica Scandinavica* 87 (3) (March 1993): 234–238.

Balsom, P.D., K. Soderlund, B. Sjodin, and B. Ekblom, "Skeletal Muscle Metabolism During Short Duration High-Intensity Exercise: Influence of Creatine Supplementation." *Acta Physiologica Scandinavica* 154 (3) (July 1995): 303–310.

Barker, E., S.F. Fujimura, M.B. Fadem, A.L. Landay, and J.A. Levy. "Immunologic Abnormalities Associated with Chronic Fatigue Syndrome." *Clinical Infectious Diseases* 18, supplement 1 (1994): S136–S141.

Barrett-Connor, E., R.T. Khaw, and S.C. Yen. "A Prospective Study of Dehydroepiandrosterone, Mortality and Cardiovascular Disease." *The New England Journal of Medicine* 315 (24) (11 December 1986): 1519–1524.

Beck, W.S. "Cobalamin and the Nervous System." Editorial. *The New England Journal of Medicine* 318 (26) (30 June 1988): 1752–1754.

Bennett, R.M., R.A. Gatter, S.M. Campbell, R.P. Andrews, S.R. Clark, and J.A. Scarola. "Cyclobenzaprine Versus Placebo in Fibromyalgia." *Arthritis and Rheumatism* 31 (12) (December 1988): 1535–1542.

Bennett, R.M., R.A. Gatter, S.M. Campbell, R.P. Andrews, S.R. Clark, and J.A. Scarola. "A Comparison of Cyclobenzaprine and Placebo in the Management of Fibrositis—A Double-Blind Controlled Study." *Arthritis and Rheumatism Primary Care Review* 2 (Supplement 4) (July-August 1990): 16–24.

Birkmayer, J.G.D. "Coenzyme Nicotinamide Adenine Dinucleotide: New Therapeutic Approach for Improving Dementia of Alzheimer's Type." *Annals of Clinical and Laboratory Science* 26 (1) (January-February 1996): 1–9.

Birkmayer, J.G.D. Interview. *Clinical Pearl News* 7 (1) (January 1997): 1–2.

Birkmayer, J.G.D. "The Coenzyme Nicotinamide Adenine Dinucleotide as a Biological Antidepressive Agent." *New Trends in Clinical Neuropharmacology* 5 (1991): 19–25.

Birkmayer, J.G.D., C. Vreko, D. Volc, and W. Birkmayer. "Nicotinamide Adenine Dinucleotide (NADH)—A New Therapeutic Approach to Parkinson's Disease. Comparison of Oral and Parenteral Application." *Acta Neurologica Scandinavica* 146 (Supplement) (1993): 32–35.

Bliznakov, E., A. Casey, and E. Premuzic. "Coenzymes Q: Stimulants of Phagocytic Activity in Rats and Immune Response in Mice." *Experientia* 26 (9) (26 September 1970): 953–954.

Bou-Holaigah, I., P.C. Rowe, J. Kan, and H. Calkins. "The Relationship Between Neurally Mediated Hypotension and the Chronic Fatigue Syndrome." *Journal of the American Medical Association* 274 (12) (27 September 1995): 961–967.

Boyne, R. *Journal of Nutrition* 116 (1982): 816–822.

Brock, M. *Acta Neurochirurgica* 47, supplement (1990): 127–128.

Burckhardt, C.S., S.R. Clark, and R.M. Bennett. "The Fibromyalgia Impact Questionnaire: Development and Validation." *Journal of Rheumatology* 18 (5) (May 1991): 728–734.

Burke, L.M., D.B. Pyne, and R.D. Telford. "Effects of Oral Creatine Supplementation on Single-Effort Sprint Performance in Elite Swimmers." *International Journal of Sports Nutrition* 6 (3) (September 1996): 222–233.

Calvani, M., A. Carta, G. Caruso, N. Benedetti, and M. Iannuccelli. "Action of Acetyl-L-Carnitine in Neurodegeneration and Alzheimer's." *Annals of the New York Academy of Sciences* 663 (21 November 1992): 483–486.

Campbell, N.R., B.B. Hasinoff, H. Stalts, B. Rao, and N.C. Wong. "Ferrous Sulfate Reduces Thyroxine Efficacy in Patients with Hypothyroidism." *Annals of Internal Medicine* 117 (12) (15 December 1992): 1010–1013.

Canaris, G.J., N.R. Manowitz, G. Mayor, and E.C. Ridgway. "The Colorado Thyroid Disease Prevalence Study." *Archives of Internal Medicine* 160 (4) (28 February 2000): 526–534.

Carette, S., M.J. Bell. W.J. Reynolds, B. Haraoui, G.A. McCain, V.P. Bykerk, S.M. Edworthy, M. Baron, B.E. Koehler, and A.G. Fam. " Comparison of Amitriptyline, Cyclobenzaprine and Placebo in the Treatment of Fibromyalgia. A Randomized, Double-Blind Clinical Trial." *Arthritis and Rheumatism* 37 (1) (January 1994): 32–40.

Carmel, R. "Pernicious Anemia—The Expected Findings of Very Low Serum Cobalamin Levels, Anemia and Macrocytosis Are Often Lacking." *Archives of Internal Medicine* 148 (8) (August 1988): 1712–1714.

Carta, A., M. Calvani, D. Bravi, and S.N. Bhuachalla. "Acetyl-L-Carnitine and Alzheimer's: Pharmacologic Considerations Beyond the Cholinergic Sphere." *Annals of the New York Academy of Sciences* 695 (24 September 1993): 324–326.

Chalmers, R.A., C.R. Roe, T.E. Stacey, and C.L. Hoppel. "Urinary Excretion of L-Carnitine and Acyl-Carnitines by Patients with Disorders of Organic Acid Metabolism: Evidence For Secondary Insufficiency of L-Carnitine." *Pediatric Research* 18 (12) (December 1984): 1325–1328.

Chandra, R.K. "Effect of Macro and Micro Nutrient Deficiencies and Excess on Immune Response." *Food Technology,* February 1985, pp. 91–93.

Chandra, R.K., et al. "NIH Workshop on Trace Element Regulation of Immunity and Infection." *Nutrition Research* 2 (1982): 721–733.

Chandra, S., et al. "Undernutrition Impairs Immunity." *Internal Medicine* 5 (December 1984): 85–99.

Chanutin, A. "The Fate of Creatine When Administered to Man." *Journal of Biological Chemistry* 67 (1926): 29–41.

Cleare, A.J., E. Heap, G.S. Malhi, S. Wessley, V. O'Keane, and J. Miell. "Low-Dose Hydrocortisone in CFS: A Randomized Crossover Trial." *The Lancet* 353 (9151) (6 February 1999): 455–458.

Cox, I.M., M.J.Campbell, and D. Dowson D. "Red Blood Cell Magnesium and Chronic Fatigue Syndrome." *The Lancet* 337 (8744) (30 March 1991): 757–760.

Cuneo, R.C., F. Salomen, C.M. Wiles, R. Hesp, and P.H. Sonksen. "Growth Hormone Treatment in Growth Hormone Deficient Adults. II. Effects on Exercise Performance." *Journal of Applied Physiology* 70 (2) (February 1991): 695–700.

Deckelbaum, R.J. "ELISA More Accurate than Microscopy for Giardia." *Infectious Diseases in Children,* October 1993, p. 30.

DeLuise, M., et al. "Reduced Activity of the Red Cell Sodium Potassium Pump in Human Obesity." *The New England Journal of Medicine* 303 (16) (30 October 30, 1980): 1017–1022.

Demitrack, M.A., K. Dale, S.E. Straus, L. Laue, S.J. Listwak, M.J. Kruesi, G.P. Chrousos, and P.W. Gold. "Evidence for Impaired Activation of the Hypothalamic-Pituitary-Adrenal Axis in Patients with Chronic Fatigue Syndrome." *Journal of Clinical Endocrinology and Metabolism* 73 (6) (December 1991): 1223–1234.

DiDonato, S., D. Pelucchetti, M. Rimoldi, M. Mora, B. Garavaglia, and G. Finocchiaro. "Systemic Carnitine Deficiency: Clinical, Biochemical and Morphological Cure with L-Carnitine." *Neurology* 34 (2) (February 1984): 157–162.

Dressing, H., and D. Riemann. "Insomnia: Are Valerian/ Melissa Combinations of Equal Value to Benzodiazepine?" *Therapiewoche* 42 (1992): 726–736.

Drewes, A.M., K.D. Nielson, S.J. Taagholt, K. Bjerregaard, L. Svendson, and J. Gade. "Slow Wave Sleep in FMS." Abstract. *Journal of Musculoskeletal Pain* 3 (Supplement 1) (1995): 29.

Dyckner, T., and P.O. Wester. "Ventricular Extrasystoles and Intracellular Electrolytes Before and After Potassium and Magnesium Infusions in Patients on Diuretic Treatment." *American Heart Journal* 97 (1) (January 1979): 12–18.

Eaton, S.B., and N. Konner. "Paleolithic Nutrition. A Consideration of Its Nature and Current Implications." *The New England Journal of Medicine* 312 (5) (31 January 1985): 283–289.

Edman, J., J.D. Sobel, and M.L. Taylor. "Zinc Status in Women with Recurrent Vulvovaginal Candidiasis." *American Journal of Obstetrics and Gynecology* 155 (5) (November 1986): 1082–1088.

Eisenger, J., *L.M.M. Medicine du-Sud-Est* 25 (7/8) (April 1989): 12371.

Eisenger, J. *Journal of Advancement in Medicine* 7 (2) (Summer 1994): 69–75.

Eisenger, J., A. Plantamura, and T. Ayavou. "Glycolysis Abnormalities in Fibromyalgia." *Journal of the American College of Nutrition* 13 (2) (April 1994): 144–148.

Eisenger, J, A. Plantamura, et al. "Biochemical Abnormalities in Fibromyalgia." Letter. *Review du Rheumatisme,* English ed. (July-September 1993): 454–455.

Eisenger, J., and T. Ayavou. "Transketolase Stimulation in Fibromyalgia." *Journal of the American College of Nutrition* 9 (1) (1990): 56–57.

Eisenger, J., H. Zakarian, et al. "Studies of Transketolase in Chronic Pain." *Journal of Advancement in Med* 5 (2) (Summer 1992): 105–113.

Ekbom, K.A. "Restless Leg Syndrome." *Neurology* 10 (1960): 868–873.

Eriksen, W., L. Sandvik, and D. Bruusgaard. "Does Dietary Supplementation of Cod Liver Oil Mitigate Musculoskeletal Pain?" *European Journal of Clinical Nutrition* 50 (10) (October 1996): 689–693.

Everson, C.A. "Sustained Sleep Deprivation Impairs Host Defense." *American Journal of Physiology* 265 (5 Part 2) (November 1993): R1148–1154.

Faglia, G., L. Bitensky, A. Pinchera, C. Ferrari, A. Paracchi, P. Beck-Peccoz, B. Ambrosi, and A. Spada. "Thyrotropin Secretion in Patients with Central Hypothyroidism: Evidence for Reduced Biological Activity of Immunoreactive Thyrotropin." *Journal of Clinical Endocrinology and Metabolism* 48 (6) (June 1979) 989–998.

Folkers, K., P. Langsjoen, Y. Nara, K. Muratsu, J. Komorowski. P.C. Richardson, and T.H. Smith. "Biochemical Deficiencies of Coenzyme Q_{10} in HIV Infection and Exploratory Treatment." *Biochemical and Biophysical Research Communications* 153 (2) (1988): 888–896.

Folkers, K., S. Shizukuishi, K. Takemura, J. Drzewoski, P. Richardson, J. Ellis, and W.C. Kuzell. "Increase in Levels of IgG in Serum of Patients Treated with Coenzyme Q_{10}." *Research Communications in Chemical Pathology and Pharmacology* 38 (2) (1982): 335–338.

Fraser, W.D., E.M. Biggart, D.J.O. O'Reilly, H.W. Gray, J.H. McKillop, and J.A. Thomson. "Are Biochemical Tests of Thyroid Function of Any Value in Monitoring Patients Receiving Thyroxine Replacement?" *British Medical Journal* 293 (6550) (27 September 1986): 808–810.

Freeman, R., and A.L. Komaroff. "Does the Chronic Fatigue Syndrome Involve the Autonomic Nervous System?" *The American Journal of Medicine* 102 (4) (April 1997): 357–363.

Friolet, R., H. Hoppeler, and S. Krahenbuhl. "Relationship Between the Coenzyme A (CoA) and the Carnitine Pools in Human Skeletal Muscle at Rest and Exhaustive Exercise Under Normal and Acutely Hypoxic Conditions." *Journal of Clinical Investigation* 94 (4) (October 1994): 1490–1495.

Fukuda, K., S.E. Straus, I. Hickie, M.C. Sharpe, J.G. Dobbins, and A. Komaroff. "The Chronic Fatigue Syndrome: A Comprehensive Approach to its Definition and Study." *Annals of Internal Medicine* 121 (12) (15 December 1994): 953–959.

Gaby, A. "Potassium-Magnesium Aspartate." *Nutrition and Healing,* October 1995, pp. 3–11.

Gaby, A. "The Role of Coenzyme Q_{10} in Clinical Medicine. Part I." *Alternative Medicine Review* 1 (1) (1996): 11–17.

Gaby, A. "The Story of L-Carnitine." *Nutrition and Healing,* April 1995, pp.3–11.

Galland, L., M. Lee, H. Bueno, and C. Heirnowitz. "Giardia as a Cause of Chronic Fatigue." *Journal of Nutritional Medicine* 1 (1990): 27–32.

Gambrell, R.D. *Consultant,* July 1994, pp. 1047–1057.

Gatter, R.A. "Pharmacotherapeutics in Fibromyalgia." *American Journal of Medicine* 81 (3A) (29 September 1986): 63–66.

Gecele, M, et al. "Acetyl-L-Carnitine in Aged Subjects With Major Depression: Clinical Efficacy and Effects on the Circadian Rhythm of Cortisol." *Dementia* 2 (1991): 333–337.

Goldenberg, D.L. "Fibromyalgia Syndrome: An Emerging but Controversial Condition." *Journal of the American Medical Association* 257 (1987): 2782–2787.

Goldenberg, D.L. "Fibromyalgia Syndrome a Decade Later: What Have We Learned?" *Archives of Internal Medicine* 159 (8) (26 April 1999): 777–785.

Goldenberg, D.L. "Treatment of Fibromyalgia Syndrome." *Rheumatic Disease Clinics of North America* 15 (1) (February 1989): 61–71.

Goldenberg, D., M. Mayskiy, R. Mossey, R. Ruthazer, and C. Schmid. "A Randomized, Double-Blind Crossover Trial of Fluoxetine and Amitriptyline in the Treatment of Fibromyalgia." *Arthritis and Rheumatism* 39 (11) (November 1996): 1852–1859.

Goldstein, J. "Fibromyalgia Syndrome: A Pain Modulation Disorder Related to Altered Limbic Function?" *Bailliere's Clinical Rheumatology* 8 (November 1994): 777–800.

Grassel, E. "Effect of Ginkgo Biloba Extract on Mental Performance." *Fortschritte der Medizin* 110 (5) (February 1992): 73–76.

Greenhaff, P.L. "Creatine and its Application as an Ergogenic Aid." *International Journal of Sports Nutrition* 5 (Supplement) (1995): S100–S110.

Greenhaff, P.L., A. Casey, A.H. Short, R. Harris, K. Soderlund, and E. Hultman. "Influence of Oral Creatine Supplementation on Muscle Torque During Repeated Bouts of Maximal Exercise in Man." *Clinical Science*; 84 (5) (May 1993): 565–571.

Greenhaff, P.L., et al. "The Influence of Oral Creatine Supplementation on Muscle Phosphocreatine Synthesis Following Intense Contraction in Man." *Journal of Physiology* 467 (1993): 75.

Greenhaff, P.L., K. Bodin, K. Soderlund, and E. Hultman. "Effect of Oral Creatine Supplementation on Skeletal Muscle Phosphocreatine Reynthesis." *Am J Physiol* 266 (5, Part 1) (May 1994): E725–E730.

Griep, E.N., J.N. Boersma, and E.R. de Kloet. "Altered Reactivity of the Hypothalamic-Pituitary Axis in the Primary Fibromyalgia Syndrome." *Journal of Rheumatology* 20 (3) (March 1993): 469–474.

Grubb, B.P., D. Samoil, D. Kosinski, K. Kip, and P. Brewster. "Use of Sertraline Hydrochloride in the Treatment of Refractory Neurocardiogenic Syncope in Children and Adolescents." *Journal of the American College of Cardiology* 24 (2) (August 1994): 490–494.

Grubb, B.P., D.A. Wolfe, D. Samoil, P. Temesy-Armos, H. Hahn, and L. Elliott. "Usefulness of Fluoxetine Hydrochloride for Prevention of Resistant Upright Tilt Induced Syncope." *Pacing and Clinical Electrophysiology* 16 (3, Part 1) (March 1993): 458–464.

Haguenauer, J.P., F. Cantenot, H. Koskas, and H. Pierart. "Treatment of Equilibrium Disturbances with Ginkgo Biloba—A Multicenter, Placebo Controlled Study." *Presse Medicale* 15 (31) (25 September 1986): 1569–1572.

Hak, A.E., H.A.P. Pols, T.J. Visser, H.A. Drexhage, A. Hofman, and J.C.M. Witteman. "Subclinical Hypothyroidism is an Independent Risk Factor for Atherosclerosis and Myocardial Infarction in Elderly Women: The Rotterdam Study." *Annals of Internal Medicine* 132 (4) (15 February 2000): 270–278.

Hallberg, L. "Does Calcium Interfere with Iron Absorption?" Editorial. *American Journal of Clinical Nutrition* 68 (1) (July 1998): 3–4.

Halpin, D., and S. Wessely. "VP-1 Antigen in Chronic Postviral Fatigue Syndrome." *The Lancet* 1 (8645) (6 May 1989):1028–1029.

Hammond, C.B. "Menopause and Hormone Replacement Therapy: An Overview." *Obstetrics and Gynecology* 87 (Supplement 2) (February 1996): 2S–15S.

Harris, R.C., K. Soderlund, and E. Hultman. "Elevation of Creatine in Resting and Exercised Muscle of Normal Subjects by Creatine Supplementation." *Clinical Science* 83 (3) (September 1992): 367–374.

Hicks, J.T. "Treatment of Fatigue: A Double Blind Study." *Clinical Medicine,* January 1964, pp. 85–90.

Hindmarch, I. "Activity of Ginkgo Biloba Extract on Short Term Memory." *Presse Medicale* 15 (31) (September 1986): 1592-1594.

Hoes, M.J. "Plasma Concentrations of Magnesium and Vitamin B$_1$ in Alcoholism and Delirium Tremens. Pathogenic and Prognostic Implications." *Acta Psychiatrica Belgica* 81 (1) (January-February 1981): 72–84.

Holmes, G.P., J.E. Kaplan, N.M. Gantz, A.L. Komaroff, L.B. Schonberger, S.E. Straus, J.F. Jones, R.E. Dubois, C. Cunningham-Rundles, and S. Pahwa. "Chronic Fatigue Syndrome: A Working Case Definition." *Annals of Internal Medicine* 108 (1988): 387–389.

Hopfenmuller, W. "Proof of the Therapeutic Effectiveness of a Ginkgo Biloba Extract—A Meta Analysis of 11 [Placebo Controlled] Trials in Aged Patients with Cerebral Insufficiency." *Arzneimittel-Forschung* 44 (9) (September 1994): 1005–1010.

Ingledew, W.J., and T. Ohnishi. "An Analysis of Some Thermodynamic Properties of Iron-Sulfur Centres in Site I of Mitochondria." *The Biochemical Journal* 186 (1) (15 January 1980): 111–117.

Ishihara, Y., Y. Uchida, S. Kitamura, and F. Takaku. "Effect of Coenzyme Q$_{10}$, a Quinone Derivative, on Guinea Pig Lung and Tracheal Tissue." *Arzneimittelforschung* 35 (6) (1985): 929–933.

Jason, L.A., J.A. Richman, A.W. Rademaker, K.M. Jordan, A.V. Plioplys, R.R. Taylor, W. McCready C.F. Huang, and S. Plioplys. "A Community-Based Study of Chronic Fatigue Syndrome." *Archives of Internal Medicine* 159 (18) (11 October 1999): 2129–2137.

Jefferies, W.M. "Low-Dosage Glucocorticoid Therapy. An Appraisal of Its Safety and Mode of Action in Clinical Disorders, Including Rheumatoid Arthritis." *Archives of Internal Medicine* 119 (3) (March 1967): 265–278.

Jenkins J.S. "The Role of Oxytocin: Present Concepts." Review. *Clinical Endocrinology* 34 (6) (June 1991): 515–525.

Jorgensen, J.O.L., S.A. Pedersen, L. Thuesen, J. Jorgensen, J. Moller, J. Muller, N.E. Skakkebaek, and J.S. Christiansen. "Long Term Growth Hormone Treatment in Growth Hormone Deficient Adults." *Acta Endocrinolica (Copenhagen)* 125 (5) (November 1991): 449–453.

Karnaze, D.S., and R. Carmel. "Low Serum Cobalamin Levels in Primary Degenerative Dementia: Do Some Patients Harbor Atypical Cobalamin Deficiency States?" *Archives of Internal Medicine* 147 (3) (March 1987): 429–431.

Keith, R.E. "Symptoms of Carnitine Like Deficiency in a Trained Runner Taking DL-Carnitine Supplements." letter, *Journal of the American Medical Association* 255 (9) (7 March 1986): 1137.

Kennes, B., I. Dumont, D. Brohee, C. Hubert, and P. Neve P "Effect of Vitamin C Supplements on Cell-Mediated Immunity in Old People." *Gerontology* 29 (1983): 305–310.

Kirn, T.F. "Do Low Levels of Iron Affect Body's Ability to Regulate Temperature, Experience Cold?" *Journal of the American Medical Association* 260 (5) (5 August 1988): 607.

Koen, F.E. "The Influence of Echinacea Purpurea On The Hypophyseal-Adrenal System;" *Arzneimittel-Forschung* 3 (1953): 133–137.

Kruse, C.A. "Treatment of Fatigue with Aspartic Acid Salts." *Northwest Medicine,* June 1961, pp. 597–603.

Kuratsune, H., K. Yamaguti, M. Takahashi, H. Misaki, S. Tagawa, and T. Kitani. "Acylcarnitine Deficiency in Chronic Fatigue Syndrome." *Clinical Infectious Disease* 18 (3 Supplement 1) (January 1994): S62–S67.

Lakshmanad, F.L., et al. "Magnesium Intakes and Balances." *American Journal of Clinical Nutrition* 60 (6 Supplement) (December 1984): 1380–1389.

Le Gal, Martine, Pascal Cathebras, Käthi Strüby. "Pharmaton Capsules in the Treatment of Functional Fatigue: A Double-Blind Study Versus Placebo Evaluated by a New Methodology." *Phytotherapy Research* 10 (1996): 10:49–53).

Lerner, A. Martin, Marcus Zervos, Howard J. Dworkin, Chug-ho Chang, James T. Fitzgerald, James Goldstein, Claudine Lawrie-Hoppen, Barry Franklin, Steven M. Korotkin, Marc Brodsky, Daniel Walsh, and William O'Neil. "New Cardiomyopathy: Pilot Study of Intravenous Ganciclovir in a Subset of the Chronic Fatigue Syndrome." *Infectious Disease in Clinical Practice* 6 (1997): 110–117.

Liebermann, J., and D.S. Bell. "Serum Angiotensin-Converting Enzyme as a Marker for the Chronic Fatigue–Immune Dysfunction Syndrome: A Comparison to Serum Angiotensin-Converting Enzyme in Sarcordosis." *American Journal of Medicine* 95 (4) (October 1993): 407–412.

Lindenbaum, J., E.B. Healton, D.G. Savage, J.C. Brust, T.J. Garrett, E.R. Podell, P.D. Marcell, S.P. Stabler, and R.H. Allen. "Neuropsychiatric Disorders Caused by Cobalamin Deficiency in the Absence of Anemia or Macrocytoses." *The New England Journal of Medicine* 318 (26) (30 June 1988): 1720–1728.

Lindenbaum, J., I.H. Rosenberg, P.W. Wilson, S.P. Stabler, and R.H. Allen. "Prevalence of Cobalamin Deficiency in the Framingham Elderly Population." *American Journal of Clinical Nutrition* 60 (1) (July 1994): 2–11.

Lockwood, K., S. Moesgaadr, T. Hanoike, and K. Folkers. "Apparent Partial Remission of Breast Cancer in "High Risk" Patients Supplemented with Nutritional Antioxidants, Essential Fatty Acids and Coenzyme Q_{10}." *Molecular Aspects of Medicine* 15 (Supplement) (1994): S231–S240.

Lockwood, K., S. Moesgaard, T. Yamamoto, and K. Folkers. "Progress on Therapy of Breast Cancer with Coenzyme Q_{10} and the Regression of Metastases." *Biochemical and Biophysical Research Communications* 212 (1) (6 July 1995): 172–177.

Loike, J.D. D.L. Zalutsky, E. Kaback, A.F. Miranda, and S.C. Silverstein. "Extracellular Creatine Regulates Creatine Transport in Rat and Human Muscle Cells." *Proceeds of the National Academy of Sciences USA* 85 (3) (February 1988): 807–811.

Lowe, J.C., A.J. Reichman, and J. Yellin. "The Process of Change During T_3 Treatment for Euthyroid Fibromyalgia: A Double-Blind, Placebo-Controlled, Crossover Study." *Clinical Bulletin of Myofascial Therapy* 2 (2/3) (1997): 91–124.

Lowe, J.C., R.L. Garrison, A.J. Reichman, J. Yellin, M. Thompson, and D. Kaufman. "Effectiveness and Safety of T₃ Therapy for Euthyroid Fibromyalgia: A Double-Blind, Placebo-Controlled Response Driven Crossover Study." *Clinical Bulletin of Myofascial Therapy* 2 (2/3) (1997): 31–58.

Lutz, E.G. "Restless Legs, Anxiety and Caffeinism." *Journal of Clinical Psychiatry* 39 (9) (September 1978): 693–698.

Marchesani, R.B. "Critical Antiviral Pathway Deficient in Chronic Fatigue Syndrome Patients." *Infectious Disease News*, August 1993, p. 4.

Marston, R.M., and B.B. Peterkin. "Nutrient Content of the National Food Supply." *National Food Review*, Winter 1980, pp. 21–25.

Mastrogiacomo, F., Bettendorff, T. Grisar, and S.J. Kish, "Brain Thiamine, Its Phosphate Esters and Its Metabolizing Enzymes in Alzheimer's Disease." *Annals of Neurology* 39 (5) (May 1996): 585–591.

May, K.P., S.G. West, M.R. Baker, and D.W. Everett. "Sleep Apnea in Male Patients with the Fibromyalgia Syndrome." *American Journal of Medicine* 94 (5) (May 1993): 505–508.

Mayer, P., H. Hamberger, and J. Drew. "Differential Effects of Ubiquinone Q₇ and Ubiquinone Analogs on Macrophage Activation and Experimental Infections in Granulocytopenic Mice." *Infection* 8 (1980): 256–261.

McCain, G.A., and K.S. Tilbe. "Diurnal Hormone Variation in Fibromyalgia Syndrome and a Comparison with Rheumatoid Arthritis." *Journal of Rheumatology* 25 (1993): 469–474.

McCully, K.K., B.H. Natelson, S. Iotti, S. Sisto, and J.S. Leigh. "Reduced Oxidative Muscle Metabolism in CFS." *Muscle and Nerve;* 15 (5) (May 1996): 621–625.

McGauley, G.A. "Quality of Life Assessment Before and After Growth Hormone Treatment in Adults With GH Deficiency." *Acta Paediatrica Scandinavica* 356 (supplement) (1989): 70–72.

McKenzie, R., A. O'Fallon A. J. Dale, M. Demitrack, G. Sharma, M. Deloria, D. Garcia-Borreguero, W. Blackwelder, and S.E. Straus. "Low-Dose Hydrocortisone for Treatment of Chronic Fatigue Syndrome: A Randomized Controlled Trial." *Journal of the American Medical Association* 280 (12) (23–30 September 1998): 1061–1066.

Meikle, A.W., R.A. Daynes, B.A. Araneo, and L.N. Parker. "Adrenal Androgen Secretion and Biologic Effects." *Endocrine and Metabolic Clinics of North America* 20 (2) (June 1991): 381–421.

Merlotti, L., T. Roehrs, G. Koshorek, F. Zorick, J. Lamphere, and T. Roth. "The Dose Effects of Zolpidem on the Sleep of Healthy Normals." *Journal of Clinical Psychopharmacology* 9 (1) (February 1989): 9–14.

Mertz, W., ed. "Beltsville 1 Year Dietary Intake Survey." *American Journal of Clinical Nutrition* 40, supplement (December 1984): 1323–1403.

Meydani, S.N., M.P. Barklund, S. Liu, M. Meydani, R.A. Miller, J.G. Cannon, F.D. Morrow, R. Rocklin, and J.B. Blumberg. "Vitamin E Supplementation Enhances Cell-Mediated Immunity in Healthy Elderly Subjects." *American Journal of Clinical Nutrition* 52 (3) (September 1990): 557–563.

Miller, S.B. "IgG Food Allergy Testing by ELISA/EIA—What Do They Really Tell Us." *Townsend Letter for Doctors and Patients*, January 1998, pp. 62–66, 106.

Millman, R.P. "Do You Ever Take A Sleep History?" *Annals of Internal Medicine* 131 (7) (October 1999): 535–536.

Moldofsky, H., and P. Scarisbrick. "Induction of Neuresthenic Musculoskeletal Pain Syndrome by Selective Sleep Stage Deprivation." *Psychosomatic Medicine* 38 (1) (January-February 1976): 35–44.

Morales, A.J., J.J. Nolan, J.C. Nelson, and S.S. Yen. "Effects of Replacement Dose of Dehydroepiandrosterone in Men and Women of Advancing Age." *Journal of Clinical Endocrinology and Metabolism* 78 (6) (June 1994): 1360–1367.

Naylor, S. "Role of Fungi in Allergic Fungal Sinusitis and Chronic Rhinosinusitis." *Mayo Clinic Proceedings* 75 (5) (May 2000):540–541.

Neeck, G., and W. Riedel. "Thyroid Function in Patients with Fibromyalgia Syndrome." *Journal of Rheumatology* 19 (7) (July 1992): 1120–1122.

Nelson, J.H., "Wheat: Its Processing and Utilization." *American Journal of Clinical Nutrition* 41, supplement (May 1985): 1070-1076.

Neri, D.F., D.Wiegmann, R.R. Stanny, S.A. Shappell, A. McCardie, and D.L. McKay. "The Effects of Tyrosine on Cognitive Performance During Extended Wakefulness." *Aviation, Space, and Environmental Medicine* 66 (4) (1995): 313–319.

Netzer, N.C., R.A. Stoohs, C.M. Netzer, K. Clark, and K.P. Strohl. "Using the Berlin Questionnaire to Identify Patients at Risk for Sleep Apnea Syndrome." *Annals of Internal Medicine* 131 (7) 5 October 1999): 485–491.

Nicolson, G.L. "Considerations When Undergoing Treatment for Chronic Infections Found in Chronic Fatigue Syndrome, Fibromyalgia, and Gulf War Illness." *Journal of Internal Medicine* 1 (1988): 115–117, 123–128.

Nicolson, G.L., M.Y. Nasralla, J. Haier, R. Irwin, N.L. Nicolson, and R. Ngwenya. "Mycoplasmal Infections in Chronic Illness: Fibromyalgia and Chronic Fatigue Syndrome, Gulf War Illness, Human Immunodeficiency Virus, and Rheumatoid Arthritis." *Medical Sentinel* 4 (1999):172–176.

Nordyke, R.A., T.S. Reppun, L.D. Madanay, J.C. Woods, A.P. Goldstein, and L.A. Miyamoto. "Alternative Sequences of Thyrotropin and Free Thyroxine Assays for Routine Thyroid Function Testing. Quality and Cost." *Archives of Internal Medicine* 158 (3) (9 February 1998): 266–272.

Norman, E.J., and J.A. Morrison. " Screening Elderly Populations for Cobalamin (Vitamin B_{12}) Deficiency Using Urinary Methylmalonic Acid Assay by Gas Chromatography Mass Spectrometry." *American Journal of Medicine* 94 (6) (June 1993): 589–594.

Norregaard, J., H. Volkmann, and B. Danneskiold-Samsoe. "A Randomized Controlled Trial of Citalopram in the Treatment of Fibromylagia." *Pain* 61 (3) (June 1995): 445–449.

O'Rourke, D., J.J. Wurtman, R.J. Wurtman, R. Chebli, and R. Gleason. "Treatment of Seasonal Depression With D-Fenluramine." *Journal of Clinical Psychiatry* 50 (9) (September 1989): 343–347.

Older, S.A., D.F. Battafarano, C.L. Danning, J.A. Ward, E.P. Grady, and S. Derman. "Delta Wave Sleep Interruption and Fibromyalgia Syndrome in Healthy Patients." abstract, *Journal of Musculoskeletal Pain* 3 (Supplement 1) (1995): 159.

Padilla, A.J. "Who Has Diabetes?" *Cortlandt Forum,* February 2000, pp. 110–111.

Parker, L.N. "Control of Adrenal Androgen Secretion." *Endocrine and Metabolic Clinics of North America* 20 (2) (June 1991): 401–421.

Parnetti, L., A. Gaiti, P. Mecocci, D. Cadini, and U. Senin. "Pharmacokinetics of IV and Oral Acetyl-L-Carnitine in a Multiple-Dose Regimen in Patients with Senile Dementia of the Alzheimer Type." *European Journal of Clinical Pharmacology* 42 (1) (1992): 89–93.

Pillemer, S., L.A. Bradley, L.J. Crofford, H. Moldofsky, and G.P. Chrousos. "The Neuroscience and Endocrinology of FMS—[An NIH] Conference Summary." *Arthritis and Rheumatism* 40 (11) (November 1997):1928–1939.

Piscopo, Gary. "Kava Kava: Gift of the Islands."*Alternative Medicine Review* 2 (5) (1997): 355–364.

Plaitakis, A., E.C. Hwang, M.H. Woert, P.E. Szilagyi, and S. Berl S Hwang EC, Woert MH, Szilagyi PE, Berl S. "Effect of Thiamine on Brain Neurotransmitter Systems." *Annals of the New York Academy of Sciences* 378 (1982): 367–381.

Plioplys, A.V., and S. Plioplys. "Amantadine and L-Carnitine Treatment of Chronic Fatigue Syndrome." *Neuropsychobiology* 35 (1) (1997): 16–23.

Posner, I.A. "Treatment of Fibromyalgia Syndrome With IV Lidocaine: A Prospective, Randomized Pilot Study." *Journal of Musculoskeletal Pain* 2 (1994): 55–65.

Postiglione, A., U. Cicerano, A. Soricelli, S. De Chiara, G. Gallotta, M. Salvatore, and M. Mancini. "Cerebral Blood Flow in Patients with Chronic Cerebrovascular Disease: Effect of Acetyl-L-Carnitine." *International Journal of Clinical Pharmacological Research*; 10 (1-2) (1990): 129–132.

Quesada, J.R., M. Talpaz, A. Rios, R. Kurzrock, and J.U. Gutterman. "Clinical Toxicity of Interferon in Cancer Patients: A Review." *Journal of Clinical Oncology* 4 (February 1986): 234–243.

Redondo, D.R. "The Effect of Oral Creatine Monohydrate Supplementation on Running Velocity." *International Journal of Sports Nutrition* 6 (3) (September 1996): 213–221.

Rees, W., B.K. Evans, and J. Rhodes. "Treating Irritable Bowel Syndrome with Peppermint Oil." *British Medical Journal* 2 (6194) (6 October 1979): 835–836.

Reeves, W.C., F.R. Stamey, J.B. Black, A.C. Mawle, J.A. Stewart, and P.E. Pellett. "Human Herpesviruses 6 and 7 in Chronic Fatigue Syndrome: A Case-Control Study." *Clinical Infectious Diseases* 31 (1) (July 2000): 48–52.

Regland, B., M. Andersson, L. Abrahamsson, J. Bagby, L.E. Dyrehag, and C.G. Gottfries. "Increased Concentrations of Homocysteine in the Cerebrospinal Fluid in Patients with Fibromyalgia and Chronic Fatigue Syndrome." *Scandinavian Journal of Rheumatology* 26 (4) (1997) 301–307.

Reid, G., K. Millsap, and A.P. Bruce. "Implantation of *Lactobacillus casei* var. Rhamnosus into Vagina." *The Lancet* 344 (8931): 1229.

Roberts, H.J. "Spontaneous Leg Cramps and Restless Legs Due to Diabetogenic (Functional) Hyperinsulinism: A Basis For Natural Therapy." *Journal of the Florida Medical Association* 60 (5) (1973): 29–31.

Rogers, S. "Chemical Sensitivity: Breaking the Paralyzing Paradigm. Part I." *Internal Medicine World Report* 7 (3): 1.

Rogers, S. "Chemical Sensitivity: Breaking the Paralyzing Paradigm. Part II." *Internal Medicine World Report* 7 (6): 8, 21–31.

Romano, T.J., and J.W. Stiller JW. "Magnesium Deficiency in Fibromyalgia Syndrome." *Journal of Nutritional Medicine* 4 (1994): 165–167.

Rosenthal, N.E. "Diagnosis and Treatment of Seasonal Affective Disorder." *Journal of the American Medical Association* 270 (22) (8 December 1993): 2717–2720.

Rowe, P.C., H. Calkins, K. DeBusk, R. McKenzie, R. Anand, G. Sharma, B.A. Cuccherini, N. Soto, P. Hohman, S. Snader, K.E. Lucas, M. Wolff, and S.E. Straus. "Fludrocortisone Acetate to Treat Neurally Mediated Hypotension in Chronic Fatigue Syndrome: A Randomized Controlled Trial." *Journal of the American Medical Association* 285 (1) (3 January 2001): 52–59.

Rowe, P.C., I. Bou-Holaigah, J.S. Kan, and H. Calkins. "Is Neurally Mediated Hypotension an Unrecognized Cause of Chronic Fatigue?" *The Lancet* 345 (8950) (11 March 1995): 623–624.

Ruhrmann, S., and S. Kasper. "Seasonal Depression. Phytotherapy and Psychopharmacologic Approaches." *Medizinische Monatsschrift TUR Pharmazeuten* 15 (10) (October 1992): 293–299.

Rushton, D.C., I.D. Ramsay, J.J. Gilkes, and M.J. Norris. "Ferritin and Fertility." Letter to the editor. *The Lancet* 337 (8757) (22 June 1991): 1554.

Saiki, I., Y. Tokushima, K. Nishimura, and I. Azuma. "Macrophage Activation with Ubiquinones and Their Related Compounds in Mice." *International Journal for Vitamin and Nutrition Research* 53 (3) (1983): 312–320.

Savolainen, J., K. Lammintausta, K. Kalimo, and M. Viander. "Candida Albicans and Atopic Dermatitis." *Journal of Clinical Experimental Allergy* 23 (4) (April 1993): 332–339.

Schroeder, H.A. "Losses of Vitamins and Trace Minerals Resulting from Processing and Preservation of Foods." *American Journal of Clinical Nutrition* 24 (5) (May 1971): 562–573.

Seelig, M.S. "The Requirement of Magnesium by the Normal Adult." *American Journal of Clinical Nutrition* 14 (June 1964): 342–390.

Shaw, D.L., et al. "Management of Fatigue." *American Journal of Medical Science,* June 1962, pp. 758–769.

Singh, Y.N., and M. Blumenthal. "Kava: An Overview." *Herbalgram* 39 (Spring 1997): 33–55.

Skinner, G.R.B., D. Holmes, A. Ahmad, J.A. Davies, and J. Benitez. "Clinical Response to Thyroxine Sodium in Clinically Hypothyroid but Biochemically Euthyroid Patients." *Journal of Nutritional and Environmental Medicine* 10 (2) (June 2000): 115–125.

Skinner, G.R., R. Thomas, M. Taylor, S. Bolt, S. Krett, and A. Wright. "Thyroxine Should be Tried in Clinically Hypothyroid but Biochemically Euthyroid Patients." *British Medical Journal* 314 (7096) (14 June 1997): 1764.

Smith, P.F., and C.L. Darlington. "Can Vestibular Compensation Be Enhanced by Drug Treatment: A Review of Recent Evidence." Review. *Journal of Vestibular Research* 4 (3) (May–June 1994): 169–179.

Smythe, H. "Fibroisitis Continues to Present Clinical Challenges." *Rheumatology for the Practicing Physician,* January 1989, pp. 13–14.

Srivastava, K.C., and T. Mustafa. "Ginger (Zingiber officinale) in Rheumatism and Musculoskeletal Disorders." *Medical Hypotheses* 39 (4) (December 1992): 342–348.

Sternberg, E.M. "Hyperimmune Fatigue Syndromes: Disease of the Stress Response?" Editorial. *Journal of Rheumatology* 20 (3) (March 1993): 418–421.

Straus, S.E., J.K. Dale, M. Tobi, T. Lawley, O. Preble, R.M. Blaese, C., Hallahan, and W. Henle. "Acyclovir Treatment of the Chronic Fatigue Syndrome. Lack of Efficacy in a Placebo-Controlled Trial." *The New England Journal of Medicine* 319 (26) (29 December 1988): 1692–1698.

Straus, S.E., S. Fritz, J.K. Dale, B. Gould, and W. Strober. "Lymphocyte Phenotype and Function in the Chronic Fatigue Syndrome." *Journal of Clinical Immunology* 13 (1) (January 1993): 30–40.

Strosberg, J.M. "Is Fibrositis a Stress Disorder?" *Rheumatology for the Practicing Physician*, January 1989, p. 12.

Susmano, A., A.S. Volgman, and T.A. Buckingham. "Beneficial Effects of Dextro-Amphetamine in the Treatment of Vasodepressor Syncope." *Pacing and Clinical Electrophysiology* 16 (6) (June 1993): 1235–1239.

Talbott, M.C. L.T. Miller, and N.I. Kerkvliet. "Pyridoxine Supplementation: Effect on Lymphocyte Responses in Elderly Persons." *American Journal of Clinical Nutrition* 46 (4) (October 1987): 659–664.

Tamborini, A., and R. Taurelle. "Value of Standardized Ginkgo Biloba Extract (EGb 761) in the Management of Congestive Symptoms of Premenstrual Syndrome." *Revue Francaise de gynecologie et d'Obstetrique* 88 (7–9) (July–September 1993): 447–457.

Tanphaichitr, V., and P. Leelahagul. "Carnitine Metabolism and Human Carnitine Deficiency". Review article. *Nutrition* 9 (3) (May–June 1993): 246–252.

Teitelbaum, J. "Estrogen and Testosterone in CFIDS/FMS." *From Fatigued To Fantastic Newsletter,* February 1997.

Teitelbaum, J. "Mitochondrial Dysfunction." *From Fatigued To Fantastic Newsletter,* July 1997.

Teitelbaum, J., and B. Bird. "Effective Treatment of Severe Chronic Fatigue: A Report of a Series of 64 Patients." *Journal of Musculoskeletal Pain* 3 (4) (1995): 91–110.

Teitelbaum, J.E., B. Bird, A. Weiss, and L. Gould. "Low Dose Hydrocortisone for Chronic Fatigue Syndrome." *Journal of the American Medical Association* 281 (1999): 1887–1888.

Teitelbaum, J.E., B. Bird, R.M. Greenfield, A. Weiss, L. Muenz, and L. Gould. "Effective Treatment of CFS and FMS: A Randomized, Double-Blind Placebo Controlled Study." *Journal of Chronic Fatigue Syndrome* 8 (2) (2001).

Thompson, C., D. Stanson, and A. Smith. "Seasonal Affective Disorder and Season-Dependent Abnormalities of Melatonin Suppression by Light." *The Lancet* 336 (8717) (22 September 1990): 703–706.

Travell, J. "Identification of Myofascial Trigger Point Syndromes: A Case of Atypical Facial Neuralgia." *Archives of Physical Medicine and Rehabilitation* 62 (1981): 100–106.

Trivellato, M., et al. "Carnitine Deficiency as the Possible Cause of Idiopathic Mitral Valve Prolapse." *Texas Heart Institute Journal* 11 (4) (1984): 370.

Vance, M.L. "Hypopituitarism." *The New England Journal of Medicine* 330 (23) (9 June 1994): 1651–1662.

Vercoulen, J.H., C.M. Swanink, F.G. Zitman, S.G. Vreden, M.P. Hoofs, J.F. Fennis, J.M. Galama, J.W. van der Meer, and G. Bleijenberg. "Randomized, Double-Blind, Placebo-Controlled Study of Fluoxetine in Chronic Fatigue Syndrome." *The Lancet* 347 (9005) (30 March 1996): 858–861.

Wainstein, M.A., and M.I. Resnick. "Managing Nosocomial Infection with C. Difficile." *Internal Medicine,* November 1995: 15–22.

Wakefield, D., A. Lloyd, J. Dwyer, S.Z. Salahuddin, and D.V. Ablashi. "Human Herpesvirus 6 and Myalgic Encephalomyelitis." *The Lancet* 1 (8593) (7 May 1988): 1059.

Walter, T., S. Arredondo, M. Arevalo, and A. Stekel. "Effect of Iron Therapy on Phagocytosis and Bactericidal Activity in Neutrophils of Iron-Deficient Infants." *American Journal of Clinical Nutrition* 44 (6) (December 1986): 877–882.

Wolbling, R.H., et al. "Local Therapy of Herpes Simplex with Dried Extract From Melisa Officianalis." *Phyto Medicine* 1 (1994): 25–31.

Wolfe, F., H.A. Smythe, M.B. Yunus, R.M. Bennett, C. Bombardier, D.L. Goldenberg, P. Tugwell, S.M. Campbell, M. Abeles, P. Clark, et al. "The American College of Rheumatology 1990 Criteria for the Classification of Fibromyalgia. Report of the Multicenter Criteria Committee." *Arthritis and Rheumatism* 33 (2) (February 1990): 160–172.

Wolfe, F., K. Ross, J. Anderson, I.J. Russell, and L. Hebert. "The Prevalence and Characteristics of Fibromyalgia in the General Population." *Arthritis and Rheumatism* 38 (1) (January 1995): 19–28.

Wolfe, F., M.A. Cathey, and D.J. Hawley. "A Double-Blind Placebo Controlled Trial of Fluoxetine in Fibromyalgia." *Scandinavian Journal of Rheumatology* 23 (5) (1994): 255–259.

Yousef, G.E., E J. Bell, G.F. Mann, V. Murugesan, D.G. Smith, R.A. McCartney, and J.F. Mowbray. "Chronic Enterovirus Infection in Patients with Postviral Fatigue Syndrome." *The Lancet,* 1 (8578) (23 January 1988): 146–147.

Yunus, M.B., and J.C. Aldag. "Restless Legs Syndrome and Leg Cramps in Fibromyalgia Syndrome: A Controlled Study," *British Medical Journal* 312 (7042) (25 May 1996): 1339.

Zelissen, P.M.J., R.J. Croughs, P.P. van Rijk, and J.A. Raymakers. "Effect of Glucocorticoid Replacement Therapy on Bone Mineral Density in Patients with Addison Disease." *Annals of Internal Medicine* 120 (3) (1 February 1994): 207–210.

Zhdanova, I.V., R.J. Wurtman, H.J. Lynch, J.R. Ives, A.B. Dollins, C. Morabito, J.K. Matheson, and D.L. Schomer. "Sleep-Inducing Effects of Low Doses of Melatonin Ingested in the Evening." *Clinical Pharmacology and Therapeutics* 57 (5) (May 1995): 552–558.

Other

Birkmayer, J.G.D. "NADH—The Energizing Coenzyme." Pamphlet. New York, NY: Menuco Corporation, 1996.

Brewer, J., K.K. Knox, and D.R. Carrigan. "Longitudinal Study of Chronic Active HHV-6 Viremia in Patients with CFS." Paper presented at IDSA Conference. Philadelphia, PA, November 1999.

Conference handout. Chronic Fatigue and Immune Dysfunction Syndrome Conference. Sponsored by the Chronic Fatigue and Immune Dysfunction Syndrome Association of America. Fort Lauderdale, FL, 7–9 October 1994.

Earnest, C.P., et al. "Effect of Creatine Monohydrate Supplementation on Muscular Strength and Endurance and Body Weight." Abstract submitted to 1994 NSCA National Conference.

Evengard, B., C.G. Nilsson, G. Astrom, G. Lindh, L. Lindqvist, R. Olin, et al. "Cerebral Spinal Fluid Vitamin B_{12} Deficiency in Chronic Fatigue Syndrome." abstract, proceedings of the American Association for Chronic Fatigue Syndrome Research Conference, San Francisco, CA, 13–14 October 1996.

Harris, M., et al. "Alterations in Leg Extension Power of Meat Eating and Non-Meat Eating (Vegetarian) Females with Creatine Supplementation. Updated" Poster presentation. Proceedings of Experimental Biology, Federation of American Societies for Experimental Biology. Anaheim, CA, 24–28 April 1994.

Hoppel, C. "Carnitine: Conditionally Essential." Ross Labs Conference Report, pp. 52–57.

Jaffe, R.M. "A Novel Treatment for Fibromyalgia Improves Clinical Outcomes in a Community-Based Study." Study presented before the American Association for the Advancement of Science. Baltimore, MD, 9 February 1996.

Jefferies, W.M. *Safe Uses of Cortisol.* Monograph. Springfield, IL: Charles C. Thomas, 1981.

Jefferies, W.M. *Safe Uses of Cortisol,* 2nd edition. Monograph. Springfield, IL: Charles C. Thomas, 1996.

Kuratsune, H., et al. "Acylcarnitine Metabolism in Mammals." Presentation before the First World Congress on CFS. Brussels, Belgium, 9–11 November 1995.

Malone, Daniel, N. Wei, and P. Hitzig. "Treatment of 76 Patients with Primary Fibromyalgia Syndrome with Combined Dopaminergic and Serotonergic Drugs." Abstract submitted to the Annual Scientific Meeting of the American College of Rheumatology, 1996.

Simons, D.G. "Myofascial Pain Syndrome Due to Trigger Points." *International Rehabilitation Medicine Association Monograph Series* 1 (November 1987).

Permissions and Credits

The cartoon on page *xx* is reprinted with the permission of Atlantic Feature Syndicate.

The "Updated CDC Criteria for Chronic Fatigue Syndrome" on page 3 is adapted from the *Annals of Internal Medicine* 121 (14 December 1994). Used with permission.

The cartoon on page 12 is by Thaves, © 1999. Used with permission.

The cartoon on page 56 is reprinted with the permission of Atlantic Feature Syndicate.

The cartoon on page 96 is reprinted with the permission of Atlantic Feature Syndicate.

The "Criteria for Fibromyalgia" and illustration on page 99 are adopted from F. Wolfe, et al., "The American College of Rheumatology 1990 Criteria for the Classification of Fibromyalgia: Report of the Multicenter Criteria Committee," *Arthritis and Rheumatology* 33 (1990). Used with permission.

The cartoon on page 104 is by Thaves, © 2000. Used by permission.

The cartoon on page 130 is reprinted with the permission of Atlantic Feature Syndicate.

The cartoon on page 176 is by Thaves, © 1999. Used with permission.

The cartoon on page 192 is by Thaves, © 1998. Used with permission.

The cartoon on page 208 is by Roy Delgado, © 1999. Used with permission.

"Effective Treatment of Severe Chronic Fatigue: A Report of a Series of 64 Patients" on pages 258–275 was originally published in the *Journal of Musculoskeletal Pain* 3 (1995). Used courtesy of Haworth Press.

"Effective Treatment of Chronic Fatigue Syndrome and Fibromyalgia: A Randomized, Double-Blind Placebo-Controlled, Intent to Treat Study" was originally published in the *Journal of Chronic Fatigue Syndrome* 8 (2) (2001).

The yeast questionnaire on pages 276–281 is adapted from W. G. Crook, M.D., *The Yeast Connection and the Woman* (Jackson, TN: Professional Books, 1995) and *The Yeast Connection Handbook* (Jackson, TN: Professional Books, 1996). Used with permission.

From Fatigued to Fantastic!

Stay on the cutting edge of CFIDS research with the *From Fatigued to Fantastic! Newsletter*. Get the latest information, critically reviewed and presented in easy-to-understand language. Features include:

- Summaries of the newest research findings
- Interviews with clinical and research experts
- Reviews of current treatments
- Questions and answers
- Resources, to help support groups reach you
- And much more!

To order, call 800-333-5287 (410-266-6958 for Maryland residents or from outside the United States) or fax to 410-266-6104, or write to Jacob Teitelbaum, M.D., 466 Forelands Road, Annapolis, MD 21401.

Please send:

☐ The *From Fatigued to Fantastic! Newsletter* (check all that apply):

For subscriptions, choose one:

___ 3-issue subscription (approximately 12-18 months) $35.00

___ No-hassle, per-issue Revolving Subscription
($9.00 will be automatically billed to your credit card
every time a new issue is printed and mailed. You can
cancel at anytime. With this revolving subscription,
you may also order back issues at $9.00 each)! $9.00 per issue

☐ Check here if this is a subscription renewal.

☐ A list of available back issues. Back issues cost is $12.00
per issue ($9.00 if you have a revolving subscription).

☐ Audiotaped interview on CFIDS/FMS
($9.00 plus $3.00 shipping) $12.00

☐ Code for website computer program to create medical
records and treatment recommendations custom-tailored
to your case (regularly $295.00 but may still be at its
introductory price of $160.00; see www.endfatigue.com). $_____

Maryland residents must add 5% sales tax. For Canadian orders, add $8.00 shipping and handling per book or video, and $6.00 per audiotape (U.S. dollars only, please). For other international orders, please add $10.00 per order for shipping and handling.

Volume discounts are available. Please call, fax or write for pricing.

Visit the *From Fatigued to Fantastic!* Website

WWW.ENDFATIGUE.COM

On it you can:

• Enter your detailed medical (and even lab) information. It will be analyzed in our educational program to create:

> –A complete and detailed medical record for your doctor;
> –A treatment protocol;
> –Detailed information sheets, all tailored to *your* case. This can save you and your doctor hours of time and guide your doctor in giving you safe and effective care. It will also guide you on many treatments you can do on your own.

• Access a list of over 700 health professionals who asked to be on our referral list (and use the "remarks" section for each).

• Access one of the most complete lists of CFIDS/FMS support groups in the world.

• Vote, and see how other people have voted, on the effectiveness of different treatments.

• Order nutritional supplements, newsletters, and other useful items.

• See updated information as it becomes available.

If you do not have Internet access and would like information on how to use the computer program, call 410–266–6958 or send a self-addressed, stamped envelope to:

FFTF, LLC
466 Forelands Road
Annapolis, MD 21401

Index